Advanced Studies in Huntington's Disease

Advanced Studies in Huntington's Disease

Edited by **Joshua Barnard**

FOSTER
ACADEMICS

New Jersey

Published by Foster Academics,
61 Van Reypen Street,
Jersey City, NJ 07306, USA
www.fosteracademics.com

Advanced Studies in Huntington's Disease
Edited by Joshua Barnard

International Standard Book Number: 978-1-63242-027-5 (Hardback)

Contents

Preface

I am honored to present to you this unique book which encompasses the most up-to-date data in the field. I was extremely pleased to get this opportunity of editing the work of experts from across the globe. I have also written papers in this field and researched the various aspects revolving around the progress of the discipline. I have tried to unify my knowledge along with that of stalwarts from every corner of the world, to produce a text which not only benefits the readers but also facilitates the growth of the field.

Huntington's is a fairly devastating neuro-degenerative disease. This condition is well studied and is, at present, incurable. It is a brain disorder that damages some specific types of neurons, leading to degeneration in several parts of the brain causing them to lose their function. This results in uncontrolled movements, loss of intellectual abilities and behavioral disturbances. Since the mutation causes have been discovered, there have been several important advancements in understanding the cellular and molecular agitations. This book consists of current knowledge on a wide variety of issues involving this disease. It will help clinicians, health care providers, researchers and graduate students to enhance their understanding and knowledge about the clinical correlates, genetic issues, neuropathological findings, cellular and molecular events and potential therapeutic interventions involved in Huntington's disease. This book not only showcases analyzed fundamental knowledge on the disease but also displays original research in various areas, which together, gives an inclusive description of the important issues in the area.

Finally, I would like to thank all the contributing authors for their valuable time and contributions. This book would not have been possible without their efforts. I would also like to thank my friends and family for their constant support.

Editor

Part 1

Metabolic Dysregulation in Huntington's Disease

Energy Metabolism in Huntington's Disease

Fabíola M. Ribeiro[1], Tomas Dobransky[3],
Eduardo A. D. Gervásio-Carvalho[1], Jader S. Cruz[1]
and Fernando A. Oliveira[2]
[1]Department of Biochemistry and Immunology,
Universidade Federal de Minas Gerais (UFMG),
[2]Department of Biological Sciences,
Universidade Federal de São Paulo (UNIFESP),
[3]DB Biotech, Kosice,
[1,2]Brazil
[3]Slovakia

1. Introduction

Neurodegenerative diseases are pathological processes characterized by neuronal death and morbid evolution leading to occupational injury and serious neuropsychiatric disorders. The natural course of neurodegenerative diseases does not show regression of symptoms or cure and current treatments are far from producing a real improvement in the quality of patient's life. Several studies have been conducted in an attempt to find causes of cellular disturbances focusing new pharmacological targets priming to successful therapeutic interventions. Studies have been directed to investigate possible changes in energy metabolism pathways. Indeed, some disturbances in glycolytic pathway and mitochondrial dysfunctions have been associated with Huntington's Disease and other neurodegenerative diseases and are often related to the events of cell death. In this section, an overview of the energy metabolism pathways will be presented and the particular aspects of energetic metabolism in Huntington's Disease will be discussed.

2. Glucose transport

Under ordinary conditions, the basic substrate for brain metabolism is glucose. In the resting state, adults use about 20% of whole-body glucose for brain metabolism. The brain has an exquisite dependence on glucose for energy production and as an important carbon source for biosynthesis of a variety of simple and complex molecules (Siegel et al., 1999). Such dependence is well demonstrated and a transient decline in the metabolism of glucose would cause a serious disruption of brain function (Oliveira et al., 2007). As glucose is a water-soluble substance its entry into brain from blood is greatly restricted (Vannucci et al., 1997). The major reason for that is the presence of an anatomical-physiological barrier – so called Blood-Brain-Barrier (BBB). The BBB is a specialized barrier made up of microvascular endothelial cells that are held together by tight junction complexes that effectively avoid the paracellular diffusion of solutes (Wilhelm et al., 2011). Even small molecules do not simply diffuse across this physical barrier. To manage this problem, not only for glucose but also for other metabolites important to brain metabolism, there are a large family of specific membrane transporters responsible to carry these molecules across the BBB by means of facilitated diffusion through the luminal and ablumenal endothelial membranes (Vannucci et al., 1997).

It is established that transport and uptake of glucose is performed by a super-family of glucose transporters belonging to the GLUT gene family. The GLUT family includes 12 genes encoding 12 GLUT proteins (Vannucci et al., 1997; Klepper and Voit, 2002). Various members of this membrane protein family have been detected in brain (GLUT-1, GLUT-3 and GLUT-5), but the initial glucose transport step across the BBB is mediated exclusively by the facilitative glucose transporter protein type 1 (GLUT-1) (Lund-Andersen, 1979; Pardridge et al., 1990; Klepper and Voit, 2002). Important to note is the fact that despite such facilitative transport mechanism, the actual concentration of glucose in brain is lower than it is in structures lacking a barrier, e.g. peripheral nerves. There is, then, no safety device to supplement carbohydrate reserve during hypoglycemia episodes making the regulation of GLUTs extremely relevant for brain physiology.

Following entry into the brain glucose is transported from the interstitial fluid into neurons primarily via GLUT-3 and into glia primarily via GLUT-1 transporters. GLUT-5 protein is known to be present in brain microglia, although its function in these cells remains unclear. This transport into the intracellular compartment is relatively rapid, making the BBB the rate-limiting step for glucose entry into brain cells (Pardridge et al., 1990).

Glucose, entering the neuronal cells, is phosphorylated irreversibly to glucose-6-phosphate (G-6~P) and metabolized in the pentose phosphate shunt or the Embden-Meyerhoff pathway, or converted to glycogen. The Embden-Meyerhoff metabolic pathway permits glycolytic conversion of glucose to pyruvate. Glycogen synthesis provides a source of fuel during periods of metabolic stress (3.3 mmol/kg rat). Evidently a decreased entry of glucose into the brain limits these three pathways and potentially contributes to the development of innumerous neuronal pathologies.

Brain metabolic needs are demanding and the way in which it circumvents this situation has long remained unclear. For the past 15 years authors are looking for a more universal explanation but it turns out to be rather complicated. The subject is controversial and the field is still very active.

Neurons and astrocytes, the two major types of brain cells, are largely responsible for the massive consumption of O_2 and glucose in the brain. Just to point out how important they are, under resting conditions, astrocytes release ~85% of the glucose they consume as lactate. On the contrary, neurons contribute minimally to glucose consumption by the brain. Thus, despite their shared localization, neurons and astrocytes exhibit a different preference for glucose consumption and utilization (Nehlig and Coles, 2007).

The ATP-dependent phosphorylation of glucose to G-6~P is the first step of glycolysis and it is catalyzed by hexokinase (HK) (Berg et al., 2006). The reaction is practically irreversible and has been recognized as a key point in the regulation of carbohydrate metabolism in brain. This whole process concomitantly generates local ADP which is important as a recycling mechanism. Important to note that hexokinase activity in neurons and in other cell types also participates in various essential processes including ATP production, apoptosis, controlling glutathione levels, and preventing neuronal oxidative unbalance (Saraiva et al., 2010). In the brain, HK-1 is the major expressed enzyme isoform. It localizes into cytosol or firmly attached to outer mitochondrial membrane. The bound enzyme is more active and the extent of binding is thought to be inversely related to the ATP/ADP ratio (Siegel et al., 1999). Interestingly, conditions where energy utilization is greater than the substrate supply there is a shift in the solubilization equilibrium towards the membrane-bound enzyme form which per se provokes a greater potential to ignite glycolysis to meet the energy demand.

The activity and specific subcellular localization of neuronal HK-1 are regulated by distinct mechanisms that act synergistically to fine-tuning glycolytic flux in response to changes in cellular environment. At this point it may be important to bring up the idea that mitochondrial-bound hexokinase 1 could be neuroprotective as has been discussed by different research groups in this field.

The reaction product of HK-1 is G-6~P which represents a major branch point in metabolism because it is a common substrate for enzymes involved in glycolytic, pentose-phosphate shunt, and glycogen-forming pathways. In glycolysis, G-6~P is the substrate of isomerase producing fructose-6-phosphate (F-6~P). This reaction is promptly reversible (small free energy change), however its equilibrium ratio in brain greatly favors G-6~P accumulation. F-6~P is phosphorylated by phosphofructokinase-1 (PFK-1), which is considered one of the most regulated catalysts of the glycolytic sequence, to form fructose-1,6-bisphosphate (F-1,6-Bis~P). As observed in other regulatory biochemical reactions it is also essentially irreversible.

A number of studies focusing into this particular metabolic reaction led to the observation that astrocytes' PFK-1 is about two fold more active than in neurons under baseline conditions (Herrero-Mendez et al., 2009). One possible reason for that is the concentration of fructose-2,6-bisphosphate (F-2,6-Bis~P), an powerful allosteric modulator of PFK-1 activity, is significantly greater in astrocytes. This dramatic difference could be ascribed to the near absence in neurons of phosphofructokinase-2/fructose-2,6-phosphatase (PFK-2/F-2,6-Pase) the bifunctional enzyme responsible for the F-2,6-Bis~P synthesis and degradation (Herrero-Mendez et al., 2009).

The question to be raised is how neurons actually control PFK-2/F-2,6-Pase activity? There are four isoforms of PFK-2/F-2,6-Pase, each encoded by a separate gene [Pfkfb1, Pfkfb2, Pfkfb3, and Pfkfb4] (Okar et al., 2001). It is reasonable to suppose that each isoform displays significantly different regulatory and kinetic features and this, in turn, determines the ratio of kinase/phosphatase activity, and as a consequence the concentration of F-2,6-Bis~P in different tissues (Yalcin et al., 2009). In a well conducted study Herrero-Mendez and colleagues (2009), using RT-PCR analysis of RNA extracts from rat cortical neurons and astrocytes, indicated that Pfkfb3 mRNA was present in neurons as well as astrocytes. Importantly, the authors demonstrated that Pfkfb3 was the most abundant mRNA expressed in both cell types. The authors expected that if neurons contained the same relative abundance of Pfkfb3 mRNA as astrocytes and lower levels of the mature enzyme that the final concentration of PFK-2/F-2,6-Bis~Pase in neurons might be regulated post-transcriptionally. Some studies exploring the mechanism of such proteasomal degradation revealed that Pfkfb3, contains a KEN box that starts at position 142 (Pesin and Orr-Weaver, 2008; Herrero-Mendez et al., 2009). This motif targets proteins for ubiquitylation by the anaphase-promoting complex/cyclosome when bound to its activator CDH1 (Pesin and Orr-Weaver, 2008). Interestingly, CDH1 silencing in neurons induced PFK-2/F-2,6-Bis~Pase accumulation and as expected increased the rate of glycolysis.

Fructose-1,6-Bis~P is split by brain aldolase to glyceraldehyde-3-phosphate (Gal-3~P) and dihydroxyacetone phosphate (DHAP). DHAP is the common substrate for both glyceraldehyde-3-phosphate dehydrogenase and triose phosphate isomerase. One important point to comment is the equilibrium between DHAP and Gal-3~P maintained by the action of triose phosphate isomerase. In brain, the equilibrium favors accumulation of DHAP. After this reaction step, glycolysis in the brain proceeds through the usual biochemical reactions to produce pyruvate (Berg et al., 2006).

As we have been discussing throughout the chapter neurons use glucose basically to maintain their antioxidant balance status. In order to do this, neurons have to downregulate glycolysis. Under this situation one the question is raised: Where does glucose go to be further metabolized? To answer this question we need to remember that pentose-phosphate pathway (PPP) uses G-6~P as substrate and that PPP is metabolic linked to glycolysis. One interesting, however somehow surprising, observation made by different laboratories is the fact that, in contrast to astrocytes, neurons do not display increased glycolytic rate upon mitochondrial inhibition as one could expect (Bolanos et al., 2008; Bolanos et al., 2010), but instead these neuronal cells entry into cell death program. These results lead us to assume that the increased glycolytic rate in astrocytes served to preserve cells from ATP depletion and cell death, most probably because glycolytic ATP was used to drive the reverse activity of ATP synthase to maintain the mitochondrial membrane potential (Nehlig and Coles, 2007; Bolanos et al., 2010; Cunnane et al., 2011). On the other hand, such treatment caused neuronal ATP depletion and apoptotic cell death (Nehlig and Coles, 2007). Based on all facts presented so far one can hypothesize that neurodegenerative diseases (including Alzheimer's Disease and Huntington's Disease) may present a diminished neuronal glycolytic activity (Oliveira et al., 2007). Data in support of this hypothesis will be discussed later.

Accumulated evidence suggest that in neurons a significant proportion of G-6~P is directed towards the PPP (Bolanos et al., 2008). Besides its role at supplying ribose-5-phosphate for nucleic acid biosynthesis, glucose oxidation through the PPP is a major component of the cytosolic NADPH regenerating cell machinery (Nelson and Cox, 2004; Bolanos et al., 2008). The rate-limiting step in PPP activity is catalyzed by glucose-6-phosphate dehydrogenase, which oxidizes G-6~P into 6-phosphogluconate, conserving the redox energy as NADPH. Next, 6-phosphogluconate is further oxidized by 6-phosphogluconate dehydrogenase, which also conserves redox energy in the form of NADPH (Nelson and Cox, 2004; Bolanos et al., 2008).

It is important to note: NADPH is a necessary cofactor in the regeneration of reduced glutathione and for the reductive reactions for lipid biosynthesis. This mechanism is not exclusive for neurons it also operates in astrocytes which have high concentrations of glutathione due to their high activity of γ-glutamyl cysteine synthetase. This enzyme catalyzes the rate-limiting step in glutathione synthesis providing a metabolic scenario to build a robust antioxidant system (Heales and Bolanos, 2002). As neurons have rather low concentrations of glutathione, and low activity of γ-glutamyl cysteine synthetase there are compelling evidence that glucose entry in the PPP is important to regenerate glutathione and provide an effective defense mechanism against oxidative stress.

The energy output and oxygen consumption in adult brain are associated with high levels of enzyme activity in the tricarboxylic acid cycle (TCA). The TCA is organized into a supramolecular complex that interacts with mitochondrial membranes and the electron transport chain (Berg et al., 2006). Therefore, mitochondria have a central role for the energetic metabolism, their main function is oxidation of acetyl-coenzyme A derived from carbohydrates, amino-acids and fatty acids to produce ATP (Nelson and Cox, 2004). These organelles provide energy for a plethora of cellular processes and the highest number of mitochondria is present in organs demanding the most of energy, such as brain, liver and muscles.

Actually, the processes responsible for energy production are recognized as oxidative phosphorylation which is coupled to the electron transport chain (ETC). The ETC is a set of five protein complexes sitting on the inner mitochondrial membrane. Three protein complexes (complex I, III and IV) work as a proton pump transferring protons through the membrane into the intermembrane space. Chemiosmotic theory predicts that most of the ATP synthesis comes from the electrochemical gradient across the inner membranes of mitochondria by ATP synthase. Energy saved in ATP is used in synaptic ion homeostasis and phosphorylation reactions. ATP is essential for the excitability and survival of neurons, oxidative phosphorylation is involved in synaptic signaling and is related to changes of neuronal structure and function.

The major role is given to complex I (NADH dehydrogenase [ubiquinone]) in controlling mitochondrial oxidative phosphorylation; its malfunctioning can result in mitochondrial dysfunction.(Davey et al., 1998; Hroudova and Fisar, 2011). Thus, many mitochondrial diseases originate from complex I deficiencies.

In adult brain, the enzyme succinate dehydrogenase (SDH), which catalysis the oxidation of succinate to fumarate, is tightly bound to mitochondrial inner membrane. In brain, SDH may also have a regulatory role when its steady state is disturbed. Important to note that the levels of succinate and isocitrate in brain tissue are little affected by changes in the flux of the TCA, as long as proper glucose supply is available. The highly unfavorable free-energy change of the malate dehydrogenase reaction is bypassed by the very rapid removal of oxaloacetate, which is maintained at low concentrations under steady-state conditions through the condensation reaction with acetyl-coenzyme A (Berg et al., 2006); Nelson and Cox, 2004).

3. Energetic metabolism deficit in Huntington's Disease

Huntington´s Disease patients face pronounced weight loss, despite sustained caloric intake, which was a first indication that alterations in energetic metabolism could play a role in Huntington´s Disease pathogenesis (O'Brien et al., 1990). In agreement with this hypothesis, Huntington´s Disease patients exhibit alterations in cerebral glucose consume, lactate levels, and mitochondrial enzymes activity involved in glucose metabolism. Moreover, ATP depletion was directly demonstrated in Huntington´s Disease brain tissue (Mochel et al., 2010a). Thus far, various mechanisms underlying energy deficit in Huntington´s Disease brain have been identified, including impaired oxidative phosphorylation (Milakovic and Johnson, 2005), altered oxidative stress (Tabrizi et al., 1999), impaired mitochondrial calcium handling (Lim et al., 2008), abnormal mitochondria trafficking (Li et al., 2010), and deregulation of the transcriptional coactivator PPARγ coactivator-1α (PGC-1α), which is a crucial factor of mitochondrial biogenesis (Cui et al., 2006), and decreased glycolysis (Powers et al., 2007).

3.1 Glucose levels are reduced in Huntington's Disease patient's brain

Positron emission tomography (PET) studies revealed that glucose metabolism in the basal ganglia and cerebral cortex is markedly reduced in Huntington´s Disease patients (Kuwert et al., 1990; Andrews and Brooks, 1998). Moreover, the decrease in glucose metabolism is specific to cortical areas, caudate and putamen, and starts in the asymptomatic phase of the disease (Kuhl et al., 1985). Regardless of the severity of symptoms and despite apparent shrinkage of brain tissue, glucose utilization appears normal throughout the rest of the brain of Huntington´s Disease patients (Kuhl et al., 1985).

Furthermore, studies performed in presymptomatic Huntington´s Disease gene carriers revealed a pattern of cerebral metabolism characterized by relative increases in thalamic, occipital, and cerebellar glucose metabolism, despite reduced caudate and putamen metabolism. Following Huntington´s Disease symptoms appearance, this pattern was altered as thalamic metabolism, which was previously elevated, was reduced (Feigin et al., 2007). These data highlights the importance of the region specific alterations in glucose metabolism for Huntington´s Disease pathology.

Interestingly, a recent report supports the idea that the hypothalamus, but not the basal ganglia, is the brain region responsible for the metabolic abnormalities that take place in Huntington´s Disease (Hult et al., 2011). Selective hypothalamic expression of a short fragment of mutant huntingtin was sufficient to recapitulate the glucose metabolic disturbances that occur in Huntington´s Disease patients. In addition, selective hypothalamic inactivation of the mutant huntingtin gene prevented the development of the metabolic phenotype in a Huntington´s Disease mouse model, BACHD mice (Hult et al., 2011). Further studies will be important to point all the regions involved in Huntington´s Disease metabolic alterations.

In addition to its role as an energetic molecule, glucose also plays a role as a signaling molecule. It has been demonstrated that increased intracellular glucose levels decreases aggregate formation and is neuroprotective in cultured cells transfected with a mutant huntingtin construct (Ravikumar et al., 2003). Glucose metabolism appears altered in Huntington´s Disease, as huntingtin transfected PC12 cells exhibit disturbed expression levels of four genes involved in glucose metabolism (Glut1, Pfkm, Aldolase A, and Enolase), as well as a reduction in cell death following over-expression of Glut1 and Pfkm (another key regulatory protein for glycolysis) (Kita et al., 2002). Glucose reduces phosphorylation of mTOR, which is a negative regulator of authophagy, and its downstream effector S6K1 (Ravikumar et al., 2003). Thus, glucose-mediated negative regulation of mTOR could induce autophagy and clearance of the mutated huntingtin protein, as well as influence other mTOR mediated activities involving cell survival, growth, and translation of protein transcripts. Furthermore, glucose can regulate Akt and GSK3, which influence cell growth and survival (Clodfelder-Miller et al., 2005). Importantly, Akt activation can protect against neuronal death (Datta et al., 1999; Kandel and Hay, 1999). Akt can also promote phosphorylation of mutated Htt protein, which functions to reduce Htt aggregate formation and neuronal cell death, providing a protective pathway in Huntington's Disease (Humbert et al., 2002; Warby et al., 2009). Highlighting the importance of Akt in Huntington's Disease pathology, both NMDA and metabotropic glutamate receptor 5 receptors can increase Akt activation in striatal neurons from Huntington's Disease mouse models (Gines et al., 2003a). These observations highlight the role of glucose as an important molecule not only for its energetic properties but also for its capacity to activate key molecules involved in cell survival and huntingtin clearance.

3.2 Enzymes involved in energetic metabolism are altered in Huntington's Disease

Mutated huntingtin protein alters the function and/or expression of a number of enzymes involved in energetic metabolism and many of these alterations can have important implications in Huntington's Disease pathology. Alteration of enzyme expression by mutated huntingtin may occur due to huntingtin-mediated regulation of transcriptional factors. For example, mutant huntingtin inhibits expression of PGC-1α, which is a transcriptional coactivator that regulates several metabolic processes, including mitochondrial biogenesis and respiration (Cui et al., 2006). Mutated huntingtin may also alter enzyme function by incorporation and sequestration of transcriptional factors and enzymes into mutated huntingtin aggregates (Yamanaka et al., 2008). The enzyme alterations caused by mutated huntingtin can have important deleterious consequence, including the metabolic deficit observed in Huntington's Disease patients.

Glyceraldehyde-3-phosphate dehydrogenase (GAPDH) and the α-ketoglutarate dehydrogenase complex can be inactivated by long polyglutamine domains, which may cause a deficit in cerebral energy metabolism (Cooper et al., 1997). Further studies have shown that the mutated huntingtin protein alters the subcellular localization of GAPDH, increasing its nuclear localization in both human fibroblasts and in neurons from a transgenic mouse model (Mazzola and Sirover, 2001, 2002; Senatorov et al., 2003). The appearance of an abnormal high molecular weight form of GAPDH in fibroblast nuclei has also been associated with decreased glycolytic activity (Mazzola and Sirover, 2001).

Pyruvate dehydrogenase activity is decreased in basal ganglia and this deficit was significantly augmented with increasing duration of illness, possibly due to a progressive loss of neurons in Huntington's Disease caudate nucleus (Butterworth et al., 1985). Activities of the complexes II, III and IV of the electron transport chain were reduced in both Huntington's Disease caudate and putamen of advanced grade (3 and 4) Huntington's Disease patients (Gu et al., 1996; Browne et al., 1997). It has been shown that lactate concentration is increased in the basal ganglia and the occipital cortex of Huntington's Disease patients (Jenkins et al., 1993; Jenkins et al., 1998). The lactate itself is not thought to be a neurotoxic metabolite, but may represent a marker for energetic changes such as reduced ATP production and excitotoxicity, which may have a direct effect on neuronal function and survival in Huntington's Disease.

A number of studies have shown that the activity of transglutaminase 2, an enzyme primarily known for cross-linking proteins, is increased in Huntington's Disease affected brain areas and that transglutaminase 2 causes an increase in huntingtin aggregation (Karpuj et al., 1999; Lesort et al., 1999; Karpuj et al., 2002). The most compelling evidence for a role of transglutaminase 2 in Huntington's Disease is provided by the work of

Mastroberardino et al. (2002). These studies reported a reduction in neuronal cell death, improved behavior and prolonged survival in R6/1 X transglutaminase 2-/-, as compared to R6/1 X transglutaminase 2+/+. In addition to affecting huntingtin aggregation, increased transglutaminase 2 activity in Huntington´s Disease caudate may contribute to mitochondrial dysfunction by incorporating aconitase into inactive polymers and dramatically decreasing aconitase activity (Kim et al., 2005).

3.3 Mitochondrial deficit in Huntington´s Disease

Studies published so far suggest that mitochondrial defects play a major role in Huntington´s Disease etiology, underlined by decreased mitochondrial biogenesis, oxidative stress, ATP deficit, increased apoptosis, and, ultimately, a central and peripheral energy deficit (Browne and Beal, 2004).

Degenerated mitochondria have been detected in the striatum of symptomatic Huntington´s Disease mice (R6/2, R6/1, N171-82Q, and Hdh150CAG mice) and could be detected before other neuronal pathological changes and concomitant with symptom onset (Yu et al., 2003). These degenerating mitochondria exhibit swelling, disruption of the cristae and mitochondrial membranes, and eventual condensation and lysosomal engulfment. Interestingly, this study shows that neuronal cell death aspects due to motichondrial alterations varied among different Huntington´s Disease mouse models (Hickey and Chesselet, 2003; Yu et al., 2003).

Mutated huntingtin protein destabilizes mitochondrial Ca^{2+} regulation (Panov et al., 2002; Choo et al., 2004). Mitochondrial Ca^{2+} abnormalities occur early in Huntington´s Disease pathogenesis and appear to be caused by a direct effect of mutant huntingtin, as incubation of normal human lymphoblast mitochondria with a fusion protein containing a long polyglutamine repeat recapitulates the mitochondrial calcium defect observed in Huntington´s Disease (Panov et al., 2002). Further studies have also demonstrated that the huntingtin protein binds to the outer membrane of mitochondria from human neuroblastoma cells and from cultured striatal cells from WT and transgenic mice (Choo et al., 2004). Moreover, binding of mutated huntingtin protein, but not of wild type, increases sensitivity to calcium-induced opening of the mitochondrial permeability transition (MPT), leading to the release of cytochrome c in normal liver mitochondria (Choo et al., 2004).

Mitochondria play an important role in buffering cytoplasmic calcium and increased neuronal calcium modifies mitochondrial ATP production by uncoupling oxidative phosphorylation (Nicholls, 2009). Calcium overload may result in discharge of the mitochondrial membrane potential, opening of the MPT pore, release of cytochrome c, and activation of cell death pathways (Nicholls, 2009). Mutated huntingtin protein causes sensitization of both the NMDA receptor and the inositol-1,4,5-triphosphate (IP3) receptor, increasing entrance of extracellular Ca^{2+} and the release of Ca^{2+} from intracellular stores, respectively (Chen et al., 1999; Sun et al., 2001; Tang et al., 2005). The final result is an increase in intracellular Ca^{2+} levels. The role of NMDA receptors on mitochondrial biogenesis has been further characterized, as the reduced mitochondrial ATP levels and decreased ATP/ADP ratio found in mutant Htt-containing striatal cells is normalized by blocking NMDA receptor-mediated calcium influx (Seong et al., 2005). Moreover, mitochondria isolated from both lymphoblasts of Huntington´s Disease patients and brains of transgenic mice have a reduced membrane potential and depolarize at lower Ca^{2+} concentrations than control mitochondria (Panov et al., 2002).

Thus, data obtained so far points to a close relationship between mitochondria deficit and NMDA-mediated excitotoxicity. The glutamatergic system plays a substantial role in neuronal cell death and there are consistent data implicating NMDA receptor activation with the excitotoxic neuronal loss that takes place in Huntington´s Disease (Zeron et al., 2002; Schiefer et al., 2004). Selective depletion of NMDA receptors has been found in Huntington´s Disease striatum, suggesting that neurons expressing NMDA receptors are preferentially vulnerable to degeneration (Dure et al., 1991). Prior to the identification of the genetic mutation responsible for Huntington´s Disease, a Huntington´s Disease mouse model was developed by the introduction of quinolinic acid, which is an NMDA receptor agonist that produces excitotoxic striatal lesions that closely resemble those seen in Huntington´s Disease brain (Beal et al., 1986). Moreover, some studies suggest that the sensitization of the NMDA receptor containing the subunit NR1/NR2B by the mutated Htt protein is responsible for causing the selective cell death of the medium sized spiny neurons present in the striatum, since these neurons express high level of this NMDA receptor subtype (Chen et al., 1999; Zeron et al., 2001).

Mitochondrial toxins that deplete ATP production can also mediate excitotoxic processes (Schulz et al., 1996; Browne and Beal, 2002). Systemic administration of 3-nitropropionic acid, which is a mitochondrial toxicant that inhibits succinate dehydrogenase, results in striatum lesions similar to those observed in Huntington´s Disease (Wullner et al., 1994). Nevertheless, 3-nitropropionic acid and malonate lesions can be prevented by NMDA antagonists, such as MK-801 and memantine (Wullner et al., 1994). Taken together these observations suggest that mitochondrial-mediated excitotoxicity is promoted by secondary mechanisms involving glutamate receptors. It has been shown that omission of glucose, exclusion of oxygen, or inclusion of inhibitors of oxidative phosphorylation or of the sodium/potassium pump, enables glutamate to express its neurotoxic effects via NMDAR (Novelli et al., 1988; Henneberry et al., 1989; Zeevalk and Nicklas, 1991). Thus, in a context of reduced intracellular energy levels an otherwise harmless amount of glutamate becomes toxic.

Studies performed with Huntington´s Disease transgenic models have implicated decreased transcription of genes regulated by cyclic adenosine 3',5'-monophosphate (cAMP) responsive element (CRE) binding protein (CREB) to Huntington´s Disease pathology (Luthi-Carter et al., 2000; Shimohata et al., 2000; Steffan et al., 2000; Nucifora et al., 2001; Wyttenbach et al., 2001). These genes include brain derived neurotrophic factor (BDNF) (Zuccato et al., 2001) and a host of others involved in diverse processes ranging from neurotransmission (Bibb et al., 2000; Luthi-Carter et al., 2000) to cholesterol metabolism (Sipione et al., 2002).

Reduced CREB dependent transcription of BDNF is a robust feature of Huntington´s Disease pathophysiology. By grades II and III of the disease, BDNF protein and mRNA levels in frontoparietal cortex are halved, and this effect can be mimicked by expressing full-length human mutant huntingtin in a rat CNS parental cell line (Ferrer et al., 2000; Zuccato et al., 2001). Reduced levels of cortical and striatal BDNF have been demonstrated in multiple mouse models of Huntington´s Disease expressing mutant Huntingtin (including

R6/2, N171-82Q, Hdh, and YAC-72 lines) (Luthi-Carter et al., 2000; Zuccato et al., 2001; Luthi-Carter et al., 2002; Gines et al., 2003b). Importantly, the diminished CREB-mediated gene transcription appears to be linked to energy impairment and deficient cAMP, which has been shown to be decreased in the cerebral spinal fluid of symptomatic Huntington´s Disease patients (Sawa et al., 1999). Furthermore, PC12 cells stimulated with forskolin, which activates adenylyl cyclases to produce cAMP from ATP, exhibit ameliorated mutant huntingtin-fragment induced phenotypes, further supporting the hypothesis that low levels of cAMP might be implicated in Huntington´s Disease pathology (Wyttenbach et al., 2001). Levels of both cAMP and CRE-signaling are decreased prior to Huntington´s Disease symptoms in Hdh^{Q111} mice (Gines et al., 2003b). These data suggest that mutant huntingtin might lead to an early metabolic deficit that amplifies the disease cascade by altering cAMP-dependent processes, including CRE-mediated gene transcription (Gines et al., 2003b).

4. Treatment options for the metabolic deficit

The presence of the mutated huntingtin gene can be detected early in life which makes substrates capable of slowing disease progression an attracting therapeutic tool. A number of energy-related therapeutic approaches have been used in preclinical models and/or Huntington´s Disease patients, such as coenzyme Q_{10}, creatine, antioxidant therapies, anaplerotic therapies, and PGC-1α agonists.

Creatine is an important energy molecule in the brain (O'Gorman et al., 1996). Creatine administration increases brain concentrations of phosphocreatine and inhibits activation of the MPT, both of which may exert neuroprotective effects (Hemmer and Wallimann, 1993; O'Gorman et al., 1996). Moreover, creatine appears to be neuroprotective in a rodent mitochondrial toxin model via enhancing cerebral energy metabolism (Koroshetz et al., 1997; Matthews et al., 1998). The R6/2 mice exhibit lower levels of creatine and ATP in the brain (Dedeoglu et al., 2003). In addition, pre-symptomatic dietary creatine supplementation extends survival in the R6/2 and N171–82Q transgenic Huntington´s Disease mice while significantly improving the clinical and neuropathological phenotype (Ferrante et al., 2000; Andreassen et al., 2001). Creatine supplementation in symptomatic R6/2 mice also has clinical benefits (Dedeoglu et al., 2003). However, so far, clinical trials have demonstrated no substantial benefit for creatine administration to Huntington´s Disease patients (Verbessem et al., 2003; Tabrizi et al., 2005). One year of creatine intake, at a rate that can improve muscle functional capacity in healthy subjects and patients with neuromuscular disease, did not improve functional, neuromuscular, and cognitive status in patients with stage I to III Huntington´s Disease (Verbessem et al., 2003). Even the low levels of cerebral creatine and phosphocreatine observed in these previous studies have been disputed, as more recent studies in which in vivo concentrations of brain metabolites were preserved found increased brain levels of creatine and phosphocreatine in the same mouse model of Huntington´s Disease used in previous studies (Tkac et al., 2007; Mochel et al., 2010a). Thus, it is still unclear whether creatine has a clinical benefit to Huntington´s Disease patients.

Q_{10} is an antioxidant and promoter of respiratory chain function that has also been tested as a treatment for Huntington´s Disease. Oral administration of Q_{10} ameliorates elevated lactate levels seen in the cortex of Huntington´s Disease patients, an effect that is reversible on withdrawal of the agent (Koroshetz et al., 1997). In addition, combination of Coenzyme

Q_{10} and creatine produces additive neuroprotective effects in reducing striatal lesion volumes produced by chronic subcutaneous administration of 3-NP to rats, improves motor performance, and extends survival in the transgenic R6/2 Huntington´s Disease mice (Yang et al., 2009). However, one large-scale study assessing the potential neuroprotective effects of coenzyme Q_{10} revealed that, at the tested dosages, Q_{10} produced no significant slowing in functional decline in early Huntington´s Disease (Huntington Study Group, 2001).

Other antioxidants, such as ascorbate and BN82451, have been shown to improve motor performance and survival of R6 mice (Klivenyi et al., 2003; Rebec et al., 2003). The level of ascorbate is significantly diminished in the striatum of Huntington´s Disease mouse models, which highlights the importance of studying the effect of ascorbate supplementation to treat Huntington´s Disease (Rebec et al., 2002; Dorner et al., 2007). However further studies will be necessary to determine whether either ascorbate or other antioxidant is capable of slowing Huntington´s Disease progression in patients.

A decrease in branched-chain amino acid (BCAA) levels has been observed in the plasma of Huntington´s Disease patients (Mochel et al., 2007). Decreased BCAA levels might occur to compensate the energetic deficit observed in Huntington´s Disease, which is caused by impaired glycolysis, citric acid cycle and/or oxidative phosphorylation, as earlier described in this chapter (Tabrizi et al., 1999; Browne and Beal, 2004; Milakovic and Johnson, 2005). Based on this hypothesis, a short-term therapeutic clinical trial was performed using triheptanoin, a triglyceride containing seven carbon fatty acids that is metabolized to acetyl-CoA and propionyl-CoA, which is an anaplerotic compound that is a precursor of the citric acid cycle intermediate, succinate (Mochel et al., 2010b). This study shows that triheptanoin therapy can improve peripheral energy metabolism in Huntington´s Disease patients, and in particular oxidative phosphorylation in skeletal muscle (Mochel et al., 2010b). However, the benefit of anaplerotic approaches to the brain energy metabolism remains to be established.

Peroxisome proliferator-activated receptor (PPAR)γ is a member of the nuclear hormone receptor family of ligand-activated transcription factors (Rosen and Spiegelman, 2001). PPARγ is the target of the insulin-sensitizing thiazolidinediones (TZDs) drugs used to treat type II diabetes and recent studies suggest that treatment of insulin resistance with a PPARγ agonist retards the development of Alzheimer's Disease (Watson and Craft, 2003; Watson et al., 2005). There is evidence suggesting that PPARγ agonists are neuroprotective and increase mitochondrial function (Schutz et al., 2005; Hunter et al., 2007). Moreover, oral treatment with rosiglitazone, which is a thiazolidinedione drug, induces mitochondrial biogenesis in mouse brain (Strum et al., 2007). Interestingly, a significant defect in the PPARγ signaling pathway has been found in mutant huntingtin-expressing cells, as compared to cells expressing wild-type huntingtin protein (Quintanilla et al., 2008). In addition, pretreatment of mutant huntingtin-expressing cells with rosiglitazone avoids the loss of mitochondrial potential, mitochondrial calcium deregulation, and oxidative stress overproduction in response to intracellular calcium overload (Quintanilla et al., 2008). Rosiglitazone also increases mitochondrial mass levels, suggesting a role for the PPARγ pathway in mitochondrial function in striatal cells (Quintanilla et al., 2008). PPARγ protein levels are decreased in the brain and peripheral tissue of R6/2 mice and in lymphocytes of Huntington´s Disease patients, probably due to a decrease in transcription as well as recruitment of PPARγ protein to huntingtin aggregates (Chiang et al., 2010). R6/2 mice treatment with TZD results in beneficial effects on energy deficiency and on several major

Huntington´s Disease phenotypes, decreasing weight loss, lessening motor deterioration, reducing mutant huntingtin aggregate formation, improving the reduced levels of two neuroprotective factor, Bcl-2 e BDNF, and increasing mouse life span (Chiang et al., 2010). Moreover, the protective effects described above appear to have been exerted, at least partially, via direct activation of PPARγ in the brain (Chiang et al., 2010).

Peroxisome proliferator-activated receptor-γ coactivator (PGC)-1α, which is a potent co-activator of PPARγ transcriptional coactivator, is a member of a family of transcription coactivators that plays a central role in the regulation of cellular energy metabolism and stimulates mitochondrial biogenesis, participating in the regulation of both carbohydrate and lipid metabolism (Liang and Ward, 2006). PGC-1α knockout mice exhibit striatum lesions resembling Huntington´s Disease, which was first evidence that this molecule could be involved in Huntington´s Disease pathology (Lin et al., 2004). Further studies have demonstrated that downregulation of PGC-1α in Huntington´s Disease striatum affects mitochondrial energy metabolism, possibly by impairing oxidative phosphorylation (Cui et al., 2006). Moreover, over-expression of exogenous PGC-1α in Huntington´s Disease striatal neurons was protective against 3-NP treatment (Weydt et al., 2006). Decreasing levels of PGC-1α were shown to parallel markers of mitochondrial dysfunction with disease progression in Huntington´s Disease patients (Kim et al., 2010). Of note, PGC-1α polymorphisms in Huntington´s Disease patients may modify Huntington´s Disease onset age (Taherzadeh-Fard et al., 2009). Interestingly, it has been shown that mutated huntingtin protein can promote transcripition repression of PGC-1alpha (Cui et al., 2006). Mutant huntingtin represses PGC-1α gene transcription by associating with the promoter and interfering with the CREB/TAF4-dependent transcriptional pathway (Cui et al., 2006). These data support a link between transcriptional deregulation and mitochondrial dysfunction in Huntington´s Disease.

Resveratrol is a polyphenol that increases the activity of SIRT1, which is an activator factor capable of increasing PGC-1α activity and mitochondrial biogenesis, as evidenced by increased oxidative-type muscle fibers, enhanced resistance to muscle fatigue, and increased tolerance to cold observed in mice treated with resveratrol (Lagouge et al., 2006). Repeated treatment with resveratrol for a period of 8 days beginning 4 days prior to 3-nitropropionic acid administration, which induces symptoms similar to Huntington´s Disease, significantly improves the 3-nitropropionic acid-induced motor and cognitive impairment (Kumar et al., 2006). When tested in the context of a transgenic mouse model of Huntington´s Disease, resveratrol increased PGC-1α mRNA levels and had protective effects in peripheral tissues, by reducing vacuolation in the brown adipose tissue and decreasing elevated blood glucose levels (Ho et al., 2010). However, there was no improvement of motor performance, weight loss, striatal atrophy and survival in Huntington´s Disease transgenic mice treated with resveratrol, which was consistent with no increase in PGC-1α mRNA levels in the striatum (Ho et al., 2010). Thus, resveratrol appears to protect against the peripheral energetic deficit in Huntington´s Disease, but it is not effective to alleviate CNS Huntington´s Disease pathology.

As stated previously, transglutaminase 2 activity appears to be increased in Huntington´s Disease, leading to huntingtin aggregation and mitochondrial aconitase inhibition (Karpuj et al., 1999; Lesort et al., 1999; Kim et al., 2005). Based on these studies, cystamine, which is a drug capable of inhibiting transglutaminase, was tested as a therapeutic tool to treat Huntington´s Disease. Cystamine treatment prolongs the lifespan and reduces associated tremor and abnormal movements in a Huntington´s Disease transgenic mice, possibly in part due to inhibition of transglutaminase 2 activity (Dedeoglu et al., 2002; Karpuj et al., 2002). However, cystamine does not inhibits transglutaminase 2 specifically, which might invalidate its therapeutic use (Jeitner et al., 2005). In addition to cystamine, there are a number of other transglutaminase inhibitors that have been tested in Huntington´s Disease, such as a set of irreversible peptidic inhibitors, the allosteric reversible small-molecule hydrazides, and inhibitors that bind to the guanosine triphosphate (GTP) binding site (Duval et al., 2005; Lai et al., 2008). However, each of these compounds was found to be inadequate for *in vivo* testing because of a general lack of selectivity or poor cellular potency (Schaertl et al., 2010).

Huntingtin-related proteomic studies represent an area of intense research. Proteins interacting with huntingtin pathological form exhibit altered patterns and metabolism. Mitochondrial metabolism alterations are observed in mouse models expressing various types of the mutated huntingtin (Browne, 2008). Moreover, knock-in mice models with pathogenic CAG repeats inserted into the murine homolog Hdh (e.g. Hdh^{Q111}, CAG 140, CAG 150) develop similar cerebral pathologies, including reduction of striatal-related dopamine receptor (Menalled, 2005). Protein-protein interaction studies resulted in the identification of many proteins interacting with huntingtin, characterizing it rather as a scaffolding, membrane-associated protein, involved in axonal trafficking of mitochondria and vesicles (Truant et al., 2006). From the large group of huntingtin-interacting proteins, the most research interest is focused on proteins that have a direct implication on its biological functions. Most of these proteins bind to the amino terminus of huntingtin near the polyglutamine domain (Holbert et al., 2001; Ferrier, 2002; McPherson, 2002). However, huntingtin-associated protein 40 (HAP40) which is affecting Rab5-mediated endosomal motility in complex with huntingtin, interacts with huntingtin through its carboxy-terminal domain (Pal et al., 2006).

Also, the first conserved 17 amino acids in the amino-terminal huntingtin represent possible membrane association signal, which may influence the polyglutamine expansion (Ross, 1997). It has been shown that specific cleavage (at the residue Arg^{167}) and related presence of defined truncation at the N-terminus of huntingtin, mediate mutant huntingtin toxicity in Huntington's Disease (Ratovitski et al., 2009). Association of huntingtin with the production of brain-derived neurotrophic factors in cortical cells, a pro-survival factor for striatal neurons, just completes the complexity of its functions (Zuccato et al., 2001). Thus, detailed studies of huntingtin-related proteome, including the role of associated proteins in regulation of basic signaling pathways of wild type protein and mutants/polyglutamine forms in Huntington´s Disease, play an important role in research for discrepancies in energetic metabolism in Huntington's Disease and other neurodegenerative disorders, alternatively. Monospecific antibodies mapping targeting well defined epitopes on huntingtin and associated proteins may play a crucial role not only in basic research and clinical diagnostics, but also in the development of an efficient treatment for Huntington's Disease.

5. Conclusion

Despite all the efforts to obtain a drug that could overcome the energetic deficit that takes place in Huntington´s Disease, no such treatment has so far been successful to treat

Huntington´s Disease patients. However, as huntingtin protein has multiple functions in cell metabolism, it is possible that combined therapeutic approaches could improve the mutated huntingtin-mediated energy debit and slow down Huntington´s Disease course.

6. Acknowledgment

CNPq – Conselho Nacional de Desenvolvimento Científico e Tecnológico; Capes – Coordenação de Aperfeiçoamento de Pessoal de Nível Superior; J.S. Cruz is a CNPq fellow researcher; F.A. Oliveira was under a Capes fellowship (postdoctoral REUNI) in the beginning of this work. E. A. D. Gervásio-Carvalho held a scholarship from FAPEMIG-SANTANDER program.

7. References

Andreassen, O.A., Jenkins, B.G., Dedeoglu, A., Ferrante, K.L., Bogdanov, M.B., Kaddurah-Daouk, R., Beal, M.F. (2001) Increases in cortical glutamate concentrations in transgenic amyotrophic lateral sclerosis mice are attenuated by creatine supplementation. *Journal of neurochemistry*, 77, 383-390; ISSN 0022-3042.

Andrews, T.C., Brooks, D.J. (1998) Advances in the understanding of early Huntington's disease using the functional imaging techniques of PET and SPET. *Molecular medicine today*, 4, 532-539; ISSN 1357-4310.

Beal, M.F., Kowall, N.W., Ellison, D.W., Mazurek, M.F., Swartz, K.J., Martin, J.B. (1986) Replication of the neurochemical characteristics of Huntington's disease by quinolinic acid. *Nature*, 321, 168-171; ISSN 0028-0836.

Berg, J.M., Tymoczko, J.L., Stryer, L., eds (2006) *Biochemistry*, 6th Edition. New York: W H Freeman; 10: 0-7167-3051-0.

Bibb, J.A., Yan, Z., Svenningsson, P., Snyder, G.L., Pieribone, V.A., Horiuchi, A., Nairn, A.C., Messer, A., Greengard, P. (2000) Severe deficiencies in dopamine signaling in presymptomatic Huntington's disease mice. *Proceedings of the National Academy of Sciences of the United States of America*, 97, 6809-6814; ISSN 0027-8424.

Bolanos, J.P., Almeida, A., Moncada, S. (2010) Glycolysis: a bioenergetic or a survival pathway? *Trends in biochemical sciences*, 35, 145-149; ISSN 0968-0004.

Bolanos, J.P., Delgado-Esteban, M., Herrero-Mendez, A., Fernandez-Fernandez, S., Almeida, A. (2008) Regulation of glycolysis and pentose-phosphate pathway by nitric oxide: impact on neuronal survival. *Biochimica et biophysica acta*, 1777, 789-793; ISSN 0006-3002.

Browne, S.E. (2008) Mitochondria and Huntington's disease pathogenesis: insight from genetic and chemical models. *Annals of the New York Academy of Sciences*, 1147, 358-382; ISSN 1749-6632.

Browne, S.E., Beal, M.F. (2002) Toxin-induced mitochondrial dysfunction. *International review of neurobiology*, 53, 243-279; ISSN 0074-7742.

Browne, S.E., Beal, M.F. (2004) The energetics of Huntington's disease. *Neurochemical research*, 29, 531-546; ISSN 0364-3190.

Browne, S.E., Bowling, A.C., MacGarvey, U., Baik, M.J., Berger, S.C., Muqit, M.M., Bird, E.D., Beal, M.F. (1997) Oxidative damage and metabolic dysfunction in Huntington's disease: selective vulnerability of the basal ganglia. *Annals of neurology*, 41, 646-653; ISSN 0364-5134.

Butterworth, J., Yates, C.M., Reynolds, G.P. (1985) Distribution of phosphate-activated glutaminase, succinic dehydrogenase, pyruvate dehydrogenase and gamma-glutamyl transpeptidase in post-mortem brain from Huntington's disease and agonal cases. *Journal of the neurological sciences*, 67, 161-171; ISSN 0022-510X.

Chen, N., Luo, T., Wellington, C., Metzler, M., McCutcheon, K., Hayden, M.R., Raymond, L.A. (1999) Subtype-specific enhancement of NMDA receptor currents by mutant huntingtin. *Journal of neurochemistry*, 72, 1890-1898; ISSN 0022-3042.

Chiang, M.C., Chen, C.M., Lee, M.R., Chen, H.W., Chen, H.M., Wu, Y.S., Hung, C.H., Kang, J.J., Chang, C.P., Chang, C., Wu, Y.R., Tsai, Y.S., Chern, Y. (2010) Modulation of energy deficiency in Huntington's disease via activation of the peroxisome proliferator-activated receptor gamma. *Human molecular genetics*, 19, 4043-4058; ISSN 0964-6906.

Choo, Y.S., Johnson, G.V., MacDonald, M., Detloff, P.J., Lesort, M. (2004) Mutant huntingtin directly increases susceptibility of mitochondria to the calcium-induced permeability transition and cytochrome c release. *Human molecular genetics*, 13, 1407-1420; ISSN 0964-6906.

Clodfelder-Miller, B., De Sarno, P., Zmijewska, A.A., Song, L., Jope, R.S. (2005) Physiological and pathological changes in glucose regulate brain Akt and glycogen synthase kinase-3. *The Journal of biological chemistry*, 280, 39723-39731; ISSN 0021-9258.

Cooper, A.J., Sheu, K.R., Burke, J.R., Onodera, O., Strittmatter, W.J., Roses, A.D., Blass, J.P. (1997) Transglutaminase-catalyzed inactivation of glyceraldehyde 3-phosphate dehydrogenase and alpha-ketoglutarate dehydrogenase complex by polyglutamine domains of pathological length. *Proceedings of the National Academy of Sciences of the United States of America*, 94, 12604-12609; ISSN 0027-8424.

Cui, L., Jeong, H., Borovecki, F., Parkhurst, C.N., Tanese, N., Krainc, D. (2006) Transcriptional repression of PGC-1alpha by mutant huntingtin leads to mitochondrial dysfunction and neurodegeneration. *Cell*, 127, 59-69; ISSN 0092-8674.

Cunnane, S., Nugent, S., Roy, M., Courchesne-Loyer, A., Croteau, E., Tremblay, S., Castellano, A., Pifferi, F., Bocti, C., Paquet, N., Begdouri, H., Bentourkia, M., Turcotte, E., Allard, M., Barberger-Gateau, P., Fulop, T., Rapoport, S.I. (2011) Brain fuel metabolism, aging, and Alzheimer's disease. *Nutrition*, 27, 3-20; ISSN 0899-9007.

Datta, S.R., Brunet, A., Greenberg, M.E. (1999) Cellular survival: a play in three Akts. *Genes & development*, 13, 2905-2927; ISSN 0890-9369.

Davey, G.P., Peuchen, S., Clark, J.B. (1998) Energy thresholds in brain mitochondria. Potential involvement in neurodegeneration. *The Journal of biological chemistry*, 273, 12753-12757; ISSN 0021-9258.

Dedeoglu, A., Kubilus, J.K., Jeitner, T.M., Matson, S.A., Bogdanov, M., Kowall, N.W., Matson, W.R., Cooper, A.J., Ratan, R.R., Beal, M.F., Hersch, S.M., Ferrante, R.J. (2002) Therapeutic effects of cystamine in a murine model of Huntington's disease. *The Journal of neuroscience : the official journal of the Society for Neuroscience*, 22, 8942-8950; ISSN 0270-6474.

Dedeoglu, A., Kubilus, J.K., Yang, L., Ferrante, K.L., Hersch, S.M., Beal, M.F., Ferrante, R.J. (2003) Creatine therapy provides neuroprotection after onset of clinical symptoms in Huntington's disease transgenic mice. *Journal of neurochemistry*, 85, 1359-1367; ISSN 0022-3042.

Dorner, J.L., Miller, B.R., Barton, S.J., Brock, T.J., Rebec, G.V. (2007) Sex differences in behavior and striatal ascorbate release in the 140 CAG knock-in mouse model of Huntington's disease. *Behavioural brain research*, 178, 90-97; ISSN 0166-4328.

Dure, L.S.t., Young, A.B., Penney, J.B. (1991) Excitatory amino acid binding sites in the caudate nucleus and frontal cortex of Huntington's disease. *Annals of neurology*, 30, 785-793; ISSN 0364-5134.

Duval, E., Case, A., Stein, R.L., Cuny, G.D. (2005) Structure-activity relationship study of novel tissue transglutaminase inhibitors. *Bioorganic & medicinal chemistry letters*, 15, 1885-1889; ISSN 0960-894X.

Feigin, A., Tang, C., Ma, Y., Mattis, P., Zgaljardic, D., Guttman, M., Paulsen, J.S., Dhawan, V., Eidelberg, D. (2007) Thalamic metabolism and symptom onset in preclinical Huntington's disease. *Brain : a journal of neurology*, 130, 2858-2867; ISSN 0006-8950.

Ferrante, R.J., Andreassen, O.A., Jenkins, B.G., Dedeoglu, A., Kuemmerle, S., Kubilus, J.K., Kaddurah-Daouk, R., Hersch, S.M., Beal, M.F. (2000) Neuroprotective effects of creatine in a transgenic mouse model of Huntington's disease. *The Journal of neuroscience : the official journal of the Society for Neuroscience*, 20, 4389-4397; ISSN 0270-6474.

Ferrer, I., Goutan, E., Marin, C., Rey, M.J., Ribalta, T. (2000) Brain-derived neurotrophic factor in Huntington disease. *Brain research*, 866, 257-261; ISSN 0006-8993.

Ferrier, V. (2002) Hip, hip, hippi! *Nature cell biology*, 4, E30; ISSN 1465-7392.

Gines, S., Ivanova, E., Seong, I.S., Saura, C.A., MacDonald, M.E. (2003a) Enhanced Akt signaling is an early pro-survival response that reflects N-methyl-D-aspartate receptor activation in Huntington's disease knock-in striatal cells. *The Journal of biological chemistry*, 278, 50514-50522; ISSN 0021-9258.

Gines, S., Seong, I.S., Fossale, E., Ivanova, E., Trettel, F., Gusella, J.F., Wheeler, V.C., Persichetti, F., MacDonald, M.E. (2003b) Specific progressive cAMP reduction implicates energy deficit in presymptomatic Huntington's disease knock-in mice. *Human molecular genetics*, 12, 497-508; ISSN 0964-6906.

Group, H.S. (2001) A randomized, placebo-controlled trial of coenzyme Q10 and remacemide in Huntington's disease. *Neurology*, 57, 397-404; ISSN 0028-3878.

Gu, M., Gash, M.T., Mann, V.M., Javoy-Agid, F., Cooper, J.M., Schapira, A.H. (1996) Mitochondrial defect in Huntington's disease caudate nucleus. *Annals of neurology*, 39, 385-389; ISSN 0364-5134.

Heales, S.J., Bolanos, J.P. (2002) Impairment of brain mitochondrial function by reactive nitrogen species: the role of glutathione in dictating susceptibility. *Neurochemistry international*, 40, 469-474; ISSN 0197-0186.

Hemmer, W., Wallimann, T. (1993) Functional aspects of creatine kinase in brain. *Developmental neuroscience*, 15, 249-260; ISSN 0378-5866.

Henneberry, R.C., Novelli, A., Cox, J.A., Lysko, P.G. (1989) Neurotoxicity at the N-methyl-D-aspartate receptor in energy-compromised neurons. An hypothesis for cell death in aging and disease. *Annals of the New York Academy of Sciences*, 568, 225-233; ISSN 0077-8923.

Herrero-Mendez, A., Almeida, A., Fernandez, E., Maestre, C., Moncada, S., Bolanos, J.P. (2009) The bioenergetic and antioxidant status of neurons is controlled by continuous degradation of a key glycolytic enzyme by APC/C-Cdh1. *Nature cell biology*, 11, 747-752; ISSN 1465-7392.

Hickey, M.A., Chesselet, M.F. (2003) Apoptosis in Huntington's disease. *Progress in neuropsychopharmacology & biological psychiatry*, 27, 255-265; ISSN 0278-5846.

Ho, D.J., Calingasan, N.Y., Wille, E., Dumont, M., Beal, M.F. (2010) Resveratrol protects against peripheral deficits in a mouse model of Huntington's disease. *Experimental neurology*, 225, 74-84; ISSN 0014-4886.

Holbert, S., Denghien, I., Kiechle, T., Rosenblatt, A., Wellington, C., Hayden, M.R., Margolis, R.L., Ross, C.A., Dausset, J., Ferrante, R.J., Neri, C. (2001) The Gln-Ala repeat transcriptional activator CA150 interacts with huntingtin: neuropathologic and genetic evidence for a role in Huntington's disease pathogenesis. *Proceedings of the National Academy of Sciences of the United States of America*, 98, 1811-1816; ISSN 0027-8424.

Hroudova, J., Fisar, Z. (2011) Connectivity between mitochondrial functions and psychiatric disorders. *Psychiatry and clinical neurosciences*, 65, 130-141; ISSN 1323-1316.

Hult, S., Soylu, R., Bjorklund, T., Belgardt, B.F., Mauer, J., Bruning, J.C., Kirik, D., Petersen, A. (2011) Mutant huntingtin causes metabolic imbalance by disruption of hypothalamic neurocircuits. *Cell metabolism*, 13, 428-439; ISSN 1550-4131.

Humbert, S., Bryson, E.A., Cordelieres, F.P., Connors, N.C., Datta, S.R., Finkbeiner, S., Greenberg, M.E., Saudou, F. (2002) The IGF-1/Akt pathway is neuroprotective in Huntington's disease and involves Huntingtin phosphorylation by Akt. *Developmental cell*, 2, 831-837; ISSN 1534-5807.

Hunter, R.L., Dragicevic, N., Seifert, K., Choi, D.Y., Liu, M., Kim, H.C., Cass, W.A., Sullivan, P.G., Bing, G. (2007) Inflammation induces mitochondrial dysfunction and dopaminergic neurodegeneration in the nigrostriatal system. *Journal of neurochemistry*, 100, 1375-1386; ISSN 0022-3042.

Jeitner, T.M., Delikatny, E.J., Ahlqvist, J., Capper, H., Cooper, A.J. (2005) Mechanism for the inhibition of transglutaminase 2 by cystamine. *Biochemical pharmacology*, 69, 961-970; ISSN 0006-2952.

Jenkins, B.G., Koroshetz, W.J., Beal, M.F., Rosen, B.R. (1993) Evidence for impairment of energy metabolism in vivo in Huntington's disease using localized 1H NMR spectroscopy. *Neurology*, 43, 2689-2695; ISSN 0028-3878.

Jenkins, B.G., Rosas, H.D., Chen, Y.C., Makabe, T., Myers, R., MacDonald, M., Rosen, B.R., Beal, M.F., Koroshetz, W.J. (1998) 1H NMR spectroscopy studies of Huntington's disease: correlations with CAG repeat numbers. *Neurology*, 50, 1357-1365; ISSN 0028-3878.

Kandel, E.S., Hay, N. (1999) The regulation and activities of the multifunctional serine/threonine kinase Akt/PKB. *Experimental cell research*, 253, 210-229; ISSN 0014-4827.

Karpuj, M.V., Becher, M.W., Springer, J.E., Chabas, D., Youssef, S., Pedotti, R., Mitchell, D., Steinman, L. (2002) Prolonged survival and decreased abnormal movements in transgenic model of Huntington disease, with administration of the transglutaminase inhibitor cystamine. *Nature medicine*, 8, 143-149; ISSN 1078-8956.

Karpuj, M.V., Garren, H., Slunt, H., Price, D.L., Gusella, J., Becher, M.W., Steinman, L. (1999) Transglutaminase aggregates huntingtin into nonamyloidogenic polymers, and its enzymatic activity increases in Huntington's disease brain nuclei. *Proceedings of the National Academy of Sciences of the United States of America*, 96, 7388-7393; ISSN 0027-8424.

Kim, J., Moody, J.P., Edgerly, C.K., Bordiuk, O.L., Cormier, K., Smith, K., Beal, M.F., Ferrante, R.J. (2010) Mitochondrial loss, dysfunction and altered dynamics in Huntington's disease. *Human molecular genetics*, 19, 3919-3935; ISSN 0964-6906.

Kim, S.Y., Marekov, L., Bubber, P., Browne, S.E., Stavrovskaya, I., Lee, J., Steinert, P.M., Blass, J.P., Beal, M.F., Gibson, G.E., Cooper, A.J. (2005) Mitochondrial aconitase is a transglutaminase 2 substrate: transglutamination is a probable mechanism contributing to high-molecular-weight aggregates of aconitase and loss of aconitase activity in Huntington disease brain. *Neurochemical research*, 30, 1245-1255; ISSN 0364-3190.

Kita, H., Carmichael, J., Swartz, J., Muro, S., Wyttenbach, A., Matsubara, K., Rubinsztein, D.C., Kato, K. (2002) Modulation of polyglutamine-induced cell death by genes identified by expression profiling. *Human molecular genetics*, 11, 2279-2287; ISSN 0964-6906.

Klepper, J., Voit, T. (2002) Facilitated glucose transporter protein type 1 (GLUT1) deficiency syndrome: impaired glucose transport into brain-- a review. *European journal of pediatrics*, 161, 295-304; ISSN 0340-6199.

Klivenyi, P., Ferrante, R.J., Gardian, G., Browne, S., Chabrier, P.E., Beal, M.F. (2003) Increased survival and neuroprotective effects of BN82451 in a transgenic mouse model of Huntington's disease. *Journal of neurochemistry*, 86, 267-272; ISSN 0022-3042.

Koroshetz, W.J., Jenkins, B.G., Rosen, B.R., Beal, M.F. (1997) Energy metabolism defects in Huntington's disease and effects of coenzyme Q10. *Annals of neurology*, 41, 160-165; ISSN 0364-5134.

Kuhl, D.E., Markham, C.H., Metter, E.J., Riege, W.H., Phelps, M.E., Mazziotta, J.C. (1985) Local cerebral glucose utilization in symptomatic and presymptomatic Huntington's disease. *Research publications - Association for Research in Nervous and Mental Disease*, 63, 199-209; ISSN 0091-7443.

Kumar, P., Padi, S.S., Naidu, P.S., Kumar, A. (2006) Effect of resveratrol on 3-nitropropionic acid-induced biochemical and behavioural changes: possible neuroprotective mechanisms. *Behavioural pharmacology*, 17, 485-492; ISSN 0955-8810.

Kuwert, T., Lange, H.W., Langen, K.J., Herzog, H., Aulich, A., Feinendegen, L.E. (1990) Cortical and subcortical glucose consumption measured by PET in patients with Huntington's disease. *Brain : a journal of neurology*, 113 (Pt 5), 1405-1423; ISSN 0006-8950.

Lagouge, M., Argmann, C., Gerhart-Hines, Z., Meziane, H., Lerin, C., Daussin, F., Messadeq, N., Milne, J., Lambert, P., Elliott, P., Geny, B., Laakso, M., Puigserver, P., Auwerx, J. (2006) Resveratrol improves mitochondrial function and protects against metabolic disease by activating SIRT1 and PGC-1alpha. *Cell*, 127, 1109-1122; ISSN 0092-8674.

Lai, T.S., Liu, Y., Tucker, T., Daniel, K.R., Sane, D.C., Toone, E., Burke, J.R., Strittmatter, W.J., Greenberg, C.S. (2008) Identification of chemical inhibitors to human tissue transglutaminase by screening existing drug libraries. *Chemistry & biology*, 15, 969-978; ISSN 1074-5521.

Lesort, M., Chun, W., Johnson, G.V., Ferrante, R.J. (1999) Tissue transglutaminase is increased in Huntington's disease brain. *Journal of neurochemistry*, 73, 2018-2027; ISSN 0022-3042.

Li, X.J., Orr, A.L., Li, S. (2010) Impaired mitochondrial trafficking in Huntington's disease. *Biochimica et biophysica acta*, 1802, 62-65; ISSN 0006-3002.

Liang, H., Ward, W.F. (2006) PGC-1alpha: a key regulator of energy metabolism. *Amerian Journal of Physiology*, 30, 145-151; ISSN 1043-4046.

Lim, D., Fedrizzi, L., Tartari, M., Zuccato, C., Cattaneo, E., Brini, M., Carafoli, E. (2008) Calcium homeostasis and mitochondrial dysfunction in striatal neurons of Huntington disease. *The Journal of biological chemistry*, 283, 5780-5789; ISSN 0021-9258.

Lin, J. et al. (2004) Defects in adaptive energy metabolism with CNS-linked hyperactivity in PGC-1alpha null mice. *Cell*, 119, 121-135; ISSN 0092-8674.

Lund-Andersen, H. (1979) Transport of glucose from blood to brain. *Physiological reviews*, 59, 305-352; ISSN 0031-9333.

Luthi-Carter, R., Hanson, S.A., Strand, A.D., Bergstrom, D.A., Chun, W., Peters, N.L., Woods, A.M., Chan, E.Y., Kooperberg, C., Krainc, D., Young, A.B., Tapscott, S.J., Olson, J.M. (2002) Dysregulation of gene expression in the R6/2 model of polyglutamine disease: parallel changes in muscle and brain. *Human molecular genetics*, 11, 1911-1926; ISSN 0964-6906.

Luthi-Carter, R., Strand, A., Peters, N.L., Solano, S.M., Hollingsworth, Z.R., Menon, A.S., Frey, A.S., Spektor, B.S., Penney, E.B., Schilling, G., Ross, C.A., Borchelt, D.R., Tapscott, S.J., Young, A.B., Cha, J.H., Olson, J.M. (2000) Decreased expression of striatal signaling genes in a mouse model of Huntington's disease. *Human molecular genetics*, 9, 1259-1271; ISSN 0964-6906.

Mastroberardino, P.G., Iannicola, C., Nardacci, R., Bernassola, F., De Laurenzi, V., Melino, G., Moreno, S., Pavone, F., Oliverio, S., Fesus, L., Piacentini, M. (2002) 'Tissue' transglutaminase ablation reduces neuronal death and prolongs survival in a mouse model of Huntington's disease. *Cell death and differentiation*, 9, 873-880; ISSN 1350-9047.

Matthews, R.T., Yang, L., Jenkins, B.G., Ferrante, R.J., Rosen, B.R., Kaddurah-Daouk, R., Beal, M.F. (1998) Neuroprotective effects of creatine and cyclocreatine in animal models of Huntington's disease. *The Journal of neuroscience : the official journal of the Society for Neuroscience*, 18, 156-163; ISSN 0270-6474.

Mazzola, J.L., Sirover, M.A. (2001) Reduction of glyceraldehyde-3-phosphate dehydrogenase activity in Alzheimer's disease and in Huntington's disease fibroblasts. *Journal of neurochemistry*, 76, 442-449; ISSN 0022-3042.

Mazzola, J.L., Sirover, M.A. (2002) Alteration of nuclear glyceraldehyde-3-phosphate dehydrogenase structure in Huntington's disease fibroblasts. *Brain research Molecular brain research*, 100, 95-101; ISSN 0169-328X.

McPherson, P.S. (2002) The endocytic machinery at an interface with the actin cytoskeleton: a dynamic, hip intersection. *Trends in cell biology*, 12, 312-315; ISSN 0962-8924.

Menalled, L.B. (2005) Knock-in mouse models of Huntington's disease. *NeuroRx : the journal of the American Society for Experimental NeuroTherapeutics*, 2, 465-470; ISSN 1545-5343.

Milakovic, T., Johnson, G.V. (2005) Mitochondrial respiration and ATP production are significantly impaired in striatal cells expressing mutant huntingtin. *The Journal of biological chemistry*, 280, 30773-30782; ISSN 0021-9258.

Mochel, F., Charles, P., Seguin, F., Barritault, J., Coussieu, C., Perin, L., Le Bouc, Y., Gervais, C., Carcelain, G., Vassault, A., Feingold, J., Rabier, D., Durr, A. (2007) Early energy deficit in Huntington disease: identification of a plasma biomarker traceable during disease progression. *PloS one*, 2, e647; ISSN 1932-6203.

Mochel, F., Durant, B., Schiffmann, R., Durr, A. (2010a) Characterization of the locoregional brain energy profile in wild-type mice and identification of an energy deficit in a neurodegenerative model. *Journal of inherited metabolic disease*, 33, S181; ISSN 0141-8955.

Mochel, F., Duteil, S., Marelli, C., Jauffret, C., Barles, A., Holm, J., Sweetman, L., Benoist, J.F., Rabier, D., Carlier, P.G., Durr, A. (2010b) Dietary anaplerotic therapy improves peripheral tissue energy metabolism in patients with Huntington's disease. *European journal of human genetics*, 18, 1057-1060; ISSN 1018-4813.

Nehlig, A., Coles, J.A. (2007) Cellular pathways of energy metabolism in the brain: is glucose used by neurons or astrocytes? *Glia*, 55, 1238-1250; ISSN 0894-1491.

Nelson, D.L., Cox, M.M., eds (2004) *Lehninger Principles of Biochemistry*, 4th Edition: W. H. Freeman; 10: 0716743396

Nicholls, D.G. (2009) Mitochondrial calcium function and dysfunction in the central nervous system. *Biochimica et biophysica acta*, 1787, 1416-1424; ISSN 0006-3002.

Novelli, A., Reilly, J.A., Lysko, P.G., Henneberry, R.C. (1988) Glutamate becomes neurotoxic via the N-methyl-D-aspartate receptor when intracellular energy levels are reduced. *Brain research*, 451, 205-212; ISSN 0006-8993.

Nucifora, F.C., Jr., Sasaki, M., Peters, M.F., Huang, H., Cooper, J.K., Yamada, M., Takahashi, H., Tsuji, S., Troncoso, J., Dawson, V.L., Dawson, T.M., Ross, C.A. (2001) Interference by huntingtin and atrophin-1 with cbp-mediated transcription leading to cellular toxicity. *Science*, 291, 2423-2428; ISSN 0036-8075.

O'Gorman, E., Beutner, G., Wallimann, T., Brdiczka, D. (1996) Differential effects of creatine depletion on the regulation of enzyme activities and on creatine-stimulated mitochondrial respiration in skeletal muscle, heart, and brain. *Biochimica et biophysica acta*, 1276, 161-170; ISSN 0006-3002.

O'Brien, C.F., Miller, C., Goldblatt, D., Welle, S., Forbes, G., Lipinski, B., Panzik, J., Peck, R., Plumb, S., Oakes, D., Kurlan, R., Shoulson, I. (1990) Extraneural metabolism in early Huntington's disease. Ann. Neurol. 28:300–301. *Annals of neurology*, 28, 300-301; ISSN 0364-5134.

Okar, D.A., Manzano, A., Navarro-Sabate, A., Riera, L., Bartrons, R., Lange, A.J. (2001) PFK-2/FBPase-2: maker and breaker of the essential biofactor fructose-2,6-bisphosphate. *Trends in biochemical sciences*, 26, 30-35; ISSN 0968-0004.

Oliveira, F.A., Galan, D.T., Ribeiro, A.M., Santos Cruz, J. (2007) Thiamine deficiency during pregnancy leads to cerebellar neuronal death in rat offspring: role of voltage-dependent K+ channels. *Brain research*, 1134, 79-86; ISSN 0006-8993.

Pal, A., Severin, F., Lommer, B., Shevchenko, A., Zerial, M. (2006) Huntingtin-HAP40 complex is a novel Rab5 effector that regulates early endosome motility and is up-regulated in Huntington's disease. *The Journal of cell biology*, 172, 605-618; ISSN 0021-9525.

Panov, A.V., Gutekunst, C.A., Leavitt, B.R., Hayden, M.R., Burke, J.R., Strittmatter, W.J., Greenamyre, J.T. (2002) Early mitochondrial calcium defects in Huntington's disease are a direct effect of polyglutamines. *Nature neuroscience*, 5, 731-736; ISSN 1097-6256.

Pardridge, W.M., Boado, R.J., Farrell, C.R. (1990) Brain-type glucose transporter (GLUT-1) is selectively localized to the blood-brain barrier. Studies with quantitative western blotting and in situ hybridization. *The Journal of biological chemistry*, 265, 18035-18040; ISSN 0021-9258.

Pesin, J.A., Orr-Weaver, T.L. (2008) Regulation of APC/C activators in mitosis and meiosis. *Annual review of cell and developmental biology*, 24, 475-499; ISSN 1081-0706.

Powers, W.J., Videen, T.O., Markham, J., McGee-Minnich, L., Antenor-Dorsey, J.V., Hershey, T., Perlmutter, J.S. (2007) Selective defect of in vivo glycolysis in early Huntington's disease striatum. *Proceedings of the National Academy of Sciences of the United States of America*, 104, 2945-2949; ISSN 0027-8424.

Quintanilla, R.A., Jin, Y.N., Fuenzalida, K., Bronfman, M., Johnson, G.V. (2008) Rosiglitazone treatment prevents mitochondrial dysfunction in mutant huntingtin-expressing cells: possible role of peroxisome proliferator-activated receptor-gamma (PPARgamma) in the pathogenesis of Huntington disease. *The Journal of biological chemistry*, 283, 25628-25637; ISSN 0021-9258.

Ratovitski, T., Gucek, M., Jiang, H., Chighladze, E., Waldron, E., D'Ambola, J., Hou, Z., Liang, Y., Poirier, M.A., Hirschhorn, R.R., Graham, R., Hayden, M.R., Cole, R.N., Ross, C.A. (2009) Mutant huntingtin N-terminal fragments of specific size mediate aggregation and toxicity in neuronal cells. *The Journal of biological chemistry*, 284, 10855-10867; ISSN 0021-9258.

Ravikumar, B., Stewart, A., Kita, H., Kato, K., Duden, R., Rubinsztein, D.C. (2003) Raised intracellular glucose concentrations reduce aggregation and cell death caused by mutant huntingtin exon 1 by decreasing mTOR phosphorylation and inducing autophagy. *Human molecular genetics*, 12, 985-994; ISSN 0964-6906.

Rebec, G.V., Barton, S.J., Ennis, M.D. (2002) Dysregulation of ascorbate release in the striatum of behaving mice expressing the Huntington's disease gene. *The Journal of neuroscience: the official journal of the Society for Neuroscience*, 22, RC202; ISSN 0270-6474.

Rebec, G.V., Barton, S.J., Marseilles, A.M., Collins, K. (2003) Ascorbate treatment attenuates the Huntington behavioral phenotype in mice. *Neuroreport*, 14, 1263-1265; ISSN 0959-4965.

Rosen, E.D., Spiegelman, B.M. (2001) PPARgamma : a nuclear regulator of metabolism, differentiation, and cell growth. *The Journal of biological chemistry*, 276, 37731-37734; ISSN 0021-9258.

Ross, C.A. (1997) Intranuclear neuronal inclusions: a common pathogenic mechanism for glutamine-repeat neurodegenerative diseases? *Neuron*, 19, 1147-1150; ISSN 0896-6273.

Saraiva, L.M., Seixas da Silva, G.S., Galina, A., da-Silva, W.S., Klein, W.L., Ferreira, S.T., De Felice, F.G. (2010) Amyloid-β Triggers the Release of Neuronal Hexokinase 1 from Mitochondria. *PloS one*, 5, e15230; ISSN 1932-6203.

Sawa, A., Wiegand, G.W., Cooper, J., Margolis, R.L., Sharp, A.H., Lawler, J.F., Jr., Greenamyre, J.T., Snyder, S.H., Ross, C.A. (1999) Increased apoptosis of Huntington disease lymphoblasts associated with repeat length-dependent mitochondrial depolarization. *Nature medicine*, 5, 1194-1198; ISSN 1078-8956.

Schaertl, S., Prime, M., Wityak, J., Dominguez, C., Munoz-Sanjuan, I., Pacifici, R.E., Courtney, S., Scheel, A., Macdonald, D. (2010) A profiling platform for the characterization of transglutaminase 2 (TG2) inhibitors. *Journal of biomolecular screening*, 15, 478-487; ISSN 1087-0571.

Schiefer, J., Sprunken, A., Puls, C., Luesse, H.G., Milkereit, A., Milkereit, E., Johann, V., Kosinski, C.M. (2004) The metabotropic glutamate receptor 5 antagonist MPEP and the mGluR2 agonist LY379268 modify disease progression in a transgenic mouse model of Huntington's disease. *Brain research*, 1019, 246-254; ISSN 0006-8993.

Schulz, J.B., Matthews, R.T., Henshaw, D.R., Beal, M.F. (1996) Neuroprotective strategies for treatment of lesions produced by mitochondrial toxins: implications for neurodegenerative diseases. *Neuroscience*, 71, 1043-1048; ISSN 0306-4522.

Schutz, B., Reimann, J., Dumitrescu-Ozimek, L., Kappes-Horn, K., Landreth, G.E., Schurmann, B., Zimmer, A., Heneka, M.T. (2005) The oral antidiabetic pioglitazone protects from neurodegeneration and amyotrophic lateral sclerosis-like symptoms in superoxide dismutase-G93A transgenic mice. *The Journal of neuroscience : the official journal of the Society for Neuroscience*, 25, 7805-7812; ISSN 0270-6474.

Senatorov, V.V., Charles, V., Reddy, P.H., Tagle, D.A., Chuang, D.M. (2003) Overexpression and nuclear accumulation of glyceraldehyde-3-phosphate dehydrogenase in a transgenic mouse model of Huntington's disease. *Molecular and cellular neurosciences*, 22, 285-297; ISSN 1044-7431.

Seong, I.S., Ivanova, E., Lee, J.M., Choo, Y.S., Fossale, E., Anderson, M., Gusella, J.F., Laramie, J.M., Myers, R.H., Lesort, M., MacDonald, M.E. (2005) HD CAG repeat implicates a dominant property of huntingtin in mitochondrial energy metabolism. *Human molecular genetics*, 14, 2871-2880; ISSN 0964-6906.

Shimohata, T., Nakajima, T., Yamada, M., Uchida, C., Onodera, O., Naruse, S., Kimura, T., Koide, R., Nozaki, K., Sano, Y., Ishiguro, H., Sakoe, K., Ooshima, T., Sato, A., Ikeuchi, T., Oyake, M., Sato, T., Aoyagi, Y., Hozumi, I., Nagatsu, T., Takiyama, Y., Nishizawa, M., Goto, J., Kanazawa I., Davidson, I., Tanese, N., Takahashi, H., Tsuji, S. (2000) Expanded polyglutamine stretches interact with TAFII130, interfering with CREB-dependent transcription. *Nature genetics*, 26, 29-36; ISSN 1061-4036.

Siegel, G.J., Agranoff, B.W., Albers, W., Fisher, S.K., Uhler, M.D., eds (1999) *Basic Neurochemistry - Molecular, Cellular and Medical Aspects*. Philadelphia: Lippincott-Raven; ISBN 10: 0-397-51820-X.

Sipione, S., Rigamonti, D., Valenza, M., Zuccato, C., Conti, L., Pritchard, J., Kooperberg, C., Olson, J.M., Cattaneo, E. (2002) Early transcriptional profiles in huntingtin-inducible striatal cells by microarray analyses. *Human molecular genetics*, 11, 1953-1965; ISSN 0964-6906.

Steffan, J.S., Kazantsev, A., Spasic-Boskovic, O., Greenwald, M., Zhu, Y.Z., Gohler, H., Wanker, E.E., Bates, G.P., Housman, D.E., Thompson, L.M. (2000) The Huntington's disease protein interacts with p53 and CREB-binding protein and represses transcription. *Proceedings of the National Academy of Sciences of the United States of America*, 97, 6763-6768; ISSN 0027-8424.

Strum, J.C., Shehee, R., Virley, D., Richardson, J., Mattie, M., Selley, P., Ghosh, S., Nock, C., Saunders, A., Roses, A. (2007) Rosiglitazone induces mitochondrial biogenesis in mouse brain. *Journal of Alzheimer's disease*, 11, 45-51; ISSN 1387-2877.

Sun, Y., Savanenin, A., Reddy, P.H., Liu, Y.F. (2001) Polyglutamine-expanded huntingtin promotes sensitization of N-methyl-D-aspartate receptors via post-synaptic density 95. *The Journal of biological chemistry*, 276, 24713-24718; ISSN 0021-9258.

Tabrizi, S.J., Blamire, A.M., Manners, D.N., Rajagopalan, B., Styles, P., Schapira, A.H., Warner, T.T. (2005) High-dose creatine therapy for Huntington disease: a 2-year clinical and MRS study. *Neurology*, 64, 1655-1656; ISSN 0028-3878.

Tabrizi, S.J., Cleeter, M.W., Xuereb, J., Taanman, J.W., Cooper, J.M., Schapira, A.H. (1999) Biochemical abnormalities and excitotoxicity in Huntington's disease brain. *Annals of neurology*, 45, 25-32; ISSN 0364-5134.

Taherzadeh-Fard, E., Saft, C., Andrich, J., Wieczorek, S., Arning, L. (2009) PGC-1alpha as modifier of onset age in Huntington disease. *Molecular neurodegeneration*, 4, 10; ISSN 1750-1326.

Tang, T.S., Slow, E., Lupu, V., Stavrovskaya, I.G., Sugimori, M., Llinas, R., Kristal, B.S., Hayden, M.R., Bezprozvanny, I. (2005) Disturbed Ca2+ signaling and apoptosis of medium spiny neurons in Huntington's disease. *Proceedings of the National Academy of Sciences of the United States of America*, 102, 2602-2607; ISSN 0027-8424.

Tkac, I., Dubinsky, J.M., Keene, C.D., Gruetter, R., Low, W.C. (2007) Neurochemical changes in Huntington R6/2 mouse striatum detected by in vivo 1H NMR spectroscopy. *Journal of neurochemistry*, 100, 1397-1406; ISSN 0022-3042.

Truant, R., Atwal, R., Burtnik, A. (2006) Hypothesis: Huntingtin may function in membrane association and vesicular trafficking. *Biochemistry and cell biology = Biochimie et biologie cellulaire*, 84, 912-917; ISSN 0829-8211.

Vannucci, S.J., Maher, F., Simpson, I.A. (1997) Glucose transporter proteins in brain: delivery of glucose to neurons and glia. *Glia*, 21, 2-21; ISSN 0894-1491.

Verbessem, P., Lemiere, J., Eijnde, B.O., Swinnen, S., Vanhees, L., Van Leemputte, M., Hespel, P., Dom, R. (2003) Creatine supplementation in Huntington's disease: a placebo-controlled pilot trial. *Neurology*, 61, 925-930; ISSN 0028-3878.

Warby, S.C., Doty, C.N., Graham, R.K., Shively, J., Singaraja, R.R., Hayden, M.R. (2009) Phosphorylation of huntingtin reduces the accumulation of its nuclear fragments. *Molecular and cellular neurosciences*, 40, 121-127; ISSN 1044-7431.

Watson, G.S., Cholerton, B.A., Reger, M.A., Baker, L.D., Plymate, S.R., Asthana, S., Fishel, M.A., Kulstad, J.J., Green, P.S., Cook, D.G., Kahn, S.E., Keeling, M.L., Craft, S. (2005) Preserved cognition in patients with early Alzheimer disease and amnestic mild cognitive impairment during treatment with rosiglitazone: a preliminary study. *The American journal of geriatric psychiatry : official journal of the American Association for Geriatric Psychiatry*, 13, 950-958; ISSN 1064-7481.

Watson, G.S., Craft, S. (2003) The role of insulin resistance in the pathogenesis of Alzheimer's disease: implications for treatment. *CNS drugs*, 17, 27-45; ISSN 1172-7047.

Weydt, P., Pineda, V.V., Torrence, A.E., Libby, R.T., Satterfield, T.F., Lazarowski, E.R., Gilbert, M.L., Morton, G.J., Bammler, T.K., Strand, A.D., Cui, L., Beyer, R.P., Easley, C.N., Smith, A.C., Krainc, D., Luquet, S., Sweet, I.R., Schwartz, M.W., La Spada, A.R. (2006) Thermoregulatory and metabolic defects in Huntington's disease transgenic mice implicate PGC-1alpha in Huntington's disease neurodegeneration. *Cell metabolism*, 4, 349-362; ISSN 1550-4131.

Wilhelm, I., Fazakas, C., Krizbai, I.A. (2011) In vitro models of the blood-brain barrier. *Acta neurobiologiae experimentalis*, 71, 113-128; ISSN 0065-1400.

Wullner, U., Young, A.B., Penney, J.B., Beal, M.F. (1994) 3-Nitropropionic acid toxicity in the striatum. *Journal of neurochemistry*, 63, 1772-1781; ISSN 0022-3042.

Wyttenbach, A., Swartz, J., Kita, H., Thykjaer, T., Carmichael, J., Bradley, J., Brown, R., Maxwell, M., Schapira, A., Orntoft, T.F., Kato, K., Rubinsztein, D.C. (2001) Polyglutamine expansions cause decreased CRE-mediated transcription and early gene expression changes prior to cell death in an inducible cell model of Huntington's disease. *Human molecular genetics*, 10, 1829-1845; ISSN 0964-6906.

Yalcin, A., Telang, S., Clem, B., Chesney, J. (2009) Regulation of glucose metabolism by 6-phosphofructo-2-kinase/fructose-2,6-bisphosphatases in cancer. *Experimental and molecular pathology*, 86, 174-179; ISSN 0014-4800.

Yamanaka, T., Miyazaki, H., Oyama, F., Kurosawa, M., Washizu, C., Doi, H., Nukina, N. (2008) Mutant Huntingtin reduces HSP70 expression through the sequestration of NF-Y transcription factor. *The EMBO journal*, 27, 827-839; ISSN 0261-4189.

Yang, L., Calingasan, N.Y., Wille, E.J., Cormier, K., Smith, K., Ferrante, R.J., Beal, M.F. (2009) Combination therapy with coenzyme Q10 and creatine produces additive neuroprotective effects in models of Parkinson's and Huntington's diseases. *Journal of neurochemistry*, 109, 1427-1439; ISSN 0022-3042.

Yu, Z.X., Li, S.H., Evans, J., Pillarisetti, A., Li, H., Li, X.J. (2003) Mutant huntingtin causes context-dependent neurodegeneration in mice with Huntington's disease. *The Journal of neuroscience : the official journal of the Society for Neuroscience*, 23, 2193-2202; ISSN 0270-6474ISSN.

Zeevalk, G.D., Nicklas, W.J. (1991) Mechanisms underlying initiation of excitotoxicity associated with metabolic inhibition. *The Journal of pharmacology and experimental therapeutics*, 257, 870-878; ISSN 0022-3565.

Zeron, M.M., Chen, N., Moshaver, A., Lee, A.T., Wellington, C.L., Hayden, M.R., Raymond, L.A. (2001) Mutant huntingtin enhances excitotoxic cell death. *Molecular and cellular neurosciences*, 17, 41-53; ISSN 1044-7431.

Zeron, M.M., Hansson, O., Chen, N., Wellington, C.L., Leavitt, B.R., Brundin, P., Hayden, M.R., Raymond, L.A. (2002) Increased sensitivity to N-methyl-D-aspartate receptor-mediated excitotoxicity in a mouse model of Huntington's disease. *Neuron*, 33, 849-860; ISSN 0896-6273.

Zuccato, C., Ciammola, A., Rigamonti, D., Leavitt, B.R., Goffredo, D., Conti, L., MacDonald, M.E., Friedlander, R.M., Silani, V., Hayden, M.R., Timmusk, T., Sipione, S., Cattaneo, E. (2001) Loss of huntingtin-mediated BDNF gene transcription in Huntington's disease. *Science*, 293, 493-498; ISSN 0036-8075.

2

The Use of the Mitochondrial Toxin 3-NP to Uncover Cellular Dysfunction in Huntington's Disease

Elizabeth Hernández-Echeagaray, Gabriela De la Rosa-López
and Ernesto Mendoza-Duarte
Laboratorio de Neurofisiología del Desarrollo y la Neurodegeneración,
Unidad de Biomedicina, FES-Iztacala,
Universidad Nacional Autónoma de México,
México

1. Introduction

Degenerative diseases that affect the nervous system are characterized by a progressive alteration of specific neuronal populations and normally end in cell death. Some neurodegenerative disorders exhibit a clear genetic origin, such as in the case of Huntington's Disease (HD); however, most neurodegenerative diseases do not have a genetic cause, suggesting that other mechanisms cause these alterations.

Even though each neurodegenerative disease exhibits specific features, many similarities in the degenerative process are also shown; the study of these similarities could provide ideas for the therapeutic management of such diseases. For example, Parkinson's, Alzheimer's, and Huntington's Diseases exhibit atypical protein assemblies, excitotoxicity, metabolic alterations, oxidative stress and mitochondrial failure (Shoffner et al., 1991; Sims et al., 1996; Kapogiannis and Mattson, 2011). All of these cellular alterations can trigger one or more forms of cell death, namely apoptosis, necrosis and/or autophagy. Normally, excitotoxicity and inflammatory activations are associated with necrosis as a type of neuronal death (Artal-Sanz and Tavernarakis, 2005); the apoptotic type of cell death is often associated with the activation of cysteine protease caspase-3 (Kroemer et al., 1998). However, in post-mortem tissue from HD patients, no clear histological or pathological data are available in support of apoptotic cell death (Vis et al., 2005), although DNA damage in the progression of degeneration was shown to be evident (Brouillet et al., 1999). Also, in animal models of neurodegeneration, oxidative stress promotes apoptotic damage, triggered by the activation of caspases (Burke et al., 1996; Krantic et al., 2005). In neurodegenration, it is important to understand which type of cell death mechanism is involved however, it is also important to be aware that the speed of cell death process in "sick" neurons is slow (Kanazawa, 2001).

2. Mitochondrial dysfunction

Studies over several decades have documented experimental evidence to support the fact that mitochondrial dysfunction and oxidative stress are part of the cellular mechanisms underlying neurodegeneration. Mitochondrial dysfunction can occur early on in the pathogenesis of several diseases, including HD (Koroshetz et al., 1997; Jenkins et al., 1993, 1998; Panov et al., 2002; Lin and Beal, 2006).

During mitochondrial respiration, reactive oxygen species (ROS) are produced as by products of respiratory chain activity; their overproduction generates oxidative stress, and is a hallmark of neurodegenerative disorders. The respiratory chain is composed of five complexes: complexes I and II collect electrons from the catabolism of fats, proteins and carbohydrates and transfer them to co-enzyme Q10, complex III and complex IV. Importantly, complexes I, III and IV utilize the energy produced by the electron gradient generated by pumping protons across the inner mitochondrial membrane; this proton gradient is used by complex V to condense Adenosine diphosphate (ADP) and inorganic phosphate into Adenosine-5'-triphosphate (ATP). Any alteration in the mitochondrial complex is expected to produce ATP deficiency (Fridovich, 1999), release of cytochrome c which activates the intrinsic pathways of neuronal death and the activation of caspases related to apoptotic damage (Maciel et al., 2004).

3. Huntington Disease

Huntington's Disease, also called Huntington's chorea because of the presence of rapid and incessant choreic movements accompanied by cognitive and psychiatric alterations, is an inherited neurodegenerative disease that affects cell projections in a specific region of the brain known as the nucleus striatum. This neurodegenerative illness was described in 1872 by George Huntington, although some features that resemble HD had already been described earlier (Walker, 2007).

The symptoms manifest in the third or fourth decade of life in most cases, and progression of the illness is slow (15 to 20 years). In comparison to other neurodegenerative diseases, the development of HD is associated with the mutation of a single gene called *Interesting Transcrip 15* (IT15), or the *Hd* gene. The mutation originates the expansion of the CAG nucleotide repeats in a single protein called huntingtin; wich is called mutant huntingtin (mhtt), when the CAG expansion is present (Taylor et al., 2002). This single mutation produces diverse cellular, physiological and anatomical changes; however, the cellular mechanisms underlying HD neurodegeneration are not yet fully understood.

A number of studies have shown that mitochondria from HD patients and animal models are damaged (Jenkings et al., 1993), suggesting that disturbances in the cellular metabolism of HD patients originate via mitochondrial dysfunction (Beal, 2005). Deficits in energy metabolism become manifest in the pre-symptomatic and symptomatic HD brain and peripheral tissues (Kuhl et al., 1982; Mazziotta et al., 1987; Grafton et al., 1990; Koroshetz et al., 1997; Lodi et al., 2000). In particular, factors related to mitochondrial functioning seem to underlie the selective vulnerability of striatal cells (Saft et al., 2005; Seong et al., 2005); for example, the reduction of the chaperone, protease and intramembrane mitochondrial molecule Omi/HTr2 (Inagaki et al., 2008), and alterations in oxidative phosphorylation functioning in general (Pickrell et al., 2011). Post-mortem studies on HD brain tissue showed decreased activity in complexes II, III and IV of the mitochondrial respiratory chain (Gu et al., 1996). Also, animal models of HD showed deficits in mitochondrial respiration (Browne et al., 1997); for example; the systemic administration of mitochondrial toxins or inhibitors generated striatal pathology and movement disorders such as chorea and dystonia, which resemble HD (Ludolph et al., 1991; Browne, 2008). In fact, accidental ingestion of the irreversible mitochondrial inhibitor 3-nitropropionic acid (3-NP) was found to cause striatal degeneration and the HD phenotype. Moreover, the systemic administration of 3-NP caused striatal cell loss and movement alterations in rats (Beal et al., 1993) and primates (Palfi et al., 1996; Dautry et al., 2000). However, an analysis of unbiased gene expression showed that changes in energy metabolism in mhtt of transgenic mice compared to 3-NP treated animals were different: while 3-NP affected mitochondrial pathway gene expression, the effects of mhtt on metabolism were extramitochondrial (Lee et al., 2007), which suggested that mitochondrial toxins such as 3-NP do not quite cause HD pathology (Olivera, 2010). However, mhtt generates mitochondrial dysfunction in HD (Grunewald & Beal 1999) and reductions in ATP generation (Seong et al., 2005), and it also alters Ca^{2+} buffering (Reddy et al., 2009) and mitochondrial trafficking (Li et al., 2010). Therefore, irrespective of whether mhtt impacts mitochondria directly or secondarily, the repercussions of mitochondrial dysfunction are devastating to cells and may underlie the disruptions in numerous cellular processes, resulting in HD pathogenesis. As a result, the identification of respiratory chain changes in complex II of respiratory chain in HD post-mortem brains led to the use of mitochondrial complex II inhibitors to generate toxicity models that replicate aspects of HD striatal pathology *in vivo*. Thus, studies on mitochondrial toxins are relevant and important for understanding defects in cellular metabolism and the energetic pathogenesis of Huntington's Disease.

4. 3-Nitropropionic acid (3-NP)

3-NP is a highly specific, time dependent and irreversible inhibitor of succinate dehydrogenase (SDH) and the Krebs cycle (Alston et al., 1977). The levels of inhibition of this enzyme by 3-NP correlate well with the levels of inhibition of the tricarboxylic acid cycle (Henry et al., 2002).

4.1 Changes in the central nervous system

3-NP treatment was found to cause striatal degeneration in rodents (Gould and Gustine 1982; Gould et al., 1985; Beal et al., 1992; Broulliet et al., 2005). In non-human primates, 3-NP produced cognitive deficits similar to those displayed by frontal-type and abnormal choreiform movements, followed by evident striatal degeneration (Palfi et al., 1998; Brouillet et al., 1999; Dautry et al., 2000).

It is known that 3-NP imitates the symptoms of dystonia, glutaric aciduria, Leber's disease and HD (Novotny et al., 1986; Janavs and Aminoff 1998; Strauss and Morton, 2003), but after discovering that the accidental ingestion of 3-NP (He et al., 1995; Ming, 1995) caused damage that was concentrated in the striatum, 3-NP was used in experimental models to study the cellular mechanisms underlying striatal neural degeneration (Alexi et al., 1998).

The initial studies suggested that excitotoxicity plays a central role in the physiological and cellular effects of 3-NP on striatal degeneration (Hamilton and Gould, 1987; Novelli et al., 1988; Zeevalk and Nicklas, 1990) because of the presence of massive glutamatergic afferents in the nuclei (Di Figlia et al., 1990); also, metabolic insults were suggested as playing a part in the mechanistic damage (Browne et al., 1997; Brouillet et al., 1999). Chronic treatment with 3-NP in rats produced astrogliosis and selective degeneration of medium-sized spiny neurons, similar to the neurochemical and histological pathology observed in post-mortem HD tissue. Interestingly, 3-NP treatment was found to retain terminals from large cholinergic interneurons and NADPH-diaphorase-positive aspiny interneurons (Beal et al., 1993; Brouillet et al., 1999).

The type of death triggered by 3-NP treatment depends on how the toxin was administered: intraparenchymal applications induce ischaemic injury features while intraperitoneal applications induce striatal degeneration, which shows more of an HD phenotype (Borlongan et al., 1997a). Another concern about the 3-NP pharmacological model of HD is related to the variations in cellular damage, which depend on whether a study is carried out *in vitro* or *in vivo*, whether rats or mice are used, whether 3-NP is administered intrastriatally or intraperitoneally, whether the treatment is acute or chronic, and whether low, sub-toxic or toxic concentrations are provided (Brouillet et al., 1999, 2005).

3-NP administered by subcutaneous (s.c.) or intraperitoneal (i.p.) injections is more toxic in rats than in mice. In rodents, the toxicity of 3-NP depends on the strain (Brouillet et al., 2005). Fisher rats, for example, are more susceptible to 3-NP toxicity than Sprague-Dawley, Wistar and Lewis strains (Ouary et al., 2000), and C57BL/6 and Balb/c mice are more resistant to 3-NP toxicity than 129SVEMS and FVB/n mice (Gabrielson et al., 2001). The strain-dependent differences observed following 3-NP intoxication are probably related to differences in elimination/detoxification of the compound (Ouary et al., 2000). Vulnerability to different agents is not restricted to animal strains; it occurs in all human groups and is due to genetic variations that give rise to different responses to drugs (Weinshilboum et al., 2003; Weinshilboum and Wang, 2006), so we need to be cautious when generalizing about the results obtained among different strains.

Other important factors are the age and gender of the animals used in experimental protocols (Brouillet et al., 1993). Interestingly, female rats are less sensitive to 3-NP than males, which suggests that oestrogen protection can affect the degree of sensitivity (Nishino et al., 1998; Mogami et al., 2002).

The method used for 3-NP delivery also influences the physiological effect; acute treatments of a single i.p. dose of 3-NP were found to lead to striatal degeneration within 6-12 h after injection (Alexi et al., 1998; Brouillet et al. 1999). Sub-chronic treatments consisting of daily repeated i.p. injections led to striatal degeneration over a few days (Beal et al., 1993; Schulz et al., 1996; Guyot et al., 1997). Chronic treatments (of more than 5 days up to 4 weeks) with the continuous systemic administration of 3-NP using subcutaneously implanted osmotic minipumps also produced striatal degeneration. Besides the mode of delivery, the treatment dose concentration also has an impact on 3-NP toxicity.

Depending on the time period over which 3-NP is administered, and the dose administered, rodents treated with 3-NP exhibit HD-like motor disorders with hyperkinetic and hypokinetic symptoms (Borlogan et al., 1997), and rats were shown to be more sensitive to the effects of 3-NP than mice (Brouillet, 2005). In rats, the administration of 3-NP (10 mg/kg i.p.) over several days was found to induce the onset of hypokinetic symptoms (Guyot et al., 1997), while its administration in two individual doses caused hyperkinetic symptoms (Borlongan et al., 1997b). However, besides the mode of delivery, the treatment dose also has an impact on 3-NP toxicity, where a 3-NP concentration of ~20 mg/kg was found to induce the expression of an HD behavioural phenotype after two injections. Nevertheless, these animals did not display extra-striatal lesions, which are frequently observed in the initial stages of HD (Beal et al., 1993; Guyot et al., 1997; Borlogan et al., 1997b). The chronic administration of low doses of 3-NP (~10 mg/kg, per day) for more than 3 weeks was found to induce sustained metabolic alterations and some other cellular features exhibited in HD patients, but did it not cause clear dyskinetic movements resembling chorea (Borlogan et al., 1997a, b; Brouillet et al., 1999).

Since there are differences in the response to 3-NP treatment among different animal strains (Ouary et al., 2000), we designed an administration plan of low concentration doses of 3-NP (15 mg/kg, i.p.) over a sub-chronic period (5 days) in C57BL/6 mice, which are known to be more resistant to 3-NP toxicity; this advantage enabled us to observe histopathological changes that mimic those found in the initial steps of the illness (Rodriguez et al., 2010), plus motor alterations such as orofacial dyskinesias and clasping behaviour (Hernández-Echeagaray et al., 2011), and spontaneous behaviours that resemblance the HD phenotype. Figure 1, shows that mice treated with low dose concentration of 3-NP displayed motor hyperactivity, as evaluated in open field tests. Hyperkinetic symptoms are exhibited in the initial steps of striatal damage in animals treated with 3-NP, whereas the hypokinetic phenotype develops later during striatal deterioration (Borlongan et al., 1997b).

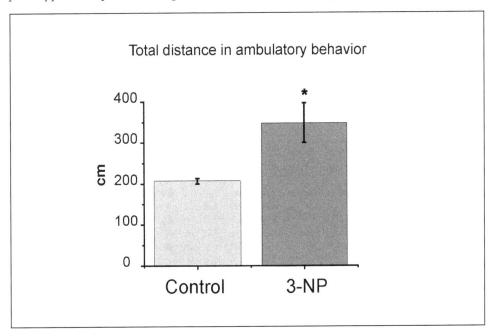

The graph shows the effects of 3-NP (15 mg / kg, per 5 days) in the spontaneous ambulatory motor behaviour of mice, scored as the total distance during 10 minutes period, evaluated in the open field test (Versadata, 3.02-1E7E software, Accuscan Instruments, INC.). There was a significant increase in locomotor activity in the 3-NP treated group (t-test, *p=0.0213). Arithmetic means and standard errors are plotted.

Fig. 1. 3-NP increases the ambulatory behavior evaluated in open field test.

We are especially interested in discerning the cellular events that take place during the beginning of the neurodegenerative process; the understanding of early dysfunctions will help in the planning of therapeutic strategies to reduce or delay cellular damage. The neuronal damage caused by low doses of 3-NP administration is restricted to striatal calbindin-positive cells (Fig. 2), leaving sparing parvalbumin and calretinin positive interneurons as previously suggested (Ferrante et al., 1987a, 1987b, Kowall et al., 1987, Massouh et al., 2008). Cellular alteration can also be initiated by caspase 3-dependent apoptosis, although necrotic cell death is also present (Rodriguez et al., 2010).

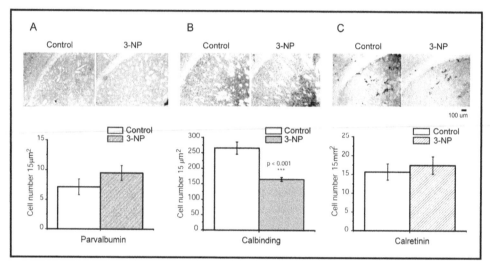

Top: light micrographs of calcium binding proteins immune localization in the neostriatal tissue. A, illustrates cells immune positive to parvalbumin. Cells were homogenously distributed in the striatum in both groups. The staining of immune positive cells was located in the soma. Graph in the bottom shows that there were no differences between groups in the number of cells expressing parvalbumin (t35 =-1.519, p=0.138). B illustrates striatal cells that were immune positive to calbinding. Calbinding positive cells were homogenously distributed a long the striatum in both groups and its localization was concentrated in the cell soma. Graph in the bottom shows that in tissue of 3-NP treated group, immune positive cells were significant reduced in comparison to control group (T99=2073.5, p<0.001). C illustrates calretinin immune positive cells. These cells were localized in dorsal striatum and staining was observed in cell body, dendrites and axonal ramifications. Interestingly tissue from 3-NP treated mice exhibited a decrease in cell ramifications but as shown in the bottom graph, the immune stained cell number did not change between groups (T82= 1686.5, p=0.523). Scale bar is 100 µm.

Fig. 2. 3-NP significantly decreases medium spiny neurons identified with the calcium binding protein calbinding.

3-NP treatment induces the abnormal production of reactive oxygen species (ROS), as well as highly reactive molecules derived from the formation of nitric oxide (NO). Succinate dehydrogenase inhibition interferes with the electron transport cascade and oxidative phosphorylation, which results in a decrease in ATP production and a cellular energy deficit (Jana et al., 2001; Lunkes et al., 2002). In studies by our group, the systemic administration of low sub-chronic doses of 3-NP did not produce a significant augmentation of NO in the brain (Rodriguez et al., 2010); however, NO and lipid peroxidation (LPO) increased in skeletal muscle (Hernández-Echeagaray et al., 2011). Previous reports looking at the involvement of NO in the toxicity of 3-NP did not draw any clear conclusions, but it has been suggested that 3-NP acts as an NO donor, increasing the levels of nitro anions (Jana et al., 2001; Lunkes et al., 2002).

Increases in NO and LPO along with signs of necrosis that manifest at the ultra-structural level in 3-NP-treated animals, like cellular oedema, are suggestive of the inflammatory process. Gene expression of the anti-inflammatory cytokine Interleukin-10 (IL-10) was found to significantly decrease whereas expression of the inflammatory cytokine Interferon-gamma (IFNγ) increased, indicating that, in low doses, 3-NP reduces the activation of anti-inflammatory cytokines (Fig. 3). This may have negative effects to prevent cellular damage.

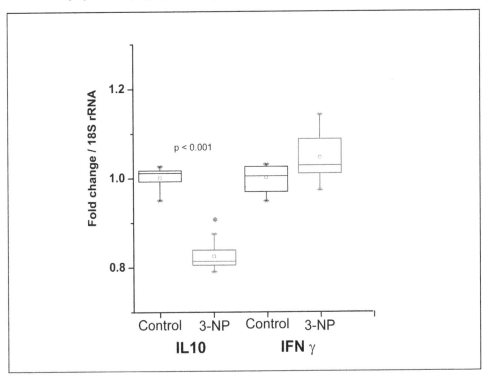

PCR products of IL-10 and INFγ in striatum of control and 3-NP treated groups are displayed. Data were analyzed by measuring continuously gene-specific PCR products and differences were assessed with the $2\_\Delta\Delta CT$ method. Data are presented as the fold increase in gene transcripts normalized to the 18S rRNA expression and relative to the control. IL-10 expression was significantly reduced in the 3-NP group (t13 = 12.904, p<0.001). INFγ exhibited a no significant increase in the 3-NP treated group (t16= 0.232, p= 0.819).

Fig. 3. Expression of striatal IL-10 and INFγ mRNA by real time RT-PCR.

Cells obtain energy from oxidative phosphorylation and from glycolysis; the glycolytic enzyme GAPDH has been implicated in neuronal degeneration (Taylor et al., 2002; Huntington's Disease Collaborative Research Group, 1993) and a reduction in GAPDH activity was demonstrated in HD patients and in a transgenic mouse model of HD (Burke et al., 1996; Matthews et al., 1997). Some studies have suggested that mitochondrial failure is secondary to striatal damage in HD (Lee et al., 2007), and then another energy source that may fail and generate damage is glycolysis. Both oxidative phosphorylation and glycolysis can be involved in the pathogenesis of neural degeneration in the striatum. However, inhibition of the glycolytic enzyme GAPDH was found to cause apoptotic damage, which is independent of the activation of caspase 3 (Rodriguez et al., 2010). Hence, alterations in glycolysis may be a critical point in neuronal death, but its inhibition activates different cellular signals than oxidative phosphorylation.

4.2 Changes in the periphery

Any deficit in energy metabolism can damage the entire physiology of an organism. Muscles metabolism is essential for locomotion and heat production (Zierath and Hawley, 2004). Patients afflicted by HD experience many deficits (Bradshaw et al., 1992; Aron et al., 2003; Abbruzzese et al., 2003), and weight loss is a characteristic feature (Robbins et al., 2006; Ciammola et al., 2011; Mochel and Haller, 2011). Transgenic mice model in an HD exhibited protein inclusions (Sathasivam et al., 1999) and mhtt aggregation in skeletal muscle (Ribchester et al., 2004). The motor impairments displayed by patients and animal models could result from central neurodegeneration, but also from alterations in muscle metabolism, reflecting peripheral disturbances as a general metabolic failure. Where metabolic collapse occurs in an organism, this could partly clarify the muscle alterations and body weight loss documented in HD patients (Stoy and McKay, 2000; Robbins et al., 2006; Ciammola et al., 2011) and transgenic HD mice (Sathasivam et al., 1999; Ribchester et al., 2004; She et al., 2011) and the alterations caused by metabolic alterations (Simoneau et al., 1995; Petersen et al., 2004).

Initially, it was thought that 3-NP did not produce major peripheral effects (Hamilton and Gould 1987). Until now, most of the studies that were carried out using 3-NP as a tool to investigate neurodegeneration focused on evaluating central damage (Beal et al., 1993; Borlongan et al., 1997; Brouillet, et al., 1999, 2005), even though in a number of them 3-NP was systemically administered. However, Gabrielson (et al., 2001) showed that 3-NP induced modifications in cardiac muscle physiology.

In addressing the possible changes that 3-NP might generate outside of the brain, our group documented modifications in skeletal muscle after uncoupling oxidative metabolism with 3-NP in low sub-chronic doses. Our hypothesis was that abnormal mitochondrial functioning during first stages of neurodegenerative disease is responsible for body weight loss in patients afflicted with HD or illness where there is a metabolic dysfunction (Stoy and McKay, 2000; Robbins et al., 2006). The systemic administration of low doses of 3-NP altered enzymatic activity in muscle, as well as the organization of the sarcomere (Hernández-Echeagaray et al., 2011), suggesting that energy failure exacerbates metabolic activity in the whole organism, producing high metabolic demands to counteract the failure of bioenergetics. When comparing muscle modifications in animals where glycolysis was inhibited, we found that iodoacetate IOA also alters the ultrastructure of the gastrocnemius muscle; this disorganization was more pronounced in animals that were treated with 3-NP (Fig. 4).

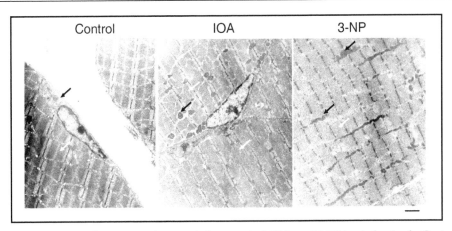

Electron microscopy of gastrocnemius muscle from control, IOA, and 3-NP treated animals. Control muscle shows normal sarcomere organization (white arrow) and mitochondria morphology (black arrow). However, sarcomere of IOA and 3-NP treated groups was altered; also the number of mithoxhondria and mitochondria morphology were modified. In particular muscles from 3-NP treated group were most affected than those from the IOA group. Micrographics magnification is 7000X. Scale bar is 500 nm.

Fig. 4. Metabolic uncoupling induces ultra structural modification in the mouse gastrocnemius muscle.

Oxidative phosphorylation or metabolic failure may generate an increase in energy consumed by muscles, as has been suggested in several degenerative disorders where alterations in oxidative phosphorylation and metabolism are compromised (Ristow, 2004). It is important to mention that in models of food restriction or malnutrition, the size and body weight of animals were affected before the nervous system became involved in the behavioural phenotype (Woodall et al., 1996; Clapham, 2004). Being aware of the peripheral and central damage due to metabolic dysfunctions might help in the clinical management of the early stages of the disease. For example, treatments designed to improve energy metabolism might modify the course of the illness and delay the progression of the disease.

5. Conclusions

The goal of this chapter was to illustrate the fact that 3-NP in low sub-chronic doses induces cellular alterations that emulate the damage exhibited in the striatum and muscle of patients afflicted by HD in the early stages of the illness. Even though 3-NP does not reproduce all signs and symptoms displayed in HD patients, it is true that it has helped in the understanding of the cellular physiology of animal models where a general failure in bioenergetics has been presumed.

6. Acknowledgements

The authors wish to thank A Ruelas for carrying out the open field test evaluation. This work was partially supported by grants from CONACyT, DGAPA-PAPIIT and Institutional support from FES-I, UNAM.

7. References

Abbruzzese G, Berardelli A (2003). Sensorimotor integration in movement disorders. Mov Disord 18; 231-40

Alston TA, Mela L, Bright HJ (1977). 3-Nitropropionate, the toxic substance of Indigofera, is a suicide inactivator of succinate dehydrogenase. Proc Natl Acad Sci USA 74; 3767-3771.

Alexi T, Hughes P E, Knusel B, Tobin A J (1998). Metabolic compromise with systemic 3-nitropropionic acid produces striatal apoptosis in Sprague–Dawley rats but not in BALB/c ByJ mice. Exp Neurol 153; 74–93.

Aron AR, Watkins L, Sahakian BJ, Monsell S, Barker RA, Robbins TW (2003). Task-set switching deficits in early-stage Huntington's disease: implications for basal ganglia function. J Cogn Neurosci 15; 629-42

Artal-Sanz M and Tavernarakis N (2005). Proteolytic mechanisms in necrotic cell death and neurodegeneration FEBS Letter 579; 3287-3296

Beal MF, Brouillet E, Jenkins BG, Ferrante RJ, Kowall NW, Miller JM, Storey E, Srivastava R, Rosen BR, Hyman BT (1993). Neurochemical and histologic characterization of striatal excitotoxic lesions produced by the mitochondrial toxin 3-nitropropionic acid. J Neurosci 13; 4181-4192

Beal MF (2005). Mitochondria take center stage in aging and neurodegeneration. Ann Neurol. 58; 495-505

Borlongan CV, Nishino H, Sanberg PR (1997a). Systemic but not intraparenquimal administration of 3-nitropropionic acid mimics the neuropathology of Huntington`s disease: a speculative explanation. Neurosci Res 28; 185-189

Borlongan CV, Koutouzis TK, Freeman TB, Hauser RA, Cahill DW, Sanberg R (1997b). Hyperactivity and hypo activity in a rat model of Huntington's Disease: The systemic 3- nitropropionic acid model. Brain Res Protoc 1; 253–257.

Bradshaw JL, Phillips JG, Dennis C, Mattingley JB, Andrewes D, Chiu E, Pierson JM, Bradshaw JA (1992). Initiation and execution of movement sequences in those suffering from and at-risk of developing Huntington's disease. J Clin Exp Neuropsychol 14;179-92.

Brouillet E, Jenkins BG, Hyman BT, Ferrante RJ, Kowall NW, Srivastava R, Roy DS, Rosen BR, Beal MF (1993). Age dependent vulnerability of the striatum to the mitochondrial toxin 3-nitropropionic acid. J Neurochem 60; 356–359.

Brouillet E, Conde F, Beal MF, Hantraye P (1999). Replicating Huntington's disease phenotype in experimental animals Prog Neurobiol 59; 427.

Brouillet E, Jacquard C, Bizat N, Blum D (2005). 3-Nitropropionic acid: A mitochondrial toxin to uncover physiopathological mechanisms underlying striatal degeneration in Huntington's disease. J Neurochem 95; 1521-1540.

Browne SE, Bowling AC, MacGarvey U, Baik MJ, Berger SC, Muqit MM, Bird ED, Beal MF (1997). Oxidative damage and metabolic dysfunction in Huntington's Disease: selective vulnerability of the basal ganglia. Ann Neurol 41; 646-653.

Browne, SE (2008). Mitochondrial and Huntington's Disease pathogenesis: Insight from genetic and chemical models. Ann NY Acad 1147; 358-382.

Burke JR, Enghild JJ, Martin ME, Jou YS, Myers RM, Roses AD, Vance JM, Strittmatter WJ (1996). Huntingtin and DRPLA proteins selectively interact with the enzyme GAPDH. Nat Med 2; 347-350

Ciammola A, Sassone J, Sciacco M, Mencacci NE, Ripolone M, Bizzi C, Colciago C, Moggio M, Parati G, Silani V, Malfatto G (2011). Low Anaerobic Threshold and Increased Skeletal Muscle Lactate Production in Subjects with Huntington's Disease. Movement Disorders, 26; 493-499.

Clapham JC (2004). Treating obesity: pharmacology of energy expenditure. Cur Drug Targets 5; 309-323.

Dautry C, Vaufrey F, Brouillet E, Bizat N, Henry PG, Conde F, Bloch G, Hantraye P (2000). Early N-acetylaspartate depletion is a marker of neuronal dysfunction in rats and primates chronically treated with the mitochondrial toxin 3-nitropropionic acid. J Cereb Blood Flow Metab 20; 789-799.

DiFiglia M (1990). Excitotoxic injury of the neostriatum: a model for Huntington's disease. TINS 13; 286-289.

Ferrante RJ, Beal MF, Kowall NW, Richardson EPJr, Martin JB (1987a). Sparing of acetylcholinesterase-containing striatal neurons in Huntington's Disease. Brain Res 411; 162-166.

Ferrante RJ, Kowall NW, Beal MF, Martin JB, Bird ED, Richardson EP Jr (1987b). Morphologic and histochemical characteristics of a spared subset of striatal neurons in Huntington's Disease. J Neuropathol Exp Neurol 46; 12-27.

Fridovich I (1999). Fundamental aspects of reactive oxygen species, or what's the matter with oxygen? Ann NY Acad Sci 893; 13–28.

Gabrielson KL, Hogue BA, Bohr VA, Cardounel AJ, Nakajima W, Kofler J, Zweier JL, Rodriguez ER, Martin LJ, de Souza Pinto NC, Bressier J (2001). Mitochondrial toxin 3-Nitropropionic acid induces cardiac and neurotoxicity differentially in mice. Am J Pathol 159; 1507-1520.

Gould DH, Gustine DL (1982). Basal ganglia degeneration,myelin alterations, and enzyme inhibition induced in mice by the plant toxin 3-nitropropanoic acid. Neuropathol Appl Neurobiol 8; 377–393.

Gould D H, Wilson MP, Hamar DW (1985). Brain enzyme and clinical alterations induced in rats and mice by nitroaliphatic toxicants. Toxicol Lett 27; 83–89.

Grafton ST, Mazziotta JC, Pahl JJ, St George-Hyslop P, Haines JL, Gusella J, Hoffman J M MD, Baxter LR, Phelps ME (1990). A comparison of neurological, metabolic, structural, and genetic evaluations in persons at risk for Huntington's disease. Ann Neurol 28; 614–621.

Grünewald T, BEAL M F (1999). Bioenergetics in Huntington's Disease. Ann NY Acad Sci 893; 203–213.

Gu M, Gash MT, Mann VM, Javoy-Agid F, Cooper JM, Schapira AH (1996). Mitochondrial defect in Huntington's disease caudate nucleus. Ann Neurol 39; 385–389.

Guyot MC, Palfi S, Stutzmann JM, Maziere M, Hantraye P, Brouillet E (1997). Riluzole protects from motor deficits and striatal degeneration produced by systemic 3-nitropropionic acid intoxication in rats. Neurosci 81; 141–149.

Hamilton BF, Gould DH (1987). Nature and distribution of brain lesions in rats intoxicated with 3-nitropropionic acid: a type of hypoxic (energy deficient) brain damage. Acta Neuropathol 72; 286–297.

He F, Zhang S, Qian F, Zhang C (1995). Delayed dystonia with striatal CT lucencies induced by a mycotoxin (3-nitropropionic acid). Neurol 45; 2178–2183.

Henry PG, Lebon V, Vaufrey F, Brouillet E, Hantraye P, Bloch G (2002). Decreased TCA cycle rate in the rat brain after acute 3-NP treatment measured by in vivo 1H-[13C] NMR spectroscopy. J Neurochem 82; 857–866.

Hernández-Echeagaray E, González N, Ruelas A, Mendoza E, Rodríguez-Martínez E, Antuna-Bizarro R (2011). Low doses of 3-nitropropionic acid in vivo induce damage in mouse skeletal muscle. Neurol Sci 32; 241-54.

Huntington's Disease Collaborative Research Group (1993). Cell; 72, 971.

Inagaki R, Tagawa K, Qi M-L, Enokido Y, Ito H, Tamura T, Shimizu S, Oyanagi K, Arai N, Kanazawa I, Wanker E E, Okazawa H (2008). Omi / Htr2 is relevant to the selective vulnerability of striatal neurons in Huntinton's disease Eur J Neurosci 28; 30-40.

Janavs J L, Aminoff M J (1998). Dystonia and chorea in acquired systemic disorders. J Neurol Neurosurg Psychiatry 65; 436–445.

Jana NR, Zemskov EA, Wang G, Nukina N (2001). Altered proteasomal function due to the expression of polyglutamine-expanded truncated N-terminal huntingtin induces apoptosis by caspase activation through mitochondrial cytochrome c release. Hum Molec Genet 10; 1049.

Jenkins BG, Koroshetz WJ, Beal MF, Rosen BR (1993). Evidence for impairment of energy metabolism in vivo in Huntington's disease using localized 1H NMR spectroscopy Neurol 43; 2689–2695.

Jenkins BG, Rosas HD, Chen YC, Makabe T, Myers R, MacDonald M, Rosen BR, Beal MF, Koroshetz WJ (1998). 1H NMR spectroscopy studies of Huntington's disease: Correlations with CAG repeat numbers. Neurology 50: 1357–1365.

Kanazawa I (2001). How do neurons die in neurodegenerative diseases? Trends in Molecular Medic 7; 339-344.

Kapogiannis D, Mattson MP (2011). Disrupted energy metabolism and neuronal circuit dysfunction in cognitive impairment and Alzheimer's disease. Lancet Neurobiol 10; 187-198.

Koroshetz WJ, Jenkins BG, Rosen BR, Beal MF (1997). Energy metabolism defects in Huntington's disease and effects of coenzyme Q10. Ann Neurol 41; 160–165.

Kowall NW, Ferrante RJ, Martin JB (1987). Patterns of cell loss in Huntington's Disease. TINS 10; 24-29.

Krantic S, Mechawar N, Reix S, Quirion R (2005). Molecular basis of programmed cell death involved in neurodegeneration. TINS, 28; 670-676.

Kroemer G, Dallaporta B, Resche-Rigon M (1998). The mitochondrial death/life regulator in apoptosis and necrosis. Annu Rev Physiol 60; 619–642.

Kuhl DE, Phelps ME, Markham CH, Metter EJ, Riege WH, Winter J (1982). Cerebral metabolism and atrophy in Huntington's disease determined by 18FDG and computed tomographic scan. Ann Neurol 12; 425–434.

Lee J M, Ivanova E V, Seong I S, Cashorali T, Kohane I, Gusella JF, MacDonald ME (2007). Unbiased gene expression analysis implicates the huntingtin polyglutamine tract in extramitochondrial energy metabolism. PLoS Genet 3; e135.

Li XJ, Orr AL, Li S (2010). Impaired mitochondrial trafficking in Huntington's disease. Biochem Biophys Acta 1802; 62–65.

Lin MT, Beal MF (2006). Mitochondrial dysfunction and oxidative stress in neurodegenerative diseases. Nat 443; 787–795.

Lodi R, Schapira AH, Manners D, Styles P, Wood NW, Taylor DJ, Warner TT (2000). Abnormal in vivo skeletal muscle energy metabolism in Huntington's disease and dentate rubropallidoluysian atrophy. Ann Neurol 48: 72–76.

Ludolph AC,He F, Spencer PS, Hammerstad J, Sabri M (1991). 3-Nitropropionic acid-exogenous animal neurotoxin and possible human striatal toxin. Can J Neuro. Sci 18; 492–498.

Lunkes A, Lindenberg KS, Ben-Haiem L, Weber C, Devys D, Landwehrmeyer GB, Mandel JL, Trottier Y (2002). Proteases acting on mutant huntingtin generate cleaved products that differentially build up cytoplasmic and nuclear inclusions. Mol Cell 10; 259-265.

Mazziotta JC, Phelps ME, Pahl JJ, Huang SC, Baxter LR, Riege WH, Hoffman JM, Kuhl DE, Lanto AB,. Wapenski JA, Markham CH (1987). Reduced cerebral glucose metabolism in asymptomatic subjects at risk for Huntington's disease. N Engl J Med 316: 357–362.

Maciel EN, Kowaltowski A J, Schwalm FD, Rodrigues J M, Souza DO, Vercesi AE, Wajner M, Castilho RF (2004). Mitochondrial permeability transition in neuronal damage promoted by Ca2+ and respiratory chain complex II inhibition. J Neurochem 90; 1025–1035.

Massouh M, Wallman MJ, Pourcher E, Parent A (2008). The fate of the large striatal interneurons expressing calretinin in Huntington's Disease. Neurosci Res 62; 216–224.

Matthews RT, Ferrante RJ, Jenkins BG, Browne SE, Goetz K, Berger S, Chen YC, Beal MF (1997). Iodoacetate produces striatal excitotoxic lesions. J Neurochem 69; 285-289.

Ming L (1995). Moldy sugarcane poisoning-a case report with a brief review. J Toxicol Clin Toxicol 33; 363–367.

Mochel F, Haller RG (2011). Energy deficit in Huntington disease: why it matters. J Clin Invest 121; 493–499.

Mogami M, Hida H, Hayashi Y, Kohri K, Kodama Y, Gyun JC, Nishino H (2002). Estrogen blocks 3-nitropropionic acid induced Ca2+ increase and cell damage in cultured rat cerebral endothelial cells. Brain Res 956; 116–125.

Nishino H, Nakajima K, Kumazaki M, Fukuda A, Muramatsu K, Deshpande SB, Inubushi T, Morikawa S, Borlongan CV, Sanberg PR (1998). Estrogen protects against while testosteroneexacerbates vulnerability of the lateral striatal artery to chemicalhypoxia by 3-nitropropionic acid. Neurosci Res 30; 303–312.

Novelli A, Reilly JA, Lysko PG, Henneberry RC (1988). Glutamate becomes neurotoxic via the N-methyl-D-aspartate receptor when intracellular energy levels are reduced. Brain Res 451; 205–212.

Novotny E JJr, Singh G, Wallace DC, Dorfman LJ, Louis A, Sogg RL, Steinman L (1986). Leber's disease and dystonia: a mitochondrial disease. Neurol 36; 1053–1060.

Oliveira JM (2010). Nature and cause of mitochondrial dysfunction in Huntington's disease: focusing on huntingtin and the striatum. J Neurochem 114; 1-12.

Ouary S, Bizat N, Altairac S, Menetrat H, Mittoux V, Conde F, Hantraye P, Brouillet E (2000). Major strain differences in response to chronic systemic administration of the mitochondrial toxin 3-nitropropionic acid in rats: implications for neuroprotection studies. Neurosci 97; 521–530.

Palfi S, Ferrante RJ, Brouillet E, Beal MF, Dolan R, Guyot MC, Peschanski M, Hantraye P (1996). Chronic 3-nitropropionic acid treatment in baboons replicates the cognitive and motor deficits of Huntington's Disease. J Neurosci 16; 3019– 3025.

Panov AV, Gutekunst CA, Leavitt BR, Hayden MR, Burke JR, Strittmatter WJ, Greenamyre JT (2002). Early mitochondrial calcium defects in Huntington's Disease are a direct effect of polyglutamines. Nat Neurosci 5; 731–736.

Petersen KF, Durour S, Befroy D, García R, Shulman GI (2004). Impaired mitochondrial activity in the insuline resistant offspring of patients with type 2 diabetes. N Engl J Med 350: 664-671.

Pickrell AM, Fukui H, Wang X, Pinto M, Moraes CT (2011). The striatum is highly susceptible to mitochondrial oxidative phosphorylation dysfunctions. J Neurosci, 31: 9895-9904.

Reddy PH, Mao P, Manczak M (2009). Mitochondrial structural and functional dynamics in Huntington's disease. Brain Res Rev 61: 33-48.

Ribchester RR, Thomson D, Wood NI, Hinks T, Gillingwater TH, Wishart TM, Court FA, Morton AJ (2004). Progressive abnormalities in skeletal muscle and neuromuscular junctions of transgenic mice expressing the Huntington's disease mutation. Eur J Neurosci 20: 3092-3114.

Ristow M (2004). Neurodegenerative disorders associated with diabetes mellitus. J Mol Med 82; 510-529.

Robbins AO, Ho AK, Barker RA (2006). Weight changes in Huntington's disease. Eur J Neurol 13; e7.

Rodríguez E, Rivera I, Astroga S, Medoza E, García F, Hernández-Echeagaray E (2010). Uncoupling Oxidative/Energy Metabolism with Low sub Chronic Doses of 3-Nitropropionic acid or Iodoacetate in vivo Produces Striatal Cell Damage. Int J Biol Sci 6; 199-212.

Saft C, Zange J, Andrich J, Muller K, Lindenberg K, Landwehrmeyer B, Vorgerd M, Kraus PH, Przuntek H, Schöls L (2005). Mitochondrial impairment in patients and asymptomatic mutation carriers of Huntington's disease. Mov Disord 20; 674-679.

Sathasivam K, Hobbs C, Turmaine M, Mangiarini L, Mahal A, Bertaux F, Wanker EE, Doherty P, Davies SW, Bates G (1999). Formation of polyglutamine inclusions in non-CNS tissue. Hum Mol Gen 8; 813-822.

Schulz JB, Henshaw DR, MacGarvey U, Beal MF (1996). Involvement of oxidative stress in 3-nitropropionic acid neurotoxicity. Neurochem Int 29; 167-171.

Seong IS, Ivanova E, Lee JM, Choo YS, Fossale E, Anderson M, Gusella JF, Laramie JM, Myers RH, Lesort M, MacDonald ME (2005). HD CAG repeat implicates a dominant property of huntingtin in mitochondrial energy metabolism. Hum Mol Genet 14; 2871-2880.

Shoffner JM, Watts RL, Juncos JL, Torroni A, Wallace DC (1991). Mitochondrial oxidative phosphorylation defects in parkinson's disease Ann Neurol 30; 332-339.

Simoneau JA, Colberg SR, Thaete FL, Kelley DE (1995). Skeletal muscle glycolytic and oxidative enzyme capacities are determinants of insulin sensitivity and muscle composition in obese women FASEB J 9; 273-278.

Sims NR (1996). Energy Metabolism, Oxidative Stress and Neuronal Degeneration in Alzheimer's Disease Neurodegeneration. Volume 5; 435-440.

Stoy N, McKay E (2000). Weight loss in Huntington's disease. Ann Neurol 48; 130-131.

Strauss KA, Morton DH (2003). Type I glutaric aciduria, part 2: a model of acute striatal necrosis. Am J Med Genet 121, 53-70.

Taylor PJ, Hardy J, Fischbeck KH (2002). Toxic proteins in neurodegenerative disease. Science 296; 1991-1995.

Vis JC, Schipper E, Boer-van Huizen RT, Verbeek MM, de Waal RMW, Wesseling P, Donkelaar H J Kremer B (2005). Expression pattern of apoptosis-related markers in Huntington's Disease Acta Neuropathol 109; 321-328.

Walker OW (2007). Huntington's disease. Lancet 369; 218-225.

Weinshilboum R (2003). Inheritance and drug response. N Engl J Med 348; 529-37.

Weinshilboum RM, Wang L (2006). Pharmacogenetics and pharmacogenomics: development, science, and translation. Annu Rev Genomics Hum Genet 7; 223-245.

Woodall SM, Breier BH, Johnston BM, Gluckman PD (1996). A model of intrauterine growth retardation caused by chronic maternal undernutrition in the rat: effects on the somatotrophic axis and postnatal growth. J Endocrinol 150; 231-242.

Zeevalk GD, Nicklas WJ (1990). Chemically induced hypoglycemia and anoxia: relationship to glutamate receptor-mediated btoxicity in retina. J Pharmacol Exp Ther 253; 1285-1292.

Zierath JR, Hawley JA (2004). Skeletal muscle fiber type: influence on contractile and metabolic properties. PLOS Biol 2; 337-348.

3

Cholesterol Metabolism in Huntington's Disease

Valerio Leoni[1], Claudio Caccia[1] and Ingemar Björkhem[2]
[1]IRCCS National Institute of Neurology "C. Besta", Milano,
[2]Karolinska Institute, Stockholm,
[1]Italy
[2]Sweden

1. Introduction

Cholesterol is present in all vertebrate cells where has several important functions. Being a structural element in plasma membranes it supports the structure and function of lipid bilayers and is regarded to be the most important "fluidity buffer" of the membrane. It is also a precursor of bile acids, steroid hormones and vitamin D. While cholesterol is involved in many cellular processes, a strong indicator of its importance is that it is the only major lipid in mammals not used in energy generation.

De novo synthesis and uptake from circulating lipoproteins cover the cholesterol needs of the cells. Almost all the mammalian cells are able to synthesize cholesterol and express the sophisticated and energy demanding enzymatic machinery required for the de novo synthesis.

In general, the cells in the body are able to release and take up cholesterol to maintain their cholesterol homeostasis: some are able to produce an excess to provide other cells, some others need exogenous cholesterol because of limited synthetic capacity.

Excess cholesterol may be toxic for the cells and a number of strategies have evolved either to export it or to store it in an esterified form. The exogenous cell supply is covered via the Low Density Lipoproteins (LDL) cycle and most of the excess is exported by the High Density Lipoprotein (HDL) mechanism (reverse cholesterol transport), mediated by members of the ATP-Binding Cassette (ABC)-transporter family.

Under normal conditions, about the 60% of the body's cholesterol is synthesized (about 700 mg/day) and the remaining is provided by the diet. The liver accounts for approximately 10% of total synthesis in humans, as does the small intestines.

The biosynthesis of cholesterol may be divided into five stages: 1) synthesis of mevalonate from acetyl-coenzymeA (CoA); 2) synthesis of isoprenoid units from mevalonate by loss of CO_2; 3) condensation of six isoprenoids units to form squalene; 4) cyclization of squalene to give the parental steroid, lanosterol; 5) formation of cholesterol by rearranging the lanosterol molecule (Fig. 1).

The most important rate limiting step is the conversion of the 3α-hydroxy-3-methylglutarylcoenzyme A (HMG-CoA) into mevalonate, catalysed by the microsomal HMG-CoA reductase (Rodwell et al., 1976). The activity of the enzyme is regulated by a negative feedback mechanism both at the protein level and at the transcriptional level. To some extent the latter effects may be mediated by oxysterols and bile acids.

Lanosterol is the first sterol formed during cholesterol biosynthesis by conversion of squalene, while lathosterol is a further precursor synthesised in later steps (Kandutsch-Russel pathway). In humans, lanosterol and lathosterol are regarded to be suitable plasma surrogate marker for whole body cholesterol synthesis (Kempen et al., 1988; Bloch et al., 1957; Matthan et al., 2000).

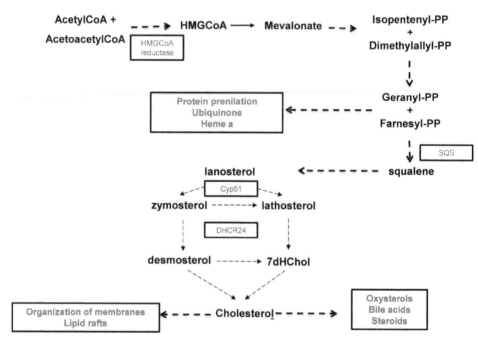

Fig. 1. Simplified diagram of cholesterol metabolism in the cells. Filled arrows mean direct enzymatic reaction, dot arrows mean metabolic reactions not presented in the figure.

Cholesterol synthesis begins with the transport of acetyl-CoA from the mitochondrion to the cytosol. Rate limiting step occurs at the 3-hydroxy-3-methylglutaryl-CoA (HMG-CoA) reducatase followed by mevalonate formation. Phosphorylation is required to solubilize the isoprenoid intermediates in the pathway (the PP abbreviation stands for pyrophosphate). Intermediates in the pathway are used for the synthesis of prenylated proteins, dolichol, coenzyme Q and the side chain of heme a. Pyrophosphated isoprenoids are condensed and ciclised by squalene synthetase (SQS) then the first sterol, lanosterol is formed. Two althernative pathways (Block and Kandush-Russel) lead to cholesterol formation. Precursor sterols can be converted by 3β-hydroxycholesterol Δ^{24} reductase (DHCR24). Cholesterol is involved in structure, organisation and function of cellular membranes and is precursor of oxysterols, bile acids and steroids.

Cholesterol is insoluble in water and is transported in the circulation associated with lipoproteins. Cholesterol is absorbed from the intestinal lumen and transported to the liver via chylomicrons. The cholesterol in these particles can be esterified, converted into bile acids or secreted into bile or collected in Very Low Density Lipoproteins (VLDL) to be transported to the extrahepatic tissues. VLDL can be remodelled by the action of lipoprotein lipase that removes triacyl-glycerol, transferring Apolipoprotein A (ApoA) and Apolipoprotein C (ApoC) from VLDL to HDL. The product of these remodelling is LDL which supplies peripheral tissues with cholesterol. The intake of cellular LDL is strictly regulated via the LDL receptors (LDLR) and Apolipoprotein B (ApoB). The influx of cholesterol inhibits HMG-CoA reductase and cholesterol synthesis and stimulates the cholesterol esterification by acylCoA:cholesterol acyltransferase (ACAT).

The reverse cholesterol transport, whereby cells from different organs eliminate excess cholesterol through the liver, is mediated by HDL. The HDL particles contain ApoA1 and acquire cholesterol directly from the plasma membrane. This transfer is mediated by members of the ABC-transporter family.

About 1 g of cholesterol is eliminated from the body every day. Approximately half of this is excreted into the faeces after conversion into bile acids; the remainder is excreted as non-metabolized cholesterol or the bacterial metabolite coprostanol. The bile acids formed have an important role in the solubilisation and absorption of fats, cholesterol, vitamins and drugs. Approximately 95% of the bile acids are reabsorbed from the intestine and reach the liver via the portal vein (entero-hepatic cycling).

There are two different major pathways in bile acid synthesis. The neutral pathway is initiated by the rate-limiting enzyme cholesterol 7α-hydroxylase which is mainly expressed in hepatocytes. Under normal conditions the neutral pathway dominates in healthy adult humans (Russel, 2003). In contrast to the acid pathway the neutral pathway is under strict metabolic control.

In many cells and organs cholesterol is eliminated by side chain oxidation as an alternative to the classical HDL-mediated reversed cholesterol transport. Thus, almost all cells in the body contain the enzyme sterol 27-hydroxylase (CYP27A1) located in the inner membrane of the mitochondria. This enzyme is particularly expressed by macrophages. At high levels of CYP27A1, 27OHC may be further oxidized by CYP27A1 into 3β-hydroxy-5-cholestenoic acid. The latter acid may be further converted into 7α-hydroxy-3-oxo-cholesten-4-cholestenoic acid and then proceed in the acidic pathway for bile acid synthesis in the liver. The latter pathway is responsible for formation of about 10 % of the daily production of bile acids in humans (Duane & Javitt, 1999; Brown & Jessup, 2009).

2. Brain cholesterol metabolism

The content of cholesterol in the brain is about 10-fold higher than in any other organ and about the 25% of the total body cholesterol is located there (Dietschy & Turley, 2004). Synthesis and storage of such a large amount of cholesterol indicates a close link between the evolution of the nervous system and a specific role for cholesterol. Within the brain about 70% of cholesterol is present in myelin. It is likely that the requirement for efficient signalling despite a small transverse diameter of axons was a key selective pressure driving the accretion of cholesterol in the mammalian brain (Dietschy & Turley, 2004; Snipe & Suter, 1997; Björkhem & Meaney, 2004). The importance of such structural role is also suggested by the long half-life of brain cholesterol: overall brain cholesterol turns over some 250-300 times slower than that in the circulation (Björkhem & Meaney, 2004).

Myelin sheath is formed by sections of plasma membrane repeatedly wrapped around an axon, with the extrusion of virtually all of the cytoplasm. Myelin is formed by two very specialized cells: the oligodendrocyte in CNS and the Schwann cell in the peripheral nervous system. As an individual axon may be ensheathed by myelin from several oligodendrocytes, periodic gaps are present in the sheath. These are called the "nodes of Ranvier" and are the site of propagation of the action potential. Myelin can thus be regarded as a discontinuous insulation that enables the saltatory conduction of the action potential (Dietschy & Turley, 2004; Snipe & Suter, 1997). In addition to a large lipid component myelin also contains many specific proteins such as proteo-lipid protein and myelin basic protein.

Recently evidence has been presented that cholesterol can regulate the correct targeting of one of the major membrane proteins of the periphery nervous system and thereby myelin compaction. These data extend the role of cholesterol in myelin from an essential structural component to a regulator of overall myelin structure (Saher et al., 2009).

Oligodendrocytes differentiate postnatally and the process of myelination both in rodents and humans occurs during the first weeks (or months) postnatally with a coordinated accumulation of cholesterol and myelin basic protein (Dietschy and Turley, 2004). During brain maturation there is a progressive accumulation of cholesterol which ends in the adulthood when the myelin formation is completed. Interestingly the rate of cholesterol synthesis is higher in the early stage of myelination and in the regions with myelin (and white matter, such as mid brain and spinal cord compared to cortex). Together with cholesterol, myelin basic protein is one of the major proteins of CNS myelin and it represents about the 30% of the brain total protein. Severe alterations to the myelin were described in case of the shiverer mutant mouse with deletion of the myelin basic protein gene (Baumann & Pham-Dinh, 2001). The remaining 30% of brain cholesterol is divided between glial cells (20%) and neurons (10%), mainly located in cellular membranes (Maxfield & Tabas, 2005). Cholesterol is organized in microdomains called lipid rafts which are involved in the maintenance of the properties of membrane proteins such as receptors and ion channels (Allen et al., 2007). In addition to its structural role, cholesterol is involved in synapthogenesis, turnover, maintenance, stabilisation and restore of synapses (Koudinov & Koudinova, 2001). In addition it is a limiting factor for outgrowth of neurites and involved in vesicle transport and exocytosis at synaptic levels (for review see also Pfrieger, 2003 a and b; Pfrieger, 2011).

According to various *in vitro* studies with cultured cells, astrocytes synthesize at least 5-10 fold more cholesterol than neurons, while oligodendrocytes have an even higher capacity for cholesterol synthesis, at least during periods of active myelination (Pitas et al., 1987; Björkhem & Meaney, 2004). According to the "outsorcing" hypothesis it was suggested that neurons down-regulate their cholesterol synthesis and rely at least in part on delivery of cholesterol from astrocytes which differentiate postnatally and release cholesterol rich lipoproteins (Pfrieger, 2011) (Fig. 2). This strategy may allow neurons to focus on generation of electrical activity rather than dispense energy on costly cholesterol synthesis. This may be of particular importance in presynaptic terminals and dendritic spines, which are distant from the soma (Dietschy & Turley, 2004; Pfrieger, 2003a; Pfrieger, 2003b; Pfrieger, 2011). ApoE is the main lipid carrier protein in the Central Nervous System (CNS) and is released by astrocytes in order to supply neurons and synaptogenesis with lipids and cholesterol (Bu, 2009; Posse de Chaves & Narayanaswam, 2008; Björkhem et al., 2010).

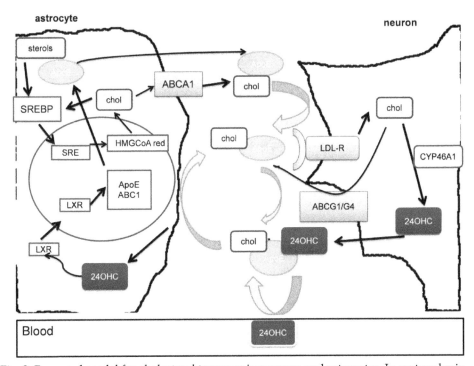

Fig. 2. Proposed model for cholesterol turnover in neurons and astrocytes. In mature brain neurons down regulate their cholesterol synthesis and relay on astrocytes delivery of cholesterol via ApoE lipoproteins. Cholesterol metabolism is a complex multisteps pathway involving endoplasmic reticulum or peroxisomes. Expression of hydroxy-methyl-glutaryl-Coenzyme A reductase (HMGCR), the rate limiting enzyme of the pathway, is regulated by feedback inhibition via the sterol-regulated element binding protein (SREBP) that binds to the sterol-regulated element (SRE-1) in the HMGCR gene. Cholesterol is loaded by astrocytes on ApoE involving also in the transport the ATP binding cassette (ABC) transporter A1 (ABCA1). The apoE-cholesterol complex is internalized via low-density lipoprotein receptors (LDLR). Excess of cholesterol is converted by neurons into the more polar 24S-hydroxycholesterol (24OHC) via the cholesterol 24-hydroxylase, CYP46. 24OHC and other oxysterols are important ligands of the liver X-activated receptor (LXR), which translocate to the nucleus (as circle in the figure) and induces expression of both the APOE and the ABCA1 genes in astrocytes. Cholesterol and 24OHC are excreted from neurons via ABC G1/G4 to ApoE particles or to CSF. 24OHC through the blood–brain barrier can be delivered into plasma for further elimination. The above proposed model is supported by a number of *in vitro* experiments with isolated neurons and astrocytes (Pfrieger, 2003a; Pfrieger, 2011; Abildayeva et al., 2006). The relation between 24OHC and ApoE is consistent with the finding of a correlation between these two factors in CSF from patients with neurodegeneration (Shafaati et al., 2007; Leoni et al., 2010). Such a relation was not found in CSF from healthy volunteers, however. The proposed model predicts a relation between levels of 24OHC and expression of LXR-target genes such as ApoE, ABCA1 and ABCG1. Such a relation was not found, however, in the brain of mice with elevated levels of 24OHC due to overexpression of CYP46A1 (Shafaati et al., 2011).

Neurons appear to produce a sufficient amounts of cholesterol to survive, to differentiate axons and dendrites and to form few and inefficient synapses. The massive formation of synapses, however, requires additional cholesterol delivered by astrocytes via ApoE-containing lipoproteins (Pfrieger 2003a; Pfrieger 2003 b; Pfrieger 2011).

Due to the efficient blood-brain barrier there is no passage of lipoprotein-bound cholesterol from the circulation into the brain (Dietschy & Turley, 2004; Snipe & Suter, 1997; Björkhem & Meaney, 2004). The blood-brain barrier thus prevents diffusion of large molecules at the level of tight junctional attachments between adjacent capillary endothelial cells. In addition to this, there is also no transvesicular movement of solution across the capillaries. It is possible that one or more members of the ATP binding cassette transporter superfamily may be involved in the exclusion of circulating cholesterol from the brain. All the cholesterol present in the brain (and in the peripheral nervous system) is thus formed by de novo synthesis. Except for active phases of specific pathological conditions, almost all (at least 99%) of the cholesterol in the nervous system is unesterified.

Cholesterol synthesis appears to be regulated by similar mechanisms both outside and inside the brain with hydroxy-methyl-glutaryl CoenzymeA reductase (HMGCR) being the most important regulatory enzyme (Snipe & Suter, 1997). However, in the brain, cholesterol synthesis via the 7-dehydrodesmosterol pathway seems to be preferred over the 7-dehydrocholesterol pathway and disruption of the gene coding for the delta 24-reductase (DHCR24) results in the accumulation of desmosterol without any accumulation of 7-dehydrodesmosterol (Wechsler et al., 2003).

In the adult brain most of the synthesis of cholesterol is balanced by formation of a hydroxylated metabolite, 24S-hydroxycholesterol (24OHC), which is able to pass across the blood-brain barrier and enter the circulation (Lütjohann et al., 1996; Björkhem & Meaney, 2004). About 6-8 mg/24h of cholesterol are released as 24OHC by the brain into the circulation (Lütjohann et al., 1996). In addition to this there is a small efflux of cholesterol from the brain in the form of ApoE containing lipoproteins via the cerebrospinal fluid (Xie et al., 2003).

Under normal conditions cholesterol 24-hydroxylase (CYP46A1), the enzyme system responsible for formation of 24S-OHC is only present in neuronal cells, mainly in cerebral cortex, hippocampus, dentate gyrus, amygdala, putamen and thalamus, i.e. associated with grey matter (Lund et al., 1999). The uptake of cholesterol by these cells may thus be balanced by the secretion of 24S-OHC. The 24S-OHC secreted from the neuronal cells may be of importance for regulation of cholesterol synthesis and secretion of this cholesterol in APOE-bound form from astroglia.

In the liver, the conversion of cholesterol into bile acids is regulated by highly sophisticated mechanisms (Russel, 2003). In the brain the expression of CYP46A1 appears to be resistant to regulatory axes known to regulate cholesterol homeostasis and bile acid synthesis. The promoter region of cholesterol 24-hydroxylase presents a high GC content, a feature often found in genes considered to have a largely housekeeping function (Ohyama et al., 2006). Oxidative stress was the only factor found to significantly affect its transcriptional activity. Cholesterol 24S-hydroxylase is localized in the neuronal cells and since these cells may depend on a flux of cholesterol from glial cells, it seems likely that substrate availability is an important regulatory factor for the enzyme under *in vivo* conditions (Björkhem, 2006).

24OHC is an endogenous regulator of the nuclear receptor Liver X Receptor (LXR). Under *in vitro* conditions 24OHC is able to regulate the expression, synthesis and secretion of ApoE (Abildayeva et al., 2006). Furthermore LXR-activation would be expected to increase expression of the sterol transporters ATP-binding cassette A1 (ABC-A1), G1 (ABC-G1) and G4 (ABC-G4) on astrocyte membranes, involved in the transport of cholesterol from glia to ApoE particles. Recently the importance of this mechanism *in vivo* was challenged by results obtained in a study on mice overexpressing CYP46A1 (Shafaati et al., 2011). Despite increased levels of 24OHC in the brain and in the circulation there was little or no increase in the expression of the different LXR target genes. In mice with combined Abcg1 and Abcg4 knockout results were obtained consistent with a role of these transporters in the efflux of cholesterol from neurons and glia in the CNS (Wang et al., 2008).

Cyp46a1 knock-out mice showed a modest reduction of hydroxy-methly-glutaryl-CoA-reductase activity and cholesterol synthesis rate while the total brain cholesterol levels were unaffected (Xie et al., 2003). Cyp46a1 (-/-) mice presented severe deficiencies in spatial, associative and motor learning associated with a delay of long lasting potential (Kotti et al., 2006). Also alterations in synaptic maturation were described. Treatment of hippocampal slices of wild type animals with an inhibitor of cholesterol synthesis essentially recapitulated the effects observed in the Cyp46a1 (-/-) mice (Russell et al., 2009).

Finally under *in vitro* conditions 24OHC is an efficient inhibitor of the formation of Aβ counteracting the positive effect of cholesterol on Amyloid Precursor Protein cleavage by β-secretase (BACE1) resulting in formation of the amyloidogenic Aβ1-42 fragment (Prasanthi et al., 2009; Bu, 2009).

In view of the fact that almost all 24OHC present in human circulation is of cerebral origin, (Björkhem et al., 2008) its plasma level is likely to be affected by the cholesterol homeostasis in the brain. It has been shown that the plasma levels are dependent both on the rate of secretion from the brain and the rate of hepatic metabolism (Bretillon et al., 2000a). Newborns have a size of the brain that is about three-fold that of the liver, whereas the size of the two organs is more or less similar in adults. As a consequence plasma levels of 24OHC are increased in children, infants and teenagers (Bretillon et al., 2000a) but are rather constant between the third to the seventh decades of life. According to one report the plasma concentrations of 24OHC are higher in males than in females (Vega et al., 2003). A similar observation was not reported by other more extensive studies. (Bretillion et al., 2000b; Leoni et al., 2008; Leoni et al., 2011; Leoni et al., 2002; Solomon et al., 2009b; van den Kommer et al., 2009; Burckhard et al., 2007).

In line with the fact that the number of metabolically active neuronal cells are decreased in the brain of patients with neurodegenerative diseases, the plasma levels of 24OHC have been reported to be decreased in Alzheimer's Disease (AD), Multiple Sclerosis (MS) and Huntington´s Disease (HD) (Papassotiropoulos et al., 2000; Kolsch et al., 2004; Solomon et al., 2009b; Koschack et al., 2009; Bretillion et al., 2000a; Bretillion et al., 2000b; Leoni et al., 2002; Teunissen et al., 2003; Danylaité Karrenbauer et al., 2006; Leoni et al., 2008; Leoni et al., 2011). Plasma levels of 24OHC may thus be regarded as a surrogate marker for the number of metabolically active neurons located in the grey matter of the brain (Björkhem, 2006).

In addition to 24OHC also 27OHC is able to pass the blood-brain barrier (Leoni et al., 2003). A continuous flux of 27OHC from the circulation into the mammalian brain has thus been demonstrated and this flux is of similar magnitude as the flux of 24OHC in the opposite direction (Heverin et al., 2005). In spite of the high influx of 27OHC into the brain the levels of this oxysterol is low, because of the rapid metabolism. It has been shown that most of the 27OHC present in CSF is derived from extracerebral 27OHC and that the levels are dependent upon the integrity of the blood-brain barrier. A damage of this barrier thus results in a higher flux of 27OHC from the circulation into the brain (Leoni et al., 2003; Heverin et al., 2005; Leoni et al., 2004). In view of the neurotoxic effect of 27OHC demonstrated in different *in vitro* experiments, the possibility has been discussed that the flux of 27OHC from the circulation into the brain could be a pathogenetic factor in the development of neurodegenerative diseases (Björkhem et al., 2009).

3. Cholesterol and neurodegenerative diseases other than Huntington´s Disease

The importance of cholesterol synthesis in the function, development and maturation of the central nervous system is very well illustrated by the consequence of genetic disorders affecting cholesterol synthesis or metabolism with prominent neurologic manifestations such as malformations, mental retardation, cognitive impairment and ataxia (Benarroch, 2008; Porter & Herman, 2011).

The most important neurodegenerative diseases in which a disturbance in cholesterol synthesis or metabolism is the primary pathogenetic factor is Smith-Lemli-Opitz syndrome and Niemann Pick Disease Type C. For details concerning these two diseases the reader should refer to the excellent review by Porter and Herman 2011.

Smith-Lemi-Opitz syndrome (SLOs) is an autosomal recessive malformation syndrome due to a mutation in the DHCR7 gene encoding 7-dehydroxycholesterol (7-DHC) reductase (Porter, 2008). Both the accumulation of 7-DHC and the reduced cholesterol synthesis participate to the SLOs phenotype, which is extremely broad, including CNS malformations such as holoprosencephaly and agenesis of the corpus callosum, mental retardation and motorial defects (Benarroch, 2008; Porter, 2008).

Niemann Pick Disease Type C (NPC) is a rare autosomal recessive neurovisceral lipid storage disease (Vanier & Millat, 2003). Mutations in the Niemann-Pick Disease, type C1 (NPC1) and Niemann-Pick Disease, type C2 (NPC2) genes have been identified as the genetic cause of the disease. NPC1 is a large membrane anchored protein with homology to HMGCR, SREBP cleavage activating protein (SCAP) and patched (PTCH1), a gene involved in Hedgehog signalling (Davies & Ioannou, 2000). In contrast, NPC2 is a small soluble glycoprotein (Storch & Xu, 2009). NPC has extreme clinical heterogeneity (Patterson, 2003; Benarroch, 2008) ranging from a rapidly fatal disorder in neonates to a neurodegenerative disorder in adults. The most common manifestations of adult NPC were cerebellar ataxia, vertical supranuclear ophthalmoplegia, dysarthria, and cognitive disturbances, followed by movement disorders (Patterson, 2003; Benarroch, 2008).

Important neurodegenerative diseases in which cholesterol metabolism is disturbed but not likely to be the primary pathogenetic factor are Alzheimer´s Disease and Parkinson´s Disease. For a detailed review see Björkhem et al. 2010. The most obvious link between Alzheimer´s Disease and cholesterol metabolism is the fact that presence of the E4 isoform of the cholesterol transporter ApoE as well as hypercholesterolemia are important risk factors for the disease.

4. Brain cholesterol in Huntington's Disease

Huntington's Disease (HD) is an inherited dominant neurodegenerative disorder characterised by a glutamine expansion within the N-terminus of the huntingtin protein (HTT) (Walker, 2007). The CAG trinucleotide repeats are located within the coding region of exon 1 of the HTT gene. HTT is widely expressed throughout the body and has been ascribed numerous roles in various intracellular functions including protein trafficking, vesicle transport, endocytosis, postsynaptic signalling, transcriptional regulation and an anti-apoptotic function (Gil & Rego, 2008). Gradual atrophy of the striatum (caudate nucleus and putamen) together with astrogliosis (Vonsattel et al., 1985) is a pathological characteristic of the disease. According to MRI investigations there is also a severe cortical atrophy combined with striatal degeneration (Aylward, 2007).

Cholesterol metabolism is affected in HD (Valenza & Cattaneo, 2011). The expression of some genes involved in the cholesterol biosynthetic pathway: hydroxy-methyl-glutaryl-CoA reductase , sterol 14-alpha demethylase (CYP51) and 7-dehydrocholesterol 7-reductase (DHCR7), were found to be reduced in inducible mutant HTT cell lines as well as in striatum and cortex of transgenic R6/2 HTT-fragment mice (Valenza et al., 2005; Valenza et al., 2007a)

Impairment of cholesterol metabolism in HD was confirmed in other additional studies.

The brain amount of the cholesterol precursors lanosterol and lathosterol, considered as markers for cholesterol synthesis (Xie et al., 2003) were found to be reduced. Also the levels of cholesterol were found to be significantly reduced in the brain of different rodent models for Huntington´s Disease such as the R6/2 mice (Valenza et al., 2007a), the yeast artificial chromosome (YAC) mice, the (HdhQ111/111) Hdh knock-in mice and others (Valenza et al., 2007b; Valenza et al., 2010).

Reduced levels of 24OHC were found in whole brain, striatum and cortex in the rodent models of Huntington's Disease, suggesting an impairment of cholesterol elimination by the metabolically active neuronal cells in the brain (Valenza et al., 2010).

The reductions of cholesterol synthesis, accumulation and turnover were found to be more marked with increasing length of the CAG repeats. In addition to the length of the repeats, the impairment of cholesterol synthesis was affected by the amount of mutated huntingtin. Finally, there was also an age-dependent effect. Thus the levels of cholesterol and cholesterol precursors were only slightly reduced in young animals during the process of maturation and much more reduced in older animals (Valenza et al., 2010).

A possible explanation for the molecular mechanism involved in the impairment of cholesterol metabolism is a mutant HTT-dependent decrease in the amount of active SREBP. The role of this factor is to translocate from the cytosolic compartment to the cell nucleus where, in presence of low cholesterol levels, it activates the transcription of SRE-controlled genes. Reduced SREBP translocation was thus found in cellular models of HD and in brain striatum collected from R6/2 mice (Valenza et al., 2005). A reduced entry of SREBP into the nucleus would be expected to lead to decreased cholesterol synthesis.

As referred to above cholesterol is critical for neurite outgrowth (Pfrieger, 2011). Neurite loss is an early manifestation of various neurodegenerative disorders, including HD, in which morphological abnormalities of the brain and defects in synaptic activity have been documented (Li et al., 2003; Levine et al., 2004; Schulz et al., 2004).

Wild type HTT is able to bind to some nuclear receptors involved in lipid metabolism: Liver-X-Receptor (LXR), PPARγ and vitamin D receptor (Futter et al., 2009). Overexpression of HTT was shown to activate LXR while a lack of HTT led to an inhibition of LXR-mediated transcription. The possibility must be considered that the mutated form of HTT is less able to up-regulate LXR and LXR-targeted genes, including SREBP. Such a mechanism could be a possible link between the HTT-mutation and the disturbances in cholesterol metabolism. Further work is needed, however, to establish this.

The mRNA levels of genes involved in cholesterol biosynthesis (hydroxy-methyl-glutaryl-CoA reductase, sterol 14-alpha demethylase, 7-dehydrocholesterol 7-reductase) and in cholesterol efflux (abca1 and abcg1) were found to be significantly reduced in primary astrocytes from both R6/2 and YAC 128 mice as compared to wild type controls or YAC18. Thus, astrocytes bearing a HTT mutation synthesized and secreted less ApoE than control cells. In accordance with this, the levels of HDL-like ApoE-lipoproteins present in CSF collected from YAC128 mice were reduced as compared to CSF from wt mice (Valenza et al., 2010). The results are consistent with a reduced ApoE mediated cholesterol transport.

In theory, the impairment of astrocyte cholesterol metabolism might be due to a combination of reduced activity of LXRs as a consequence of the reduced levels of 24OHC (Valenza et al., 2010) and a reduced SREBP activation. According to the study by Shafaati et al., however, the levels of 24OHC may be less important for LXR activation under *in vivo* conditions (Shafaati et al., 2011). It seems likely that there are other yet uncovered HTT-sensitive mechanisms that are of importance for synthesis, transport and delivery of cholesterol from astrocytes to neurons .

Both MRI and pathological investigations demonstrated abnormalities in oligodendrocytes and white matter in HD brains (Myers et al., 1991; Gomez-Tortosa et al., 2001; Fennema-Notestine et al., 2004; Paulsen et al., 2008; Tabrizi et al., 2009; Nopoulos et al., 2011; Rosas et al., 2010) even in pre manifesting subjects (Gomez-Tortosa et al., 2001; Bartzokis et al., 2007; Tabrizi et al., 2009). Pathological alteration of white matter may represent an early event in HD pathogenesis.

In primary oligodendrocytes, mutant HTT was found to inhibit the regulatory effect of Peroxisome-proliferator-activated receptor-gamma co-activator 1 alpha (PGC1α) on HmgCoA synthetase and HmgCoA reductase, expression of myelin basic protein and cholesterol metabolism (Xjiang et al., 2011). Brains from R6/2 and BACHAD mice had abnormal myelination, reduced expression of myelin basic protein and PGC1α (Xjiang et al., 2011). In a PGC1α knock out mice model defective myelination, reduced expression of myelin basic protein and reduction of cholesterol synthesis and accumulation has been demonstrated. The expression of HMGCoA reductase and HMGCoA synthetase and myelin basic protein was found to be reduced in this model (Xjiang et al., 2011). Peroxisome-proliferator-activated receptor gamma co-activator 1 alpha (PGC1α) plays a role in the transcriptional regulation of energy metabolism and has been implicated in several neurodegenerative disorders (Finck & Kelly, 2006), including HD (Cui et al., 2006; Weydt et al., 2006; Chaturvedi et al., 2009; Chaturvedi et al., 2010; McConoughey et al., 2010). PGC1α knockout mice exhibited vacuolar abnormalities in the CNS that were primarily associated with the white matter (Lin et al., 2006; Leone et al., 2005). It is likely that PGC1α is involved in regulation of cholesterol synthesis by direct or indirect interaction with SREBP and LXR affecting, thus, myelination.

5. Study of peripheral and cerebral cholesterol metabolism in neurodegenerative disorders

5.1 Huntington's Disease

Plasma concentration of 24OHC was found reduced in HD patients compared to healthy subjects. Both in two populations (an Italian and an English cohort), as well as in the combined two cohorts, 24OHC levels were significantly reduced at any disease stage (Leoni et al., 2008). The reduction of plasma 24OHC was found to parallel the degree of caudate atrophy (measured as reduction of caudate volume at MRI). A significant positive correlation was found between 24OHC levels and degree of caudate atrophy as measured by morphometric MRI (Leoni et al., 2008). These results support that reduction of plasma 24S-hydroxycholesterol is related to the loss of metabolically active neuronal cells in the brain and thus to the degree of brain athrophy (see also Leoni & Caccia, 2011).

Total plasma cholesterol was found to be reduced in pre-manifesting subjects and in HD patients compared to controls (Markianos et al., 2008). In other studies (Leoni et al., 2008; Leoni et al., 2011) a slight reduction was found with the progress of the disease stage. A significant reduction of cholesterol levels were however found only in the mast advanced cases (stage 3-5).

In a more detailed study on cholesterol homeostasis in HD it was reported that the cholesterol precursors lanosterol and lathosterol were reduced in plasma collected from HD patients at any disease stage. Also the level of the bile acid precursor 27-hydroxycholesterol was significantly reduced. Thus both whole-body and brain cholesterol homeostasis appear to be impaired in HD (Leoni et al., 2011).

HD gene positive carriers (named pre-manifest individuals) have been shown to present significant cognitive and neuropsychiatric dysfunction in parallel with changes in whole-brain volume, regional grey and white matter, at a stage prior to motor onset of disease. (Paulsen et al., 2008; Tabrizi et al., 2009). The plasma levels of 24OHC in pre-manifest subjects were similar to those of controls and higher than those of HD patients. However the gene positive pre-manifest subjects were heterogeneous: some subjects were very close to the motor onset with advanced neurodegeneration, others were far from onset. In subjects close to motor onset, 24OHC levels were found to be lower compared to those far from onset, and similar to the levels observed in manifest HD patients (Leoni et al., 2008). Interestingly, the markers of cholesterol synthesis lathosterol and lanosterol, and the marker of cholesterol elimination (27-hydroxycholesterol) were found to be reduced in pre-manifest subjects while the levels of 24S-hydroxycholesterol were reduced in patients proportionally to the degree of brain atrophy observed at MRI.

Presence of huntingtin mutations appears the be associated with a general global effect on cholesterol synthesis. Thus it is tempting to suggest that the huntingtin protein has a regulatory role in the normal cerebral as well as extracerebral biosynthesis of cholesterol (Valenza & Cattaneo, 2011). The production of 24OHC by the neuronal cells is likely to be dependent both on the numbers of such cells and on availability of substrate cholesterol. Both these factors are likely to be affected by HTT mutations.

5.2 Plasma sterols and oxysterols in neurodegenerative disease

Impairment of cholesterol metabolism were described also in animal models and patients affected by Multiple Sclerosis and Alzheimer's Disease.

Multiple Sclerosis (MS) is the most common autoimmune and demyelinating disorder of the CNS. Axonal damage and neurodegeneration is commonly found in the brains of patients with MS in both lesions and in normal-appearing white matter (Miller et al., 2002). Substantial neuronal loss and volume loss were demonstrated in grey matter, resulting in brain atrophy measured at Magnetic Resonance Imaging (MRI) (Cifelli et al., 2002). Plasma 24OHC was significantly reduced in relapsing-remitting and in primary progressive MS patients with a long story of disease (Leoni et al., 2002; Teunissen et al., 2003). The reduction of plasma 24OHC may reflect the total spatiotemporal burden of disease (i.e. the cumulative effects of its dissemination in space and its duration in time) since a significant correlation between plasma 24OHC and the volume of T2-weighted hyperintense lesions in relapsing-remitting and in primary progressive patients (Danylaité Karrenbauer et al., 2006). A significant direct correlation was observed between the plasma 24S-hydroxycholesterol and the Grey Matter Fraction (MRI marker of brain atrophy) of MS patients (Leoni & Caccia, 2011) . Lathosterol was found reduced in patients affected by MS (Teunissen, 2003) as well in animal model of MS (Teunissen et al., 2007). Also 27-hydroxycholesterol was found reduced in plasma collected from patients (Leoni et al., 2002; Teunissen et al., 2003) suggesting that whole body cholesterol metabolism may be altered in MS.

In AD the annual rate of global brain atrophy is 2-3% as compared with 0.2-0.5% in healthy controls (Fox et al., 1999; Jack et al., 2010). There is a prominent early involvement of medial temporal lobe structures, especially the enthorineal cortex and hippocampus (Jack et al., 1998). The progressive extensive atrophy is associated to a progressive reduction of the brain (Heverin et al., 2004) and plasma levels of 24OHC, and the latter is negatively correlated to the Mini Mental Score (Papassotiropoulos et al., 2000; Solomon et al., 2009b). A significant correlation of 24OHC with the hippocampal volume (Koschack et al., 2009) or the direct or fractional volumes of grey matter was found in mid-age or aged individuals (Solomon et al., 2009b). Such correlation was missed in case of Mild Cognitive Impairment (MCI) or AD patients: a possible explanation could be the abnormal expression of the CYP46 enzyme in glial cells that was shown in the brain of patients affected by AD (Brown et al., 2004; Bogdanovic et al., 2001), which occurs as a compensatory mechanism in neuronal degeneration.

Finally it was found that the reduction of plasma 24OHC correlated with the severity of dementia or the degree of brain atrophy (Papassotiropoulos et al, 2000; Solomon et al., 2009b).

Epidemiological studies showed an association between elevated total cholesterol at midlife and increased risk of AD (Kivipelto & Salomon, 2006). Long-term studies reported that a decline in plasma total cholesterol levels from midlife to late-life is associated with early stages in dementia development. It is likely that while high midlife cholesterol is a risk factor for AD, decreased cholesterol later in life may instead reflect an going pathological processes in the brain and should be considered as a frailty marker, predictive of worse cognitive functioning (Stewart et al., 2007; Mielke et al., 2005; Solomon et al., 2009a; Solomon et al., 2009b). A large 21- year follow-up study presented an association between serum total cholesterol changes from midlife to late-life and late-life cognitive status: a moderate decrease is associated with increased risk of a more impaired late-life cognitive status after adjusting for major confounders (Solomon et al., 2007).

No correlation between serum total cholesterol or LDL-C and CSF biomarkers was reported (Solomon et al., 2009a). No significant differences about total or LDL-cholesterol were found between aging individuals, MCI and AD patients but significant reductions of cholesterol precursors lathosterol and lanosterol and 27-hydroxycholesterol were instead observed in AD patients compared to MCI and aging individuals. As expected Aβ1-42 changed in the same way while tau and P-tau in the opposite one. Thus, the CSF biomarkers signature in aging population with cognitive decline was found associated with reduction of whole body cholesterol metabolism (Solomon et al., 2009a). In AD patients (but not in case of MCI or control individuals) lower plasma total cholesterol and LDL-C were found related to lower brain volumes/higher CSF volumes (Solomon et al., 2009a). In contrast, in the control group lower levels of the cholesterol precursors lanosterol and lathosterol (considered as marker of a lower rate of endogenous cholesterol synthesis) were related to higher brain volumes/lower CSF volumes. The positive correlations between lanosterol, lathosterol, total cholesterol and LDL-C with brain volumes in patients with AD compared to MCI and controls are consistent with the hypothesis of a central nervous system (CNS)-induced depressing effect of neurodegeneration on extracerebral cholesterol metabolism (Solomon et al., 2009).

Very recent studies on patients with Parkinson's Disease have reported a markedly decreased level of 24OHC in the plasma, which is consistent with the finding of correlation between brain atrophy, CNS neuronal mass and its plasma levels (Björkhem et al., 2009).

In addition to the above diseases, brain tumours and some severe central nervous system infections also have reduced levels of 24OHC in the circulation (Bretillon et al., 2000b).

6. Conclusion

A clear link has been established between the glutamine expansion in the huntingtin gene and cholesterol metabolism. The mechanism behind this is still unknown. Since the effect on cholesterol synthesis is global it seems likely that the huntingtin gene is of regulatory importance for cholesterol synthesis also under normal conditions. It should be noted that unexplained global effect on cholesterol homeostasis has been observed also in other neurodegenerative diseases such as Alzheimer´s Disease.

Liver integrity and clearance, presence of CNS pathology, therapies, cholesterol recommended levels, body mass index, diet were found to affect significantly the whole body cholesterol metabolism and plasma levels of 24OHC (Bretilion et al., 2000; Björkhem et al., 2009; Björkhem, 2006; Brown & Jessup, 2009; Leoni & Caccia, 2011). The criteria of selection of the control population, the pre-analytical factors of sample collection and handling, the methodology used for the study of sterols and oxysterols may affect the final findings. The use of sterols and side-chain oxidised cholesterol as biomarker for the diagnosis of neurodegenerative diseases seems to be still limited. However, the plasma level of a neuronal metabolite of cholesterol, 24S-hydroxycholesterol, appears to be a valuable biomarker for the progression of Huntington´s Disease.

7. Acknowledgments

The authors wish to gratefully acknowledge the collaboration along the years of Dr. A. Salomon, Prof. M. Kivipelto, Dr. T. Mastermann, Dr. M. Shafaati at Karolinska Insitutet, Stockholm, Sweden; Dr. C. Mariotti and Dr. S. Di Donato, IRCCS Istituo Neurologico "C. Besta", Milano, Italy; Dr. M. Valenza at University of Milano, Italy.

Financial support: Italian Mininster of Health, Fondi per giovani Ricercatori 2008, to V. Leoni; Swedish Science Council and the Swedish Brain Power to I. Björkhem.

8. References

Abildayeva, K., Jansen, P. J., Hirsch-Reinshagen, V., Bloks, V. W., Bakker, A. H., Ramaekers, J. de Vente, F. C., Groen, A. K., Wellington, C. L. , Kuipers, F., & Mulder, M. (2006). 24(S)-hydroxycholesterol participates in a liver X receptor-controlled pathway in astrocytes that regulates apolipoprotein E-mediated cholesterol efflux. *J. Biol. Chem.*, Vol.281, No.18, (May 2006), pp. 12799-12808, ISSN 0021-9258

Allen, J.A., Halverson-Tamboli, R.A., & Rasenick, M.M. (2007). Lipid raft microdomains and neurotransmitter signalling. *Nat. Rev. Neurosci.*, Vol.8, No.2, (February 2007), pp. 128–140, ISSN 1471-003X

Aylward, E.H. (2007). Change in MRI striatal volumes as a biomarker in preclinical Huntington's disease. *Brain Res. Bull.*, Vol.72, No.2-3, (April 2007), pp. 152-158, ISSN 0361-9230

Bartzokis, G., Lu, P.H., Tishler, T.A., Fong, S.M., Oluwadara, B., Finn, J.P., Huang, D., Bordelon, Y., Mintz, J., & Perlman, S. (2007). Myelin breakdown and iron changes in Huntington's disease: pathogenesis and treatment implications. *Neurochem. Res.*, Vol.32, No.10, (October 2007), pp. 1655-1664, ISSN 0364-3190

Baumann. N., & Pham-Dinh, D. (2001). Biology of oligodendrocyte and myelin in the mammalian central nervous system. *Physiol. Rev.*, Vol.81, No.2, (April 2001), pp. 871-927, ISSN 0031-9333

Benarroch, E.E. (2008). Brain cholesterol metabolism and neurologic disease. *Neurology*, Vol.71, No.17, (October 2008), pp. 1368-1373, ISSN 0028-3878

Björkhem, I. (2006). Crossing the barrier, oxysterols as cholesterol transporters and metabolic modulators in the brain. *J. Intern. Med.*, Vol.260, No.6, (November 2006), pp. 493-508, ISSN 0954-6820

Bjorkhem, I., & Meaney, S. (2004). Brain cholesterol: long secret life behind a barrier. *Arterioscler. Thromb. Vasc. Biol.*, Vol.24, No.5, (May 2004), pp. 806-815, ISSN 1079-5642

Björkhem, I., Cedazo-Minguez, A., Leoni, V., & Meaney, S. (2009). Oxysterols and neurodegenerative diseases. *Mol. Aspects Med.*, Vol.30, No.3, (June 2009), pp. 171-179, ISSN 0098-2997

Björkhem, I., Leoni, V., & Meaney, S. (2010). Genetic connections between neurological disorders and cholesterol metabolism. *J. Lipid Res.*, Vol.51, No.9, (September 2010), pp. 2489-2503, ISSN 0022-2275

Bloch, K., Clayton, R.B., & Schneider, P.B. (1957) Synthesis of lanosterol in vivo. *J. Biol. Chem.*, Vol.224, No1, (January1957), pp. 175–183, ISSN 0021-9258

Bogdanovic, N., Bretillon, L., Lund, E.G., Diczfalusy, U., Lannfelt, L., Winblad, B., Russell, D.W., & Björkhem, I. (2001). On the turnover of brain cholesterol in patients with Alzheimer's disease. Abnormal induction of the cholesterol-catabolic enzyme CYP46 in glial cells. *Neurosci. Lett.* Vol 314, No1-2 (November 2001), pp. 45-48. ISSN 0304-3940

Bretillon, L., Lütjohann, D., Stahle, L., Widhe, T., Bindl, L., Eggersten, G., Diczfalusy, U., & Bjorkhem, I., (2000a). Plasma levels of 24S-hydroxycholesterol reflect the balance between cerebral production and hepatic metabolism and are inversely related to body surface. *J. Lipid Res.*, Vol.41, No.5, (May 2000), pp. 840-845, ISSN 0022-2275

Bretillon, L., Siden, Å., Wahlund, L.O., Lütjohann, D., Minthon, L., Crisby, M., Hillert, J., Groth, G.C., Diczfalusy, U., & Björkhem, I. (2000b). Plasma levels of 24S-hydroxycholesterol in patients with neurological diseases. *Neurosci. Lett.*, Vol.293, No.2, (October 2000), pp. 87-90, ISSN 0304-3940

Brown, A.J., & Jessup, W. (2009). Oxysterols, Sources, cellular storage and metabolism, and new insights into their roles in cholesterol homeostasis. *Mol. Aspects Med.*, Vol.30, No.3, (June 2009), pp. 111-122, ISSN 0098-2997

Brown, J. 3rd, Theisler, C., Silberman, S., Magnuson, D., Gottardi-Littell, N., Lee, J.M., Yager, D., Crowley, J., Sambamurti, K., Rahman, M.M., Reiss, A.B., Eckman, C.B., & Wolozin, B. (2004). Differential expression of cholesterol hydroxylases in Alzheimer's disease. *J. Biol. Chem.* Vol 279, No 33 (August 2004), pp. 34674-34681. ISSN 0021-9258

Bu, G. (2009). Apolipoprotein E and its receptors in Alzheimer's disease, pathways, pathogenesis and therapy. *Nat. Rev. Neurosci.*, Vol.10, No.5, (May 2009), pp. 333-344, ISSN 1471-003X

Burkard, I., von Eckardstein, A., Waeber, G., Vollenweider, P., & Rentsch, K.M. (2007). Lipoprotein distribution and biological variation of 24S- and 27-hydroxycholesterol in healthy volunteers. *Atherosclerosis*. Vol.194, No.1 (September 2007), pp. 71-78. ISSN 0021-9150

Chaturvedi, R.K., Adhihetty, P., Shukla, S., Hennessy, T., Calingasan, N., Yang, L., Starkov, A., Kiaei, M., Cannella, M., Sassone, J., Ciammola, A., Squitieri, F., & Beal, M.F. (2009). Impaired PGC-1alpha function in muscle in Huntington's disease. *Hum. Mol. Genet.*, Vol.18, No.16, (August 2009), pp. 3048-3065, ISSN 0964-6906

Chaturvedi, R.K., Calingasan, N.Y., Yang, L., Hennessey, T., Johri, A., & Beal, M.F. (2010). Impairment of PGC-1alpha expression, neuropathology and hepatic steatosis in a transgenic mouse model of Huntington's disease following chronic energy deprivation. *Hum. Mol. Genet.*, Vol.19, No.16, (August 2010), pp. 3190-3205, ISSN 0964-6906

Cifelli, A., Arridge, M., Jezzard, P., Esiri, M.M., Palace, J., & Matthews, P.M. (2002). Thalamic neurodegeneration in multiple sclerosis. *Ann. Neurol.* Vol.52, No.5, (November 2002), pp. 650-653. ISSN 0364-5134

Cui, L., Jeong, H., Borovecki, F., Parkhurst, C.N., Tanese, N., & Krainc, D. (2006). Transcriptional repression of PGC-1alpha by mutant huntingtin leads to mitochondrial dysfunction and neurodegeneration. *Cell*, Vol.127, No.1, (October 2006), pp. 59-69, ISSN 0092-8674

Danylaité Karrenbauer, V., Leoni, V., Lim, E.T., Giovannoni, G., Ingle, G.T., Sastre-Garriga, J., Thompson, A.J., Rashid, W., Davies, G., Hillert, J., Miller, D.H., Björkhem, I., & Masterman, T. (2006). Plasma cerebrosterol and magnetic resonance imaging measures in multiple sclerosis. *Clin. Neurol. Neurosurg.*, Vol.108, No.5, (July 2006), pp. 456-460, ISSN 0303-8467

Davies, J. P., & Ioannou, Y. A. (2000). Topological analysis of Niemann-Pick C1 protein reveals that the membrane orientation of the putative sterol-sensing domain is identical to those of 3-hydroxy-3-methylglutaryl-CoA reductase and sterol regulatory element binding protein cleavage-activating protein. *J. Biol. Chem.*, Vol.275, No.32, (August 2000), pp. 24367-24374, ISSN 0021-9258

Dietschy, J.M., & Turley, S.D. (2004). Thematic review series, brain lipids. Cholesterol metabolism in the central nervous system during early development and in the mature animal. *J. Lipid Res.*, Vol.45, No.8, (August 2004), pp. 1375–1397, ISSN 0022-2275

Duane, W.C., & Javitt, N.B. (1999). 27-hydroxycholesterol: production rates in normal human subjects. *J. Lipid Res.*, Vol.40, No.7, (July 1999), pp. 1194-1199, ISSN 0022-2275

Fennema-Notestine, C., Archibald, S.L., Jacobson, M.W., Corey-Bloom, J., Paulsen, J.S., Peavy, G.M., Gamst, A.C., Hamilton, J.M., Salmon, D.P., & Jernigan, T.L. (2004). In vivo evidence of cerebellar atrophy and cerebral white matter loss in Huntington disease. *Neurology*, Vol.63, No.6, (September 2004), pp. 989-995, ISSN 0028-3878

Finck, B.N., & Kelly, D.P. (2006). PGC-1 coactivators: inducible regulators of energy metabolism in health and disease. *J. Clin. Invest.*, Vol.116, No.3, (March 2006), pp. 615-622, ISSN 0021-9738

Fox, N.C., Scahill, R.I., Crum, W.R., & Rossor, M.N. (1999). Correlation between rates of brain atrophy and cognitive decline in AD. *Neurology*, Vol.52, No.8, (May 1999), pp. 1687-1689, ISSN 0893-0341

Futter, M., Schoenmakers, H., Sadiq, O., Chatterjee, K., & Rubinsztein, D.C. (2009). Wild-type but not mutant huntingtin modulates the transcriptional activity of liver X erceptors. J. Med. Genetic., Vol.46, No.7, (July 2009), pp. 438-446, ISSN 0022-2593

Gil, J.M., & Rego A.C. (2008). Mechanisms of neurodegeneration in Huntington's disease. *Eur. J. Neurosci.*, Vol.27, No.11, (June 2008), pp. 2803-2820, ISSN 0953-816X

Gomez-Tortosa, E., MacDonald, M.E., Friend, J.C., Taylor, S.A., Weiler, L.J., Cupples, L.A., Srinidhi, J., Gusella, J.F., Bird, E.D., Vonsattel, J.P., & Myers, R.H. (2001). Quantitative neuropathological changes in presymptomatic Huntington's disease. *Ann. Neurol.*, Vol.49, No.1, (January 2001), pp. 29-34, ISSN 0364-5134

Heverin, M., Bogdanovic, N., Lütjohann, D., Bayer, T., Pikuleva, I., Bretillon, L., Diczfalusy, U., Winblad, B., & Björkhem, I. (2004). Changes in the levels of cerebral and extracerebral sterols in the brain of patients with Alzheimer's disease. *J. Lipid Res.*, Vol.45, No.1, (January 2004), pp. 186–193, ISSN 0022-2275

Heverin, M., Meaney, S., Lütjohann, D., Diczfalusy, U., Wahren, J., & Björkhem, I. (2005). Crossing the barrier, net flux of 27-hydroxycholesterol into the human brain. *J. Lipid Res.*, Vol.46, No.5, (May 2005), pp. 1047-1052, ISSN 0022-2275

Jack, C.R. Jr., Knopman, D.S., Jagust, W.J., Shaw, L.M., Aisen, P.S., Weiner, M.W., Petersen, R.C., & Trojanowski, J.Q. (2010). Hypothetical model of dynamic biomarkers of the Alzheimer's pathological cascade. *Lancet Neurol.*, Vol.9, No.1, (January 2010) pp. 119-128, ISSN 1474-4422

Jack, C.R.Jr., Petersen, R.C., Xu, Y., O'Brien, P.C., Smith, G.E., Ivnik, R.J., Tangalos, E.G., & Kokmen, E. (1998). Rate of medial temporal lobe atrophy in typical aging and Alzheimer's disease. *Neurology*, Vol.51, No.4, (October 1998), pp. 993-999, ISSN 0028-3878

Kempen, H.J., Glatz, J.F., Gevers Leuven, J.A., van der Voort, H.A., & Katan, M.B. (1988). Serum lathosterol concentration is an indicator of whole-body cholesterol synthesis in humans. *J. Lipid Res.*, Vol.29, No.9, (September 1988), pp. 1149–1155, ISSN 0022-2275

Kivipelto, M., & Solomon, A. (2006). Cholesterol as a risk factor for Alzheimer's disease - epidemiological evidence. *Acta Neurol. Scand. Suppl.*, Vol.114, No.s185, (August 2006), pp. 50-57, ISSN 0065-1427

Kolsch, H., Heun, R., Kerksiek, A., Bergmann, K.V., Maier, W., & Lutjohann, D. (2004). Altered levels of plasma 24S- and 27-hydroxycholesterol in demented patients. *Neurosci. Lett.*, Vol.368, No.3, (September 2004), pp. 303-308, ISSN 0304-3940

Koschack, J., Lütjohann, D., Schmidt-Samoa, C., & Irle, E. (2009). Serum 24S-hydroxycholesterol and hippocampal size in middle-aged normal individuals. *Neurobiol. Aging.*, Vol.30, No.6, (June 2009), pp. 898-902, ISSN 0197-4580

Kotti, T.J., Ramirez, D.M., Pfeiffer, B.E., Huber, K.M., & Russell, D.W. (2006). Brain cholesterol turnover required for geranylgeraniol production and learning in mice. *Proc. Natl. Acad. Sci. U.S.A.*, Vol.103, No.10, (March 2006), pp. 3869–3874, ISSN 0027-8424

Koudinov, A.R., & Koudinova, N.V.(2001). Essential role for cholesterol in synaptic plasticity and neuronal degeneration. *FASEB J.*, Vol.15, No.10, (August 2001), pp. 1858 –1860, ISSN 0892-6638

Leone, T.C., Lehman, J.J., Finck, B.N., Schaeffer, P.J., Wende, A.R., Boudina, S., Courtois, M., Wozniak, D.F., Sambandam, N., Bernal-Mizrachi, C., Chen, Z., Holloszy, J.O., Medeiros, D.M., Schmidt, R.E., Saffitz, J.E., Abel, E.D., Semenkovich, C.F., & Kelly, D.P. (2005). PGC-1alpha deficiency causes multi-system energy metabolic derangements: muscle dysfunction, abnormal weight control and hepatic steatosis. *PloS. Biol.*, Vol.3, No.4, (April 2005), e101, ISSN 1545-7885

Leoni, V., & Caccia, C. (2011). Oxysterols as biomarkers in neurodegenerative diseases. *Chem. Phys. Lipids*, Vol.164, No.6, (September 2011), pp. 515-524, ISSN 0009-3084

Leoni, V., Mariotti, C., Nanetti, L., Salvatore, E., Squitieri, F., Bentivoglio, A.R., Bandettini Del Poggio, M., Piacentini, S., Monza, D., Valenza, M., Cattaneo, E., & Di Donato, S. (2011). Whole body cholesterol metabolism is impaired in Huntington's disease. *Neurosci. Lett.*, Vol.494, No.3, (May 2011), pp. 245-249, ISSN 0304-3940

Leoni, V., Mariotti, C., Tabrizi, S.J., Valenza, M., Wild, E.J., Henley, S.M., Hobbs, N.Z., Mandelli, M.L., Grisoli, M., Björkhem, I., Cattaneo, E., & Di Donato, S. (2008). Plasma 24S-hydroxycholesterol and caudate MRI in pre-manifest and early Huntington's disease. *Brain*, Vol.131, No.11, (November 2008), pp. 2851-2859, ISSN 0006-8950

Leoni, V., Masterman, T., Diczfalusy, U., De Luca, G., Hillert, J., & Björkhem, I., (2002). Changes in human plasma levels of 24S-hydroxycholesterol during progression of multiple sclerosis. *Neurosci. Lett.*, Vol.331, No.3, (October 2002), pp. 163-166, ISSN 0304-3940

Leoni, V., Masterman, T., Patel, P., Meaney, S., Diczfalusy, U., & Björkhem, I. (2003). Side-chain oxidised oxysterols in cerebrospinal fluid and integrity of blood-brain barrier. *J. Lipid Res.*, Vol.44, No.4, (April 2003), pp. 793-799, ISSN 0022-2275

Leoni, V., Mastermann, T., Mousavi, F.S., Wretlind, B., Wahlund, L.O., Diczfalusy, U., Hillert, J., & Björkhem, I. (2004). Diagnostic use of cerebral and extracerebral oxysterols. *Clin. Chem. Lab. Med.*, Vol.42, No.2, (February 2004), pp.186-191, ISSN 1434-6621

Leoni, V., Solomon, A., & Kivipelto, M. (2010). Links between ApoE, brain cholesterol metabolism, tau and amyloid beta-peptide in patients with cognitive impairment. *Biochem. Soc. Trans.*, Vol.38, No.4, (August 2010), pp. 1021-1025, ISSN 0300-5127

Levine, M.S., Cepeda, C., Hickey, M.A., Fleming, S.M., & Chesselet, M.F. (2004). Genetic mouse models of Huntington's and Parkinson's diseases: illuminating but imperfect. *Trends Neurosci.*, Vol.27, No.11, (November 2004), pp. 691-697, ISSN 0166-2236

Li, J.Y., Plomann, M., & Brundin, P. (2003). Huntington's disease: a synaptopathy? *Trends Mol. Med.*, Vol.9, No.10, (October 2003), pp. 414-420, ISSN 1471-4914

Lin, T., Xiang, Z., Cui, L., Stallcup, W., & Reeves, S.A. (2006). New mouse oligodendrocyte precursor (mOP) cells for studies on oligodendrocyte maturation and function. *J. Neurosci. Methods.*, Vol.157, No.2, (October 2006), pp. 187-194, ISSN 0165-0270

Lund, E.G., Guileyardo, J.M., & Russell, D.W. (1999). cDNA cloning of cholesterol 24-hydroxylase, a mediator of cholesterol homeostasis in the brain. *Proc. Natl. Acad. Sci. U.S.A.*, Vol.6, No.13, (June 1999), pp. 7238–7243, ISSN 0027-8424

Lütjohann, D., Breuer, O., Ahlborg, G., Nennesmo, I., Siden, Å., Diczfalusy, U., & Björkhem, I. (1996). Cholesterol homeostasis in human brain, evidence for an age-dependent flux of 24S-hydroxycholesterol from the brain into the circulation. *Proc. Natl. Acad. Sci. U.S.A.*, Vol. 93, No.18, (September 1996), pp. 9799–9804, ISSN 0027-8424

Markianos, M., Panas, M., Kalfakis, N., & Vassilopoulos, D. (2008). Low plasma total cholesterol in patients with Huntington's disease and first-degree relatives. *Mol. Genet. Metab.*, Vol. 93, No. 3, (March 2008), pp. 341-346, ISSN 1096-7192

Matthan, N.R., Raeini-Sarjaz, M., Lichtenstein, A.H., Ausman, L.M., & Jones, P.J. (2000). Deuterium uptake and plasma cholesterol precursor levels correspond as methods for measurement of endogenous cholesterol synthesis in hypercholesterolemic women. *Lipids*, Vol.35, No.9, (September2000), 1037-1044, ISSN 0024-4201

Maxfield, F.R., & Tabas, I. (2005). Role of cholesterol and lipid organization in disease. *Nature*, Vol.438, No.7068, (December 2005), pp. 612–621, ISSN 0028-0836

McConoughey, S.J., Basso, M., Niatsetskaya, Z.V., Sleiman, S.F., Smirnova, N.A., Langley, B.C., Mahishi, L., Cooper, A.J., Antonyak, M.A., Cerione, R.A., Li, B., Starkov, A., Chaturvedi, R.K., Beal, M.F., Coppola, G., Geschwind, D.H., Ryu, H., Xia, L., Iismaa, S.E., Pallos, J., Pasternack, R., Hils, M., Fan, J., Raymond, L.A., Marsh, J.L., Thompson, L.M., & Ratan, R.R. (2010). Inhibition of transglutaminase 2 mitigates transcriptional dysregulation in models of Huntington disease. *EMBO Mol. Med.*, Vol.2, No.9, (September 2010), pp. 349-370, ISSN 1757-4676

Mielke, M.M., Zandi, P.P., Sjogren, M., Gustafson, D., Ostling, S., Steen, B., & Skoog, I. (2005). High total cholesterol levels in late-life associated with a reduced risk of dementia. *Neurology*, Vol.64, No.10, (May 2005), pp. 1689–1695, ISSN 0028-3878

Miller, D.H. (2002). MRI monitoring of MS in clinical trials. *Clin. Neurol. Neurosurg.*, Vol.104, No.3, (July 2002), pp. 236-243, ISSN 0303-8467

Myers, R.H., Vonsattel, J.P., Paskevich, P.A., Kiely, D.K., Stevens, T.J., Cupples, L.A., Richardson, E.P.Jr., & Bird E.D. (1991). Decreased neuronal and increased oligodendroglial densities in Huntington's disease caudate nucleus. *J. Neuropathol. Exp. Neurol.*, Vol.50, No.6, (November 1991), pp. 729-742, ISSN 0022-3060

Nopoulos, P.C., Aylward, E.H., Ross, C.A., Mills, J.A., Langbehn, D.R., Johnson, H.J., Magnotta, V.A., Pierson, R.K., Beglinger, L.J., Nance, M.A., Barker, R.A., & Paulsen, J.S. (2011). Smaller intracranial volume in prodromal Huntington's disease: evidence for abnormal neurodevelopment. *Brain*, Vol.134, No.1, (January 2011), pp. 137-142, ISSN 0006-8950

Ohyama, Y., Meaney, S., Heverin, M., Ekstrom, L., Brafman, A., Shafir, M., Andersson, U., Olin, M., Eggertsen, G., Diczfalusy, U., Feinstein, E., & Bjorkhem, I. (2006). Studies on the transcriptional regulation of cholesterol 24-hydroxylase (CYP46A1): marked insensitivity toward different regulatory axes. *J. Biol. Chem.*, Vol.281, No.7, (February 2006), pp. 3810-3820, ISSN 0021-9258

Papassotiropoulos, A., Lütjohann, D., Bagli, M., Locatelli, S., Jessen, F., Rao, M.L., Maier, W., Björkhem, I., von Bergmann, K., & Heun, R. (2000). Plasma 24S-hydroxycholesterol, a peripheral indicator of neuronal degeneration and potential state marker for Alzheimer's disease. *Neuroreport*, Vol.11, No.9, (June 2000), pp. 1959-1962, ISSN 0959-4965

Patterson, M.C. (2003). A riddle wrapped in a mystery: understanding Niemann-Pick disease, type C. *Neurologist*, Vol.9, No.6, (November 2003), pp. 301-310, ISSN 1074-7931

Paulsen, J.S., Langbehn, D.R., Stout, J.C., Aylward, E., Ross, C.A., Nance, M., Guttman, M., Johnson, S., MacDonald, M., Beglinger, L.J., Duff, K., Kayson, E., Biglan, K., Shoulson, I., Oakes, D., & Hayden, M. (2008). Detection of Huntington's disease decades before diagnosis: the Predict-HD study. *J. Neurol. Neurosurg. Psychiatry.*, Vol.79, No.8, (August 2008), pp. 874-880, ISSN 0022-3050

Pfrieger F.W. (2003a). Cholesterol homeostasis and function in neurons of the central nervous system. *Cell. Mol. Life Sci.*, Vol.60, No.6, (June 2003), pp. 1158-1171, ISSN 1420-682X

Pfrieger, F.W. (2003b). Outsourcing in the brain, do neurons depend on cholesterol delivery by astrocytes? *Bioessays*, Vol.25, No.1, (January 2003), pp. 72–78, ISSN 0265-9247

Pfrieger, F.W., & Ungerer, N. (2011). Cholesterol metabolism in neurons and astrocytes. Prog. Lipid. Res., Vol.50, No.4, (October 2011), pp. 357-371, ISSN 0163-7827

Pitas, R. E., Boyles, J. K., Lee, S. H., Foss, D., & Mahley, R. W. (1987). Astrocytes synthesize apolipoprotein E and metabolize apolipoprotein E-containing lipoproteins. *Biochim. Biophys. Acta*, Vol.917, No.1, (January 1987), pp. 148-161, ISSN 0006-3002

Porter, F.D. & Herman, G.E. (2011). Malformation syndromes caused by disorders of cholesterol synthesis. *J. Lipid Res.* Vol.52, No.1, (January 2011), pp. 6-34, ISSN 0022-2275

Porter, F.D. (2008). Smith-Lemli-Opitz syndrome: pathogenesis, diagnosis and management. *Eur. J. Hum. Genet.*, Vol.16, No.5, (May 2008), pp. 535-541, ISSN 1018-4813

Posse de Chaves, E., & Narayanaswami, V. (2008). Apolipoprotein E and cholesterol in aging and disease in the brain. *Future Lipidol.*, Vol.3, No.5, (October 2008), pp. 505–530, ISSN 1746-0875

Prasanthi, J.R., Huls, A., Thomasson, S., Thompson, A., Schommer, E., & Ghribi, O. (2009). Differential effects of 24-hydroxycholesterol and 27-hydroxycholesterol on beta-amyloid precursor protein levels and processing in human neuroblastoma SH-SY5Y cells. *Mol. Neurodegener.*, Vol.4, No.1, (January 2009), ISSN 1750-1326

Rodwell, V.W., Nordstrom, J.J., & Mitschelen, J.J. (1976). Regulation of HMG-CoA reductase. *Adv. Lipid Res.*, Vol.14, (1976), pp. 1-74, ISSN 0065-2849

Rona-Voros, K., & Weydt, P. (2010). The role of PGC-1alpha in the pathogenesis of neurodegenerative disorders. *Curr. Drug. Targets.*, Vol.11, No.10, (October 2010), pp. 1262-1269, ISSN 1389-4501

Rosas, H.D., Lee, S.Y., Bender, A.C., Zaleta, A.K., Vangel, M., Yu, P., Fischl, B., Pappu, V., Onorato, C., Cha, J.H., Salat, D.H., & Hersch, S.M. (2010). Altered white matter microstructure in the corpus callosum in Huntington's disease: implications for cortical "disconnection". *Neuroimage*, Vol.49, No.4, (February 2010), pp. 2995-3004, ISSN 1053-8119

Russell, D. W., Halford, R. W., Ramirez, D. M., Shah, R., & Kotti, T. (2009). Cholesterol 24-hydroxylase: an enzyme of cholesterol turnover in the brain. *Annu. Rev. Biochem.*, Vol.78, (July 2009), pp. 1017-1040, ISSN 0066-4154

Russell, D.W. (2003). The enzymes, regulation, and genetics of bile acid synthesis. *Annu. Rev. Biochem.*, Vol.72, (July 2003), pp. 137-174, ISSN 0066-4154

Saher, G., Quintes, S., Mobius, W., Wehr, M. C., Kramer-Albers, E. M., Brugger, B., & Nave, K. A. (2009). Cholesterol regulates the endoplasmic reticulum exit of the major membrane protein P0 required for peripheral myelin compaction. *J. Neurosci.*, Vol.29, No.19, (May 2009), pp. 6094-6104, ISSN 0270-6474

Schulz, J.G., Bosel, J., Stoeckel, M., Megow, D., Dirnagl, U., & Endres, M. (2004). HMG-CoA reductase inhibition causes neurite loss by interfering with geranylgeranylpyrophosphate synthesis. *J. Neurochem.*, Vol.89, No.1, (April 2004), pp. 24-32, ISSN 0022-3042

Shafaati, M., Olin, M., Båvner, A., Pettersson, H., Rozell, B., Meaney, S., Parini, P., & Björkhem, I. (2011). Enhanced production of 24S-hydroxycholesterol is not sufficient to drive liver X receptor target genes in vivo. *J. Intern. Med.*, (April 2011), [Epub ahead of print], ISSN 1365-2796

Snipe, G., & Suter, U. (1997). Cholesterol and myelin.In : Bitmaan R.ed. *Cholesterol*. New York:Plenum Press; 1998.

Solomon, A., Kåreholt, I., Ngandu, T., Winblad, B., Nissinen, A., Tuomilehto, J., Soininen, H., & Kivipelto, M. (2007). Serum cholesterol changes after midlife and late-life cognition: twenty-one-year follow-up study. *Neurology*, Vol.68, No.10, (November 2007), pp. 751-756, ISSN 0893-0341

Solomon, A., Kivipelto, M., Wolozin, B., Zhou, J., & Whitmer, R.A. (2009 b). Midlife serum cholesterol and increased risk of Alzheimer's and vascular dementia three decades later. Dement. *Geriatr. Cogn. Disord.*, Vol.28, No.1, (August 2009), pp. 75-80, ISSN 1420-8008

Solomon, A., Leoni, V., Kivipelto, M., Besga, A., Oksengård, A.R., Julin, P., Svensson, L., Wahlund, L.O., Andreasen, N., Winblad, B., Soininen, H., & Björkhem, I. (2009a). Plasma levels of 24S-hydroxycholesterol reflect brain volumes in patients without objective cognitive impairment but not in those with Alzheimer's disease. *Neurosci. Lett.*, Vol.462, No.1, (September 2009), pp. 89-93, ISSN 0304-3940

Stewart, R., White, L.R., Xue, Q.L., & Launer, L.J. (2007). Twenty-six-year change in total cholesterol levels and incident dementia: the Honolulu-Asia Aging Study. *Arch. Neurol.*, Vol.64, No.1, (January 2007), pp. 103–107, ISSN 0003-9942

Storch, J., & Xu, Z. (2009). Niemann-Pick C2 (NPC2) and intracellular cholesterol trafficking. *Biochim. Biophys. Acta*, Vol.1791, No.7, (July 2009), pp. 671-678, ISSN 0006-3002

Tabrizi, S.J., Langbehn, D.R., Leavitt, B.R., Roos, R.A., Durr, A., Craufurd, D., Kennard, C., Hicks, S.L., Fox, N.C., Scahill, R.I., Borowsky, B., Tobin, A.J., Rosas, H.D., Johnson, H., Reilmann, R., Landwehrmeyer, B., Stout, J.C., TRACK-HD investigators (2009). Biological and clinical manifestations of Huntington's disease in the longitudinal TRACK-HD study, cross-sectional analysis of baseline data. *Lancet Neurol.*, Vol.8, No.8, (September 2009), pp. 791-801, ISSN 1474-4422

Teunissen, C.E., Dijkstra, C.D., Polman, C.H., Hoogervorst, E.L., von Bergmann, K., & Lütjohann, D. (2003). Decreased levels of the brain specific 24S-hydroxycholesterol and cholesterol precursors in serum of multiple sclerosis patients. *Neurosci. Lett.*, Vol.347, No.3, (August 2003), pp. 159-162, ISSN 0304-3940

Teunissen, C.E., Floris, S., Sonke, M., Dijkstra, C.D., De Vries, H.E., & Lütjohann, D. (2007). 24S-hydroxycholesterol in relation to disease manifestations of acute experimental autoimmune encephalomyelitis. *J. Neurosci. Res.*, Vol.85, No.7, (May 2007), pp. 1499-1505, ISSN 1097-4547

Valenza, M., & Cattaneo, E. (2011). Emerging roles for cholesterol in Huntington's disease. *Trends Neurosci.*, (July 2011), [Epub ahead of print], ISSN 1878-108X

Valenza, M., Carroll, J.B., Leoni, V., Bertram, L.N., Bjorkhem, I., Singaraja, R.R., Di Donato, S., Lutjohann, D., Hayden, M.R., & Cattaneo, E. (2007b). Cholesterol biosynthesis pathway is disturbed in YAC128 mice and is modulated by huntingtin mutation. *Hum. Mol. Genet.*, Vol.16, No.18, (September 2007), pp. 2187-2198, ISSN 0964-6906

Valenza, M., Leoni, V., Karasinska, J.M., Petricca, L., Fan, J., Carroll, J., Pouladi, M.A., Fossale, E., Nguyen, H.P., Riess, O., MacDonald, M., Wellington, C., DiDonato, S., Hayden, M., & Cattaneo, E. (2010). Cholesterol defect is marked across multiple rodent models of Huntington's disease and is manifest in astrocytes. *J. Neurosci.*, Vol.30, No.32, (August 2010), pp. 10844-10850, ISSN 0270-6474

Valenza, M., Leoni, V., Tarditi, A., Mariotti, C., Bjorkhem, I., Di Donato, S., & Cattaneo, E. (2007a). Progressive dysfunction of the cholesterol biosynthesis pathway in the R6/2 mouse model of Huntington's disease. *Neurobiol. Dis.*, Vol.28, No.1, (October 2007), pp. 133-142, ISSN 0969-9961

Valenza, M., Rigamonti, D., Goffredo, D., Zuccato, C., Fenu, S., Jamot, L., Strand, A., Tarditi, A., Woodman, B., Racchi, M., Mariotti, C., Di Donato, S., Corsini, A., Bates, G., Pruss, R., Olson, J.M., Sipione, S., Tartari, M., & Cattaneo, E. (2005). Dysfunction of the cholesterol biosynthetic pathway in Huntington's disease. *J. Neurosci.*, Vol.25, No.43, (October 2005), pp. 9932-9939, ISSN 0270-6474

van den Kommer, T.N., Dik, M.G., Comijs, H.C., Fassbender, K., Lütjohann, D., & Jonker, C. (2009).Total cholesterol and oxysterols: early markers for cognitive decline in elderly? *Neurobiol. Aging*, Vol.30, No.4, (april 2009), pp. 534-545, ISSN 0197-4580

Vanier, M. T., & Millat, G. (2003). Niemann-Pick disease type C. *Clin. Genet.*, Vol.64, No.4, (October 2003), pp. 269-281, ISSN 0009-9163

Vega, G.L., Weiner, M.F., Lipton, A.M., Von Bergmann, K., Lutjohann, D., Moore, C., & Svetlik, D. (2003). Reduction in levels of 24S-hydroxycholesterol by statin treatment in patients with Alzheimer disease. *Arch. Neurol.*, Vol.60, No.4, (April 2003), pp. 510-515, ISSN 0003-9942

Vonsattel, J.P., Myers, R.H., Stevens, T.J., Ferrante, R.J., Bird, E.D., & Richardson, E.P.Jr. (1985). Neuropathological classification of Huntington's disease. *J. Neuropathol. Exp. Neurol.*, Vol.44, No.6, (November 1985), pp. 559-577, ISSN 0022-3069

Walker, F.O. (2007). Huntington´s disease. *Lancet.*, Vol.369, No.9557, (January 2007), pp. 218-228, ISSN 0140-6736

Wang, N., Yvan-Charvet, L., Lütjohann, D., Mulder, M., Vabmierlo, T., Kim, T.W., & Tall, A.R. (2008). ATP-binding cassette transporters G1 and G4 mediate cholesterol and desmosterol efflux to HDL and regulate sterol accumulation in the brain. *FASEB J.*, Vol.22, No.4, (April 2008), pp. 1073–1082, ISSN 0892-6638

Wechsler, A., Brafman, A., Shafir, M., Heverin, M., Gottlieb, H., Damari, G., Gozlan-Kelner, S., Spivak, I., Moshkin, O., Fridman, E., Becker, Y., Skaliter, R., Einat, P., Faerman, A., Bjorkhem, I., & Feinstein, E. (2003). Generation of viable cholesterol-free mice. *Science*, Vol.302, No.5653, (December 2003), pp. 2087, ISSN 0036-8075

Weydt, P., Pineda, V.V., Torrence, A.E., Libby, R.T., Satterfield, T.F., Lazarowski, E.R., Gilbert, M.L., Morton, G.J., Bammler, T.K., Strand, A.D., Cui, L., Beyer, R.P., Easley, C.N., Smith, A.C., Krainc, D., Luquet, S., Sweet, I.R., Schwartz, M.W., & La Spada, A.R. (2006). Thermoregulatory and metabolic defects in Huntington's disease transgenic mice implicate PGC-1alpha in Huntington's disease neurodegeneration. *Cell Metab.*, Vol.4, No.5, (November 2006), pp. 349-362, ISSN 1550-4131

Xiang, Z., Valenza, M., Cui, L., Leoni, V., Jeong, H.K., Brilli, E., Zhang, J., Peng, Q., Duan, W., Reeves, S.A., Cattaneo, E., & Krainc, D. (2011). Peroxisome-proliferator-activated receptor gamma coactivator 1 α contributes to dysmyelination in experimental models of Huntington's disease. *J. Neurosci.*, Vol.31, No.26 (June 2011), pp. 9544-9553, ISSN 0270-6474

Xie, C., Lund, E.G., Turley, S.D., Russell, D.W., & Dietschy, J.M. (2003). Quantification of two pathways for cholesterol excretion from the brain in normal mice and mice with neurodegeneration. *J. Lipid Res.*, Vol.44, No.9, (September 2003), pp. 1780-1789, ISSN 0022-227

4

Consequences of Mitochondrial Dysfunction in Huntington's Disease and Protection via Phosphorylation Pathways

Teresa Cunha-Oliveira[1]*, Ildete Luísa Ferreira[1]* and A. Cristina Rego[1,2]
1CNC-Center for Neuroscience and Cell Biology, University of Coimbra,
2Faculty of Medicine, University of Coimbra,
Portugal

1. Introduction

Huntington's Disease (HD) is an autosomal dominant neurodegenerative disorder clinically characterized by psychiatric disturbances, progressive cognitive impairment and choreiform movements. These symptoms are associated with the selective atrophy and neuronal loss in the striatum, cortex and hypothalamus. The disease is caused by a mutation at the 5' terminal of the huntingtin (*HTT*) gene involving the expansion of CAG triplet, which encodes for glutamine. Mutant huntingtin (mHtt) may be cleaved by proteases originating neurotoxic fragments, and also undergoes conformational changes that lead to the formation of protein aggregates (Gil and Rego 2008, for review). Among several mechanisms of neurodegeneration, mHtt is related to mitochondrial dysfunction and relevant changes in energy metabolism in both central and peripheral cells, which may underlie cell death (Gil and Rego 2008, for review).

In this review chapter we emphasize the role of mitochondrial dysfunction in neurodegeneration in HD, particularly centering on loss of mitochondrial activity and the regulation of intrinsic apoptosis in central and peripheral HD human tissue or cells, and in animal models of HD. We focus on the changes in energy metabolism, oxidative stress, the link to transcriptional dysfunction and the regulation of intrinsic apoptosis. We further explore the therapeutic role of promoting phosphorylation pathways through selective inhibition of phosphatases (e.g. with FK506) and/or activation of kinase signaling cascades mediated by neurotrophins, namely brain-derived neurotrophic factor (BDNF) and nerve growth factor (NGF).

2. Mitochondrial dysfunction and apoptosis in HD

2.1 Mitochondrial dysfunction

The mechanisms by which neurons die in HD are uncertain, however, mitochondrial dysfunction and apoptosis have been implicated. Mitochondria are important organelles

---

*These authors contributed equally

that regulate the life and death of cells and neurons are particularly dependent on these organelles due to their high energy requirements.

Mitochondrial dysfunction is considered a common feature in the pathogenesis of neurodegenerative disorders like HD (Kim *et al.* 2010;Oliveira 2010;Parker, Jr. *et al.* 1990), and constitutes a cellular hallmark for neurodegeneration, occurring as a consequence of defective mitochondrial composition, trafficking to synapses, calcium handling, ATP production, transcription abnormalities and/or electron transport chain (ETC) impairment (Rosenstock *et al.* 2010, for review). Moreover, cell and animal models of HD exhibit mitochondrial impairment and metabolic deficits similar to those found in HD patients (reviewed in Damiano *et al.* 2010;Quintanilla and Johnson 2009). mHtt may cause mitochondrial dysfunction by directly interacting with the organelle (Panov et al. 2002) by evoking defects in mitochondrial dynamics, organelle trafficking and fission and fusion, which, in turn, may result in bioenergetic failure, or indirectly by perturbing transcription of nuclear-encoded mitochondrial proteins (Bossy-Wetzel *et al.* 2008, for review).

The hypothesis that mitochondrial dysfunction contributes to the pathogenesis of HD was first tested pharmacologically by using 3-nitropropionic acid (3-NP) and malonate, irreversible and reversible inhibitors of succinate dehydrogenase (a component of both the tricarboxylic acid cycle and the complex II of the ETC), respectively. Administration of these inhibitors to animals results in pathological characteristics of HD, such as marked increases in striatal lactate concentration, striatal lesions and motor disturbances (Beal *et al.* 1993;Brouillet *et al.* 1993;Frim *et al.* 1993), involving an immediate ATP drop and secondary increase in reactive oxygen species (ROS), which is correlated with profound mitochondrial fragmentation (Brouillet *et al.* 1999). Selective striatal neurodegeneration induced by 3-NP appears to be related to the early expression and activation of matrix metalloproteinase-9 by ROS which can digest the endothelial basal lamina, leading to the disruption of the blood–brain barrier and to progressive striatal damage (Kim *et al.* 2003). Concordant with 3-NP mimicking the disease, in 1974 a defect in succinate dehydrogenase was reported in the caudate and, to a lesser extent, in the cortex of postmortem HD brains (Stahl and Swanson 1974). Moreover, yeast expressing mHtt showed a significant reduction in oxidative phosphorylation due to a decrease in complexes II and III activities (Solans *et al.* 2006).

Furthermore, early studies of cortical biopsies obtained from patients with either juvenile or adult onset HD showed abnormal mitochondria morphology and function (Goebel *et al.* 1978;Tellez-Nagel *et al.* 1974). Functional changes in mitochondrial ETC were also observed in HD, namely decreased mitochondrial complexes II/III activity and succinate oxidation in striatal tissue from HD patients (Stahl and Swanson 1974;Gu *et al.* 1996;Browne *et al.* 1997;Benchoua *et al.* 2006). Moreover, a decrease in complex IV activity was found in HD striatum (Browne *et al.* 1997;Gu *et al.* 1996).

In skeletal muscle, mHtt was reported to affect the activity of mitochondrial complex I (Arenas *et al.* 1998) and also complexes II/III (Ciammola *et al.* 2006;Turner *et al.* 2007), along with mitochondrial depolarization, cytochrome c release and caspases activation (Ciammola *et al.* 2006;Turner *et al.* 2007). In platelets from HD patients, some authors also found a decrease in complex I activity (Parker, Jr. *et al.* 1990), whereas others reported no changes in the activity of mitochondrial complexes (Gu *et al.* 1996;Powers *et al.* 2007a). A decrease in mitochondrial complex II/III activity was also found in lymphoblasts of HD patients (Sawa *et al.* 1999). No significant differences were observed in complexes I and IV but a correlation was found between complex II/III activity and disease duration and progress and inclusion formation in muscle (Turner *et al.* 2007).

Cybrids, an *ex-vivo* human peripheral cell model in which the contribution of mitochondrial defects from patients may be isolated, are an interesting approach to study mitochondrial dysfunction (King and Attardi 1989). Results from our laboratory showed that HD cybrids, prepared from the fusion of HD human platelets with NT2 rho0 cells, depleted of mitochondrial DNA, did not exhibit significant modifications in the activity of ETC complexes I–IV or specific mitochondrial DNA (mtDNA) sequence variations, suggestive of a primary role in mitochondrial susceptibility in the subpopulation of HD carriers studied (Ferreira et al. 2010). In accordance, Swerdlow and collaborators (1999) showed that HD cybrids did not present changes in ETC activity, oxidative stress or calcium homeostasis. Despite unchanged activity of mitochondrial complexes, this cell model presented evidences of mitochondrial dysfunction based on significant changes on mitochondrial membrane potential and increased ROS generation (Ferreira et al. 2010). The presence of mtDNA variations, including an 8656A N G variant in one patient, was previously shown in a screening study for mutations in the tRNA(leu/lys) and MTATP6 genes of 20 patients with HD (Kasraie *et al.* 2008). However, the nucleotides 8915-9207 of the same gene did not present any sequence variation in our HD cybrids (Ferreira et al. 2010). One of our HD cybrid lines carried the 3394T N C mutation with status "unclear" (Ferreira et al. 2010), previously described in cases suffering from Leber Hereditary Optic Neuropathy (LHON), which was shown to be related with HD features (Morimoto *et al.* 2004). In addition, a decrease in mitochondrial DNA content was found in cerebral cortex of HD patients (Horton *et al.* 1995).

It is accepted that mHtt not only impairs mitochondrial function, but also compromises cytosolic and mitochondrial calcium homeostasis, which contributes to neuronal dysfunction and death in HD (Damiano *et al.* 2010;Quintanilla and Johnson 2009, for review). Multiple changes in mitochondrial calcium handling (Panov *et al.* 2002;Oliveira *et al.* 2007), metabolism (Damiano *et al.* 2010), and susceptibility to apoptosis (Sawa *et al.* 1999) were suggested to be related with mitochondrial localization of mHtt (Orr *et al.* 2008). Indeed, mHtt interaction with neuronal mitochondria of YAC72 transgenic mice (Panov et al. 2002) was directly linked to mitochondrial calcium abnormalities (Choo et al. 2004;Panov et al. 2002). In this respect our group has also demonstrated changes in calcium handling linked to mitochondrial dysfunction in striatal neurons from YAC128 HD mice and cells derived from knock-in mice (Oliveira *et al.* 2006). Interestingly, increased vulnerability of striatal mitochondria to calcium loads was found to be present in both intact neurons and astrocytes, when compared with their cortical counterparts. Moreover, a lower mitochondrial calcium buffering capacity in intact striatal *versus* cortical astrocytes, associated with increased cyclosporin A-dependent permeability transition, suggested that the striatum is at higher risk for disturbed interactions between neurons and astrocytes (Oliveira and Goncalves 2009).

Various mitochondrial abnormalities observed in human patient samples, postmortem HD brains, cellular, invertebrate and vertebrate models of the disease, cooperate with mitochondrial ETC dysfunction in the genesis of HD (Pandey *et al.* 2010, for review). These include imbalance of calcium buffering capacity and oxidative stress, impaired axonal transport and abnormal fission and fusion of mitochondria, which are further described in this Chapter.

2.2 Altered mitochondrial trafficking and dynamics

Mitochondrial shape and structure are maintained by mitochondrial fission and fusion and disruption of mitochondrial dynamics was shown to be involved in HD (Chen and Chan 2009, for review). Fission is controlled by dynamin-related protein 1 (Drp1), mostly localized in the cytoplasm and in the mitochondrial outer membrane (MOM), and fission 1 (Fis1), localized to the MOM. On the other hand, mitochondrial fusion is ruled by mitofusin 1 (Mfn1) and mitofusin 2 (Mfn2), localized in the MOM, and optic atrophy-1 (Opa1), localized in the mitochondrial inner membrane (MIM) (Chen and Chan 2009, for review). In a healthy neuron, fission and fusion mechanisms balance equally and mitochondria alter their shape and size to move from cell body to the axons, dendrites, and synapses, and back to the cell body through mitochondrial trafficking. Recently, a role for abnormal mitochondrial networking in HD pathogenesis was described, involving mitochondrial fragmentation and cristae alterations, in different cellular models of HD (lymphoblasts from HD patients, striatal progenitor cell lines isolated from knock-in HdhQ111 mouse embryos and in YAC128 primary striatal neurons), explaining their increased susceptibility to apoptosis (Costa *et al.* 2010). Thus, increased cytotoxicity induced by overexpression of Htt proteins containing expanded polyglutamine (polyQ) tracts is likely mediated, at least in part, by an alteration in normal mitochondrial dynamics, which results in increased mitochondrial fragmentation (Wang *et al.* 2009). In striatal neurons from moderate-to-severe grade HD patients, both mitochondrial loss and altered mitochondrial morphogenesis have been described, with increased mitochondrial fission and reduced fusion (Kim *et al.* 2010). Indeed, mHtt was recently shown to bind the mitochondrial fission Drp-1 and increase its enzymatic activity (Song *et al.* 2011). Furthermore, overexpression of proteins that stimulate mitochondrial fusion attenuates the toxicity of Htt proteins containing expanded polyQ tracts in both HeLa cells and *C. elegans* (Wang *et al.* 2009).

Efficient mitochondrial trafficking is especially important in neurons with long axons and dendrites, to ensure high metabolic energy requirements for neuronal signaling, plasticity and neurotransmitter release. mHtt impairs axonal transport of mitochondria, decreases mitochondrial function and damages neurons in affected regions of HD patients' brains (Shirendeb *et al.* 2011). In particular, specific N-terminal fragments of mHtt (produced before aggregate formation) were shown to preferentially associate with mitochondria *in vivo*, in an age-dependent way, directly affecting the mitochondrial traffic in an HD-knock-in mouse model (Orr *et al.* 2008). In rat cortical neurons expressing full-length mHtt, an early event in HD pathophysiology is the aberrant mobility and trafficking of mitochondria caused by cytosolic Htt aggregates (Chang *et al.* 2006). Sequestration of mitochondrial proteins along with defective trafficking might lead to failure of ATP synthesis, energy depletion, and ultimately cell death in striatal neurons isolated from transgenic mice expressing mHtt with 72 glutamines (Trushina et al. 2004). Thus, disruption of mitochondrial trafficking in neurodegenerative diseases and abnormal mitochondrial dynamics, due to the perturbation of balance between fission and fusion, may mediate and amplify mitochondrial dysfunction in HD, compromising the supply of energy for normal neuronal function (Bossy-Wetzel *et al.* 2008, for review).

2.3 Changes in energy metabolism

Neurons are largely dependent on ATP to perform their functions and, thus, a decrease in mitochondrial energy metabolism may highly contribute to neurodegeneration. Moreover, mitochondria in striatal neurons, especially in the GABAergic medium-sized spiny neurons (MSNs), seem to be selectively vulnerable to metabolic stress, which may contribute to the selective loss of these neurons in HD (Jin and Johnson 2010, for review). Evidences of altered energy metabolism in HD include a decrease in glucose metabolism, observed in the caudate, putamen and cortex of symptomatic and pre-symptomatic HD patients (Kuhl *et al.* 1982;Kuwert *et al.* 1990). Modified glycolytic energy metabolism, in particular, has been described in HD patients, both in central and in peripheral tissues. This includes elevated levels of lactate in the striatum (Jenkins *et al.* 1993) and in the cortex (Jenkins *et al.* 1993;Koroshetz *et al.* 1997), and increased lactate/pyruvate ratio in the CSF (Koroshetz *et al.* 1997). However, decreased astrocytic glucose metabolism, with preserved oxygen metabolism, was described in the striatum of early symptomatic HD patients (Powers *et al.* 2007b). A significant decrease in phosphocreatine/inorganic phosphate ratio was found in resting muscle (Koroshetz *et al.* 1997) of HD patients, evidencing bioenergetic changes in HD peripheral tissues. Previous studies showed low levels of phosphocreatine/inorganic phosphate ratio in muscle of HD patients, compared to control subjects (Lodi *et al.* 2000), and a delayed recovery of phosphocreatine levels in HD patients in response to exercise (Saft *et al.* 2005). Moreover, reduced ATP production was observed in muscle of both presymptomatic and symptomatic HD patients (Lodi *et al.* 2000). In fact, the onset of energy-related manifestations at the presymptomatic stages of the disease, such as alterations in brain and muscle metabolism and weight loss, suggest that the energy deficit is likely to be an early phenomenon in the cascade of events leading to HD pathogenesis (Mochel and Haller 2011). Conversely, in HD N171-82Q mice model, increased glucose metabolism and ATP levels were found in brain tissue, suggesting that the neuronal damage in HD tissue may be associated with increased energy metabolism at the tissue level, leading to modified levels of various intermediary metabolites (Olah *et al.* 2008). Interestingly, we observed that HD cybrid lines exhibited increased glycolytic ATP levels compared to control cybrids, which were correlated with increased lactate/pyruvate levels (Ferreira *et al.* 2011). In these cybrids, the activity of G6PD, a key enzyme of the pentose phosphate pathway, was decreased (Ferreira *et al.* 2011), suggesting that glucose metabolization occurs primarily through the glycolytic pathway. Furthermore, mitochondrial NADH/NADt ratio was decreased (Ferreira *et al.* 2011), which was further correlated with a large decrease in the activity and protein levels of pyruvate dehydrogenase (PDH) (Ferreira *et al.* 2011). Nevertheless, the activity of alpha-ketoglutarate dehydrogenase (KGDH), another NADH producer in the tricarboxylic acid cycle, was increased, suggesting a compensatory mechanism to counterbalance the decrease in NADH production through the PDH. Decreased PDH activity was also previously observed in the caudate and putamen of HD patients (Sorbi *et al.* 1983), which was correlated with increasing duration of the illness (Butterworth *et al.* 1985). Moreover, PDH expression was shown to decrease with age in the striatum of R6/2 transgenic mice (Perluigi *et al.* 2005). A decrease in mitochondrial alanine and an increase in mitochondrial glutamate levels observed in these cybrids may be interpreted as an attempt to recover ketoglutarate levels and thus mitochondrial NADH (Ferreira *et al.* 2011). Alanine levels were also found to be decreased in the CSF of HD patients, along with decreased pyruvate levels and increased lactate/pyruvate ratio (Koroshetz *et al.* 1997). Our results demonstrated that HD cybrid lines possess inherent bioenergetically dysfunctional mitochondria derived from HD patients' platelets in the presence of a functional nuclear background (Ferreira et al. 2011). Mitochondrial dysfunction at the level of PDH, upstream the oxidative phosphorylation, affected amino acid metabolic fluxes and the cellular bioenergetics through glycolysis stimulation, which assumed a greater importance in promoting ATP production (Ferreira et al. 2011).

2.4 Oxidative stress

Oxidative phosphorylation at the level of mitochondrial ETC is a major source of ROS, such as superoxide anion (the radical formed from the direct reduction of oxygen due to electron leakage at the ETC), hydrogen peroxide and hydroxyl radical (the most reactive and unstable radical). In the absence of effective antioxidants, ROS generated by dysfunctional mitochondria may attack mitochondrial components, promoting intracellular oxidative stress and leading to protein, lipid and DNA oxidation, further contributing to mitochondrial dysfunction.

Oxidative damage was shown to play an important role in the pathogenesis and progression of HD in the R6/2 transgenic mouse model (Perluigi *et al.* 2005) and also in post-mortem samples obtained from the striatum and cortex of human HD brain (Sorolla *et al.* 2010). An increase in DCF fluorescence, indicative of an increase in hydroperoxide levels, was also described in the striatum of R6/1 mice 11-35 weeks (Perez-Severiano *et al.* 2004). In accordance, we demonstrated that, under basal conditions, HD cybrids were endowed with a significant higher production of hydroperoxides when compared to control cybrids (Ferreira et al., 2010). These data differ from a previous study showing no evidence of ROS generation in untreated HD cybrids (Swerdlow *et al.* 1999); however, these authors did not exclude a subtle mitochondrial pathology in these cells. In agreement, we showed that HD cybrids are more vulnerable than control cybrids to produce superoxide upon exposure to 3-NP or staurosporine (STS), whereas increased hydroperoxide production was mainly evoked by STS, suggesting that the presence of higher amounts of hydroperoxides in untreated HD cybrids masks the effect caused by 3-NP-induced mitochondrial inhibition (Ferreira *et al.* 2010).

Several biomarkers of oxidative stress, such as oxidized macromolecules, were found in HD patients and in HD models. Oxidized DNA was found in the caudate of HD patients (Browne *et al.* 1997), whereas oxidized mtDNA was reported in the parietal cortex of late stage (grade 3-4) HD patients (Polidori *et al.* 1999). 8-Hydroxy-deoxyguanosine was also found in peripheral blood of HD patients (Chen *et al.* 2007;Hersch *et al.* 2006). Moreover, oxidized DNA markers were also found in forebrain, striatum (Tabrizi *et al.* 2000;Bogdanov *et al.* 2001), urine, plasma and striatal dialysates of R6/2 mice at 12 and 14 weeks of age (Bogdanov *et al.* 2001). An increase in lipid peroxidation markers was also found in HD human blood (Chen *et al.* 2007;Stoy *et al.* 2005) or brain (Browne *et al.* 1999) and in R6/2 mouse brain (Tabrizi *et al.* 2000;Perez-Severiano *et al.* 2000). Protein oxidation markers, such as carbonyl levels, were also found to be increased in mitochondrial enzymes, resulting in decreased mitochondrial activity in the striatum of Tet/HD94 conditional HD mice (Sorolla *et al.* 2010).

Decreased activities of the antioxidant enzymes Cu–Zn-superoxide dismutase and glutathione peroxidase in erythrocytes (Chen *et al.* 2007), and decreased catalase activity were found in skin fibroblasts from HD patients (del Hoyo *et al.* 2006). A decrease in the antioxidant enzyme Cu/Zn-superoxide dismutase was also observed in R6/1 mice at 35 weeks (Santamaria *et al.* 2001). Moreover, the antioxidant agents lipoic acid and BN-82451 are neuroprotective in HD mice (R6/2 and N171–82Q lines), increasing survival and delaying striatal atrophy in these genetic models of HD (Andreassen *et al.* 2001;Klivenyi *et al.* 2003), further evidencing participation of oxidative damage in the process of neurodegeneration in HD. However, 3-NP *in vivo* exposure induced antioxidant response element (ARE)-dependent gene expression in cultured astrocytes through the transcription factor nuclear factor (erythroid-derived 2)-like 2 (Nrf2), leading to gene expression of antioxidant and detoxification genes (Shih *et al.* 2005).

2.5 Transcriptional deregulation

Nuclear localization of mHtt was shown to play a role in toxicity (Saudou *et al.* 1998), possibly due to interference of the mutant protein with nuclear transcription factors and co-factors (Benn *et al.* 2008;Zhai *et al.* 2005). Moreover, mitochondrial dysfunction in HD has been related to transcriptional deregulation.

Mitochondrial gene expression is regulated in the nucleus by the transcriptional co-activator peroxisome proliferative activated receptor gamma coactivator 1 alpha (PGC-1alpha) (Lin *et al.* 2004;Lin *et al.* 2005), and in the mitochondria, by the nuclear-encoded mitochondrial transcription factor A (Tfam) (Kaufman *et al.* 2007), which also regulate mitochondrial function and biogenesis.

Abnormal PGC-1alpha function was shown to result in significant mitochondrial impairment (Kim *et al.* 2010). The levels of PGC-1alpha and Tfam were found to be reduced in HD (Cui et al. 2006;Chaturvedi et al. 2009). Moreover, both proteins have been reported to be significantly reduced in brain lysates from HD patients, which was correlated with HD progression (Kim et al. 2010). A significant decrease in PGC-1alpha mRNA was found in the caudate nucleus in asymptomatic HD patients, accompanied by reduced expression of genes involved in energy metabolism (Cui *et al.* 2006). Interestingly, decreased expression of PGC-1alpha was observed in MSNs (largely affected in HD), whereas striatal interneurons showed increased mRNA levels for PGC-1alpha (Cui *et al.* 2006) which could, at least partially, explain the different vulnerability of these striatal neuronal populations. PGC-1alpha and Tfam were also reduced in muscle biopsies and myoblast cultures from HD subjects (Chaturvedi *et al.* 2009). Transcriptional repression of PGC-1alpha by mHtt leads not only to mitochondrial dysfunction, but also to neurodegeneration, suggesting a key role for PGC-1alpha in the control of energy metabolism in the early stages of HD pathogenesis (Cui *et al.* 2006). Thermoregulatory and metabolic defects in HD transgenic mice also implicate PGC-1alpha in HD neurodegeneration (Weydt *et al.* 2006), and polymorphisms at the PGC-1alpha gene modify the age at onset in HD (Weydt *et al.* 2009). In accordance, activation of PGC-1alpha/peroxisome proliferator-activated receptor gamma (PPARgamma) seems to protect against neurodegeneration (St-Pierre *et al.* 2006).

PGC-1alpha controls many aspects of oxidative metabolism, including respiration and mitochondrial biogenesis by co-activating and enhancing the expression and activity of several transcription factors, including the nuclear respiratory factors (NRF)-1 and NRF-2 (also known as GA-binding protein, GABP), PPARgamma and the estrogen related receptor alpha (ERRalpha) (Scarpulla 2002;Scarpulla 2011). It was recently shown that PGC-1alpha downstream transcription factors NRF-1 and Tfam are genetic modifiers of HD

(Taherzadeh-Fard *et al.* 2011). PGC-1alpha is indirectly involved in regulating the expression of mtDNA transcription *via* increased expression of Tfam, which is co-activated by NRF-1 (Scarpulla 2002;Kelly and Scarpulla 2004). Moreover, mitochondrial-dependent generation of ROS in HD seems to be due, at least in part, to suppression of PGC-1alpha in the presence of mHtt, as this transcription coactivator is required for the induction of ROS-detoxifying enzymes, namely Mn-superoxide dismutase and glutathione peroxidase (St-Pierre *et al.* 2006), implicating PGC-1alpha as an important protector against oxidative damage in HD. Importantly, activation of PPARgamma was recently shown to rescue mitochondrial dysfunction in HD (Chiang *et al.* 2011).

An important and key event in the signaling cascade that regulates PGC-1alpha expression is related with mitogen- and stress-activated protein kinase 1 (MSK-1) activation (Martin *et al.* 2011). MSK1 induces neuroprotection in HD, involving chromatin remodeling at the PGC-1 alpha promoter (Martin *et al.* 2011).

cAMP response element-binding (CREB) is a major transcription factor for PGC-1alpha (Cui *et al.* 2006). CREB is widely expressed and has a well-established role in neuronal protection (Lee *et al.* 2005). mHtt was shown to interfere with CREB transcriptional processes, through direct interaction with CREB-binding protein (CBP) (Steffan *et al.* 2000) and with TATA box-binding protein (TBP)-associated factor TAF4/TAFII130 (Dunah *et al.* 2002;Shimohata *et al.* 2000), leading to an increase in mHtt-induced cytotoxicity (Steffan *et al.* 2001). TAFII130 is a co-factor for CREB-dependent transcriptional activation that binds to polyQ, strongly suppressing CREB-mediated transcription (Shimohata *et al.* 2000). Reduction in cAMP levels in HD mice and HD patients likely contributes to the significant reduction in CREB activation (Gines *et al.* 2003). Moreover, CBP co-localizes with mHtt (Nucifora, Jr. *et al.* 2001), being found in nuclear inclusions in HD mice (Nucifora, Jr. *et al.* 2001;Steffan *et al.* 2001) and human brain (Nucifora, Jr. *et al.* 2001). In accordance, CRE-response genes such as corticotrophin-releasing hormone, proenkephalin, substance P were found to be reduced in brain tissue in HD patients (Augood *et al.* 1996;De Souza 1995) and R6/2 mice (Luthi-Carter *et al.* 2002).

Our group has previously shown that dysregulation of CREB activation and histone acetylation occurs in 3-NP-treated cortical neurons (Almeida *et al.* 2010), an *in vitro* model of mitochondrial complex II inhibition in HD. The phosphorylation status of CREB is critical for its activity and several protein kinases, such as calcium/calmodulin-dependent kinase II and IV, protein kinase C, PI3K, Akt, MAPK, and Rsk2, have been reported to promote the activation of CREB (Yamamoto *et al.* 1988;Matthews *et al.* 1994;Du and Montminy 1998;Bito *et al.* 1996;Impey *et al.* 1998;Perkinton *et al.* 2002). Phosphorylation on Ser133 leads to CREB activation and promotes the transcription of a large number of genes, through interaction with its nuclear partner CBP (Mayr and Montminy 2001). Results from our laboratory showed that 3-NP treatment of cortical neurons decreased both CREB phosphorylation on Ser133 and CBP levels (Almeida *et al.* 2010), strongly suggesting reduced CREB-dependent gene expression/activation. The decrease in CREB phosphorylation was possibly due to the activation of phosphatases in response to 3-NP exposure. Several studies have shown that calcineurin, whose expression is regulated by 3-NP (Napolitano *et al.* 2004), also regulate the duration of CREB phosphorylation (Bito *et al.* 1996). However, the concentration of 3-NP used in our study did not significantly alter calcineurin (Almeida *et al.* 2004). The decrease in total CBP levels after 3-NP exposure could be explained by an independent mechanism, related with caspase-3 (Almeida *et al.* 2010), but not calpain activation (Almeida *et al.* 2004). CBP has previously been reported to be specifically targeted for cleavage by caspases (and also by calpains) at the onset of neuronal apoptosis (Rouaux *et al.* 2003). A decrease in CBP was correlated with reduced acetylation of histones H3 and H4 and with a reduction in CBP/p300 HAT activity, even while total HAT activity remained unchanged (Rouaux *et al.* 2003). Similarly, we showed that 3-NP did not alter total HAT activity, but significantly decreased overall HDAC activity, likely explaining why we did not observe a reduction in H3 or H4 acetylation (Almeida *et al.* 2010). Instead, we observed an increase in both H3 and H4 acetylation in cortical neurons upon exposure to 3-NP. Because 3-NP induces caspase-3 activation (Almeida *et al.* 2004), we hypothesized that caspase-3 plays a role in inactivating HDACs. On the other hand, inhibition of HDAC may constitute a mechanism of protection of cells exposed to mild metabolic stress. Indeed, neuroprotection induced by HDAC inhibitors in HD striatal cells involves more efficient calcium handling, thus improving the neuronal ability to cope with excitotoxic stimuli (Oliveira *et al.* 2006).

mHtt was previously reported to bind p53 and upregulate its expression and transcriptional activity (Bae *et al.* 2005). It was demonstrated that some of the alterations induced by mHtt in mitochondrial homeostasis and cell death were dependent on p53 (Bae *et al.* 2005). Recently, mHtt expression was correlated with an increase in phosphorylated p53 at Ser15, a decrease in acetylation at Lys382, altered ubiquitination pattern, and oligomerization activity. The lack of a proper p53-mediated signaling cascade or its alteration in the presence of DNA damage may contribute to the slow progression of cellular dysfunction which is a hallmark of HD pathology (Illuzzi *et al.* 2011).

Specific protein-1 (Sp1) is another transcription factor that was found to bind mHtt, resulting in inhibition of Sp1-mediated transcription of genes in post-mortem brain tissue of pre-symptomatic and symptomatic HD patients (Dunah *et al.* 2002), such as NGF receptor (Li *et al.* 2002). Sp1 is a regulatory protein that binds to guanine-cytosine boxes and mediates transcription through its glutamine-rich activation domains which target components of the basal transcriptional complex, such as TAFII130 (Sugars and Rubinsztein 2003,for review). Furthermore, it has also been shown that, despite normal protein levels and nuclear binding activity, the binding of Sp1 to specific promoters of susceptible genes is significantly decreased in transgenic HD mouse brains, striatal HD cells and human HD brains, suggesting that mHtt dissociates Sp1 from target promoters, inhibiting the transcription of specific genes (Chen-Plotkin *et al.* 2006). Sequestration of Sp1 and TAFII130 into nuclear inclusions leads to the inhibition of Sp1-mediated transcription (Dunah *et al.* 2002;Li *et al.* 2002). Moreover, shorter N-terminal Htt fragments, which are more prone to misfold and aggregate, are more competent to bind and inhibit Sp1 (Cornett *et al.* 2006). Interestingly, this effect was reversed *in vitro* by HSP40, a molecular chaperone that reduces mHtt misfolding (Cornett *et al.* 2006).

mHtt may also lose the ability to bind and interact with other transcription factors regulated by wild-type huntingtin (Htt), as is the case of the neuron-restrictive silencer element (NRSE)-binding transcription factors, in which the failure of mHtt to interact with transcriptional factor complex repressor-element-1 transcription factor (REST)/neuron-restrictive silencer factor (NRSF) in the cytoplasm leads to its nuclear accumulation. There, it binds to NRSE sequences and promotes histone deacetylation, leading to the remodeling of the chromatin into a closed structure, resulting in the suppression of NRSE-containing genes, including the bdnf gene (Zuccato *et al.* 2003). In this case, the loss of the normal Htt function may have profound effects, leading to decreased levels of BDNF, an important survival factor for striatal neurons (section 2.2). Indeed, BDNF-knockout models were shown to largely recapitulate the expression profile of human HD (Strand *et al.* 2007), suggesting that striatal MSNs suffer similar insults in HD and BDNF-deprived environments.

2.6 Regulation of mitochondrial-driven apoptosis

Neurodegeneration in HD has been associated with increased cell death by apoptosis, particularly by the intrinsic pathway, highly regulated by mitochondria. Previous studies demonstrated the presence of caspases cleavage sites in Htt, a mechanism that may also contribute to apoptotic death by generating truncated toxic fragments of this protein (Wellington *et al.* 1998), although the CAG length does not seem to modulate the susceptibility for cleavage. mHtt is a substrate for several caspases and calpains (Kim *et al.* 2001) and the polyglutamine fragments of Htt may present enhanced toxicity, promoting caspases activation by interfering with mitochondrial function, thus amplifying the generation of toxic truncated mHtt (Graham *et al.* 2010). Moreover, sequestration of pro-caspases in the aggregates is thought to promote their activation, triggering an intracellular cascade of proteolytic events (Gil and Rego 2008, for review). Interestingly, wild-type Htt was found to have antiapoptotic properties against a variety of apoptotic stimuli, including serum withdrawal, death receptors, and proapoptotic Bcl-2 homologs (Rigamonti *et al.* 2000), namely through inhibition of cytochrome c-dependent procaspase-9 processing and activity (Rigamonti *et al.* 2001). Furthermore, calpain (Gafni and Ellerby 2002), caspase-1 (Ona *et al.* 1999) and caspase-8 (Sanchez *et al.* 1999) activities are increased in HD human brains, suggesting that an apoptotic mechanism is responsible for HD neuronal loss (Gil and Rego 2008, for review). Moreover, cultured blood cells from patients homozygous for CAG repeat mutations and heterozygous with high size mutations causing juvenile onset presented significantly increased caspases -2, -3, -6, -8 and -9 activities, decreased cell viability and pronounced mitochondria morphological abnormalities, compared with cells from HD patients carrying low mutation size and controls (Squitieri *et al.* 2011).

Cell death by necrosis and apoptosis, along with energy deficiency, were previously described in striatal, cortical and hippocampal cells exposed to 3-NP (Behrens *et al.* 1995;Pang and Geddes 1997;Almeida *et al.* 2004;Almeida *et al.* 2006;Brouillet *et al.* 2005), and both processes of cell damage have been proven to involve mitochondria (Kroemer and Reed 2000). Concordantly with a higher role of intrinsic apoptosis in HD, Ferrer and collaborators (2000) found a reduction in Fas and FasL expression levels in the caudate and putamen of HD patients. Mitochondria has been largely recognized to play a critical role in cell death by releasing apoptogenic factors, such as cytochrome c and apoptosis-inducing factor (AIF), from the intermembrane space into the cytoplasm.

As described before, by directly interacting with the mitochondria (Panov *et al.* 2002), mHtt may cause mitochondrial abnormalities in HD, leading to cytochrome c release (Panov *et al.* 2002), and a decrease in mitochondrial membrane potential (Sawa *et al.* 1999). Release of cytochrome *c* along with the activation of caspases -1, -8, and -9 have been demonstrated in HD (Ona *et al.* 1999;Sanchez *et al.* 1999;Kiechle *et al.* 2002), and increased Bcl-2 and Bax were also reported in HD patients' brain, especially in the most severely affected (Vis *et al.* 2005).

Overexpression of mHtt, but not the normal protein, increases oxidative stress-induced mitochondrial fragmentation in HeLa cells, which correlates with increased caspase-3 activation and cell death (Wang *et al.* 2009). Results from our laboratory highly suggested that 3-NP induces both caspase-dependent and -independent cell death (Almeida *et al.* 2006). Our group also showed that exposure of HD cybrid cell lines to 3-NP or STS caused DNA fragmentation and moderate caspase-3 activation, evidencing an increased susceptibility of HD cybrids to apoptosis (Ferreira *et al.* 2010). In contrast, 3-NP-treated control cybrids died predominantly by necrosis, not involving caspase-3 activation (Ferreira *et al.* 2010), suggesting that HD mitochondria are endowed with pro-apoptotic machinery and thus more susceptible to this type of cell death. Moreover, preserved ATP in HD cybrids compared to control cybrids (Ferreira et al. 2011) may facilitate apoptotic cell death. Mitochondrial-dependent apoptosis in HD cybrids subjected to 3-NP was correlated with increased release of mitochondrial cytochrome c, AIF, Bax translocation, caspase-3 activation and ROS formation (Ferreira *et al.* 2010). Increased mitochondrial Bim and Bak levels, and a slight release of cytochrome c in untreated HD cybrids further explained their moderate susceptibility to mitochondrial-dependent apoptosis under basal conditions (Ferreira et al. 2010). These data appear to be consistent with possible subtle effects of mHtt in the mitochondria of HD cybrids. 3-NP has been also shown to collapse mitochondrial membrane potential and to downregulate striatal Bcl-2 levels (Zhang *et al.* 2009b), promoting cytochrome c release from mitochondria, transient caspase-9 processing, activation of calpains and subsequent striatal apoptosis (Bizat *et al.* 2003;Zhang *et al.* 2009b). 3-NP-induced decrement in Bcl-2 may also play a role in mitochondrial-dependent autophagy activation (through the release of Beclin 1 from hVps34 complex), which was also involved in striatal neuronal apoptosis (Zhang *et al.* 2009a).

Our group has also reported that 3-NP causes mitochondrial-dependent apoptotic neuronal death through the release of cytochrome c and consequent activation of caspases, or the release of AIF in cortical neurons, depending on the concentration of 3-NP (Almeida *et al.* 2004;Almeida *et al.* 2006;Almeida *et al.* 2009). Enhanced mitochondrial-dependent apoptosis was also observed in 3-NP-treated cortical neurons as a result of decreased Bim turnover (Almeida *et al.* 2004). mHtt fragments were previously shown to directly induce the opening of the mitochondrial permeability transition pore (PTP) in isolated mouse liver mitochondria, with the consequent release of cytochrome c (Choo *et al.* 2004), which evokes caspase cascade activation. Choo and collaborators (2004) also described that mitochondria from liver of knock-in mouse model of HD and from homozygous ST*Hdh*^Q111 cells were more sensitive to calcium-induced cytochrome c release, swelling at lower calcium loads. An increased striatal mitochondrial susceptibility to the induction of permeability transition (Brustovetsky *et al.* 2003) may be responsible to the striatal selectivity for energy deficit associated with mHtt. An age- and polyQ-dependent decrease in the amount of calcium necessary to induce permeability transition in striatal mitochondria was observed in severe (R6/2 mice) and in mild (*HdhQ92* knock-in mice) HD mouse models (Brustovetsky *et al.* 2003). Moreover, increased mitochondrial calcium loading capacity, previously shown in isolated mitochondria from 12-13 week-old R6/2 and 12 month-old YAC mice brain (Oliveira *et al.* 2007) could constitute a compensatory mechanism, to extend neuronal function and survival or, alternatively, it could simply reflect an artifact resulting from mitochondria isolation, as it was not observed in neuronal *in situ* experiments following exposure to excitotoxic stimuli (Oliveira *et al.* 2007).

Myoblasts obtained from presymptomatic and symptomatic HD subjects also showed mitochondrial depolarization, cytochrome c release and increased activities of caspases -3, -8 and -9 (Ciammola *et al.* 2006). In addition, peripheral blood cells, in particularly B lymphocytes from HD patients, may reflect changes observed in HD brain. Our group previously found increased Bax expression in B and T lymphocytes, and monocytes from HD patients, with no alterations in Bcl-2 expression levels, and decreased mitochondrial membrane potential in B lymphocytes (Almeida *et al.* 2008), further suggesting that an adverse effect of mHtt is not limited to neurons. Moreover, mitochondria from lymphoblasts of HD patients have been shown to present increased susceptibility to apoptotic stimuli due to an abnormal mitochondrial transmembrane potential (Sawa et al. 1999). Lymphoblasts derived from HD patients also showed increased stress-induced apoptotic cell death associated with caspase-3 activation, abnormal calcium homeostasis and mitochondrial dysfunction (Panov *et al.* 2002;Sawa *et al.* 1999).

3. Protective effects involving modulation of phosphorylation pathways — The case of FK506 and the neurotrophins BDNF and NGF

Even though HD has a single genetic cause, the multiplicity of pathogenic mechanisms involved suggests that several different targets must be taken into account in order to slow down HD progression. Despite important advances in elucidating the molecular pathways involved in HD neurodegeneration, there is currently no therapy that delays the onset of the disease. In this respect, stimulation of phosphorylation pathways by neurotrophins or calcineurin inhibitors (such as FK506) may be a promising strategy.

3.1 FK506 — An inhibitor of calcineurin

It is well accepted that mHtt is associated with calcium handling abnormalities (Quintanilla and Johnson 2009, for review). Calcineurin can be activated by abnormal calcium levels occurring in HD. Classically, calcineurin (or protein phosphatase 3, formerly known as protein phosphatase 2B) can promote apoptosis through dephosphorylation of Bad at Ser112 and Ser136 (Wang *et al.* 1999), a proapoptotic member of the Bcl-2 family. Dephosphorylated Bad translocates from the cytosol to the mitochondria, where it inhibits antiapoptotic activity of Bcl-2 and Bcl-xL, ultimately leading to cell death. Calcineurin couples intracellular calcium to the dephosphorylation of other selected substrates, which include transcription factors [nuclear factor of activated T-cells (NFAT)], ion channels (inositol-1,4,5 triphosphate receptor), proteins involved in vesicular trafficking (amphyphysin, dynamin), scaffold proteins (AKAP79), and phosphatase inhibitors (DARPP-32 inhibitor-1) (Aramburu *et al.* 2000).

Calcineurin was recently shown to be involved in the dephosphorylation of Drp1, thus increasing Drp1 association with mitochondria and promoting fission, cristae disruption, cytochrome c release and apoptosis (Costa *et al.* 2010;Cereghetti *et al.* 2010). Concordantly, the calcineurin inhibitor PPD1 blocked Drp1 translocation to mitochondria and fragmentation of the organelle, delaying intrinsic apoptosis by preventing fragmentation and release of cytochrome *c*, suggesting an important function of calcineurin in mitochondrial fragmentation and in the amplification of cell death (Cereghetti *et al.* 2010).

FK506, also known as tacrolimus, is a selective inhibitor of calcineurin (Griffith *et al.* 1995) that has shown to exert neuroprotective effects in several cellular and animal models of HD. Kumar and Kumar (2009) showed that systemic treatment with FK506 significantly improved cognitive function in a 3-NP rodent model. In the 3-NP neuronal model, we have previously shown that FK506 precludes cytochrome c release, activation of caspase-3 and DNA fragmentation in cultured cortical neurons (Almeida *et al.* 2004). FK506 neuroprotection against 3-NP-induced apoptosis was associated with the redistribution of Bcl-2 and Bax in the mitochondrial membrane of cortical neurons (Almeida *et al.* 2004). Moreover, FK506 significantly attenuated oxidative stress as evidenced by restoring glutathione levels and acetylcholinesterase activity in 3-NP treated animals (Kumar and Kumar 2009), highlighting the therapeutic potential of this compound. In a recent study from our laboratory FK506 has shown neuroprotective effects against apoptosis and necrosis under mild cell death stimulus, in the presence of full-length mHtt, in 3-NP-treated primary striatal neurons and immortalized striatal cells derived from HD knock-in mice (ST*Hdh*$^{Q111/Q111}$ mutant cells) (Rosenstock *et al.* 2011).

In the context of mHtt expression, intraperitoneal injection of calcineurin inhibitors was shown to accelerate the neurological phenotype in R6/2 mice (Hernandez-Espinosa and Morton 2006), which are resistant to excitotoxicity (Hansson *et al.* 1999). Interestingly, reduced calcineurin protein levels and activity were observed in this HD animal model (Xifro *et al.* 2009). In contrast, calcineurin is involved in cell death induced by activation of N-methyl-D-aspartate receptors (NMDARs) in knock-in striatal cells expressing full-length mHtt (Xifro *et al.* 2008). Moreover, FK506 and the genetic inactivation of calcineurin protected against mHtt toxicity through increased phosphorylation of Htt (Pardo *et al.* 2006) and further ameliorated the defect in BDNF axonal transport (Pineda *et al.* 2009).

3.2 BDNF and NGF — Activators of survival pathways

Trophic support to neurons largely influences neuronal survival and function. BDNF, a pro-survival factor that is produced by cortical neurons, is necessary for the survival of striatal neurons in the brain. This is particularly relevant in HD since its transcription (Zuccato *et al.* 2001) and axonal transport (Gauthier *et al.* 2004) are decreased by the presence of mHtt, affecting the survival of both striatal and cortical neurons. Members of the neurotrophin family, namely BDNF and NGF, have been suggested as therapeutic candidates to treat neurodegenerative disorders because they promote neuronal survival in different lesion models (Connor and Dragunow 1998). Indeed, implantation of NGF-secreting fibroblasts was found to reduce the size of adjacent striatal 3-NP lesions (Frim *et al.* 1993).

Wild-type Htt was demonstrated to promote the expression of BDNF by interacting with the REST/NRSF in the cytoplasm, preventing this complex from translocating into the nucleus and binding to NRSE present in the promoter of the bdnf gene (Zuccato *et al.* 2003). Wild-type Htt also promoted the vesicular transport of BDNF along the microtubules through a mechanism involving Htt -associated protein 1 (HAP1) and the p150 subunit of dynactin (Gauthier *et al.* 2004). Thus, wild-type Htt controls neurotrophic support and survival of striatal neurons by promoting BDNF transcription and vesicular transport along microtubules (Gauthier *et al.* 2004).

In contrast, mHtt decreases transcription of BDNF, which results in decreased production of cortical BDNF in HD (Zuccato *et al.* 2001), leading to insufficient neurotrophic support for striatal neurons, which then die. Accordingly, a reduction in cortical BDNF mRNA levels was shown to correlate with the progression of the disease in a mouse model of HD (Zuccato *et al.* 2005). In addition, BDNF-knockout models were shown to largely recapitulate the expression profiling of human HD (Strand *et al.* 2007), suggesting that striatal MSNs suffer similar insults in HD and BDNF-deprived environments. Moreover, mHtt appears to be responsible for altering the wild-type Htt /HAP1/p150 complex, causing an impaired association between motor proteins and microtubules, and attenuating BDNF transport, which results in loss of neurotrophic support (Gauthier *et al.* 2004). Thus, restoring wild-type Htt activity and increasing BDNF production are promising therapeutic approaches for treating HD (Zuccato *et al.* 2001).

BDNF was previously shown to prevent the death of different populations of striatal projection neurons in a quinolinic acid model of HD (Perez-Navarro *et al.* 2000;Kells *et al.* 2004) and in striatal neurons exposed to 3-NP (Ryu *et al.* 2004). The effects of BDNF are mainly mediated by TrkB receptor-induced activation of key signaling pathways, including phosphoinositide phospholipase C (PLC-γ), rat sarcoma GTPase (Ras)/MEK/ Ras–mitogen-activated protein kinase (MAPK) and PI3K/Akt pathways (Huang and Reichardt 2003), which have been shown to regulate apoptotic cell death by increasing the transcription of neuroprotective proteins such as Bcl-2 (Pugazhenthi *et al.* 2000) and/or by posttranslational modifications of proteins such as Bad and Bim (Scheid et al. 1999;Luciano et al. 2003). Bim phosphorylation by MAPK promotes its subsequent ubiquitination and degradation (Ley *et al.* 2003), whereas serine phosphorylation of Bad is associated with protein 14-3-3 binding and inhibition of Bad-induced cell death (Masters *et al.* 2001). Data from our laboratory support an important role for BDNF in protecting cortical neurons against apoptotic cell death caused by 3-NP through the activation of PI3K and MEK1/2 intracellular signaling pathways and the regulation of Bim turnover (Almeida et al. 2009). Moreover, signaling of BDNF and NGF culminates in the transcription of neuroprotective proteins through the activation of critical transcription factors such as CREB and nuclear factor-kB (NFkB) (Huang and Reichardt 2003). As described in section 1.5, when activated by phosphorylation, CREB binds to its co-activator CBP and the complex is competent to initiate gene transcription (Mayr and Montminy 2001). Similarly, phosphorylation of IkB releases the p65:p50 NFkB heterodimers, which then translocate to the nucleus to initiate transcription. Pro-survival proteins whose expression is dependent on these transcription factors include proteins such as Bcl-2, Mn-superoxide dismutase and BDNF (Saha et al. 2006). A recent study from our laboratory also suggested that BDNF and NGF induce positive changes in the levels and activities of CREB and NFkB, and both neurotrophins counteracted 3-NP-induced chromatin-bound histone acetylation modifications. The latter finding was correlated with BDNF-induced hyperphosphorylation of HDAC2, explaining the neuroprotective role of this neurotrophin in the context of mitochondrial dysfunction (Almeida *et al.* 2010).

4. Conclusions

In summary, biochemical studies support the view that mitochondrial dysfunction, including impaired oxidative phosphorylation, tricarboxylic acid cycle dysfunction, and oxidative stress are important determinants of altered energy metabolism in HD. Bioenergetic changes in HD may be related with impaired intracellular transport and transcriptional deregulation in the disease (Mochel and Haller 2011). Impaired bioenergetics in HD likely represents downstream effects of both a mHtt toxic gain-of-function and a loss-of-function of the wild-type protein. Thus, therapeutic strategies designed to improve energy metabolism and survival pathways dependent on kinase signaling in the HD brain will possibly impact the course of the disease, delaying its onset and the rate of progression. BDNF support (which can be rescued by wild-type Htt) and FK506 may have important therapeutic effects as enhancers of phosphorylation pathways, preventing mitochondrial dysfunction caused by mHtt and mitochondrial-dependent apoptosis.

5. Acknowledgements

T.C.O. holds a postdoctoral fellowship from 'Fundação para a Ciência e a Tecnologia' (FCT), Portugal (SFRH/BPD/34711/2007). A.C.R. acknowledges financial support from FCT Grant PTDC/SAU-FCF/108056/2008.

6. References

Almeida S., Brett A. C., Gois I. N., Oliveira C. R. and Rego A. C. (2006) Caspase-dependent and -independent cell death induced by 3-nitropropionic acid in rat cortical neurons. *J. Cell Biochem.* 98, 93-101. ISSN: 0730-2312 (Print); ISSN: 0730-2312 (Linking)

Almeida S., Cunha-Oliveira T., Laco M., Oliveira C. R. and Rego A. C. (2010) Dysregulation of CREB activation and histone acetylation in 3-nitropropionic acid-treated cortical neurons: prevention by BDNF and NGF. *Neurotox. Res.* 17, 399-405. ISSN: 1476-3524 (Electronic); ISSN: 1029-8428 (Linking)

Almeida S., Domingues A., Rodrigues L., Oliveira C. R. and Rego A. C. (2004) FK506 prevents mitochondrial-dependent apoptotic cell death induced by 3-nitropropionic acid in rat primary cortical cultures. *Neurobiol. Dis.* 17, 435-444. ISSN: 0969-9961 (Print); ISSN: 0969-9961 (Linking)

Almeida S., Laco M., Cunha-Oliveira T., Oliveira C. R. and Rego A. C. (2009) BDNF regulates BIM expression levels in 3-nitropropionic acid-treated cortical neurons. *Neurobiol. Dis.* 35, 448-456. ISSN:1095-953X (Electronic); ISSN: 0969-9961 (Linking)

Almeida S., Sarmento-Ribeiro A. B., Januario C., Rego A. C. and Oliveira C. R. (2008) Evidence of apoptosis and mitochondrial abnormalities in peripheral blood cells of Huntington's disease patients. *Biochem. Biophys. Res. Commun.* 374, 599-603. ISSN: 1090-2104 (Electronic); ISSN: 0006-291X (Linking)

Andreassen O. A., Ferrante R. J., Dedeoglu A. and Beal M. F. (2001) Lipoic acid improves survival in transgenic mouse models of Huntington's disease. *Neuroreport* 12, 3371-3373. ISSN: 0959-4965 (Print); ISSN: 0959-4965 (Linking)

Aramburu J., Rao A. and Klee C. B. (2000) Calcineurin: from structure to function. *Curr. Top. Cell Regul.* 36, 237-295. ISSN: 0070-2137 (Print); ISSN: 0070-2137 (Linking)

Arenas J., Campos Y., Ribacoba R., Martin M. A., Rubio J. C., Ablanedo P. and Cabello A. (1998) Complex I defect in muscle from patients with Huntington's disease. *Ann. Neurol.* 43, 397-400. ISSN: 0364-5134 (Print); ISSN: 0364-5134 (Linking)

Augood S. J., Faull R. L., Love D. R. and Emson P. C. (1996) Reduction in enkephalin and substance P messenger RNA in the striatum of early grade Huntington's disease: a detailed cellular in situ hybridization study. *Neuroscience* 72, 1023-1036. ISSN: 0306-4522 (Print); ISSN: 0306-4522 (Linking)

Bae B. I., Xu H., Igarashi S., Fujimuro M., Agrawal N., Taya Y., Hayward S. D., Moran T. H., Montell C., Ross C. A., Snyder S. H. and Sawa A. (2005) p53 mediates cellular dysfunction and behavioral abnormalities in Huntington's disease. *Neuron* 47, 29-41. ISSN: 0896-6273 (Print); ISSN: 0896-6273 (Linking)

Beal M. F., Brouillet E., Jenkins B., Henshaw R., Rosen B. and Hyman B. T. (1993) Age-dependent striatal excitotoxic lesions produced by the endogenous mitochondrial inhibitor malonate. *J. Neurochem.* 61, 1147-1150. ISSN: 0022-3042 (Print); ISSN: 0022-3042 (Linking)

Behrens M. I., Koh J., Canzoniero L. M., Sensi S. L., Csernansky C. A. and Choi D. W. (1995) 3-Nitropropionic acid induces apoptosis in cultured striatal and cortical neurons. *Neuroreport* 6, 545-548. ISSN: 0959-4965 (Print); ISSN: 0959-4965 (Linking)

Benchoua A., Trioulier Y., Zala D., Gaillard M. C., Lefort N., Dufour N., Saudou F., Elalouf J. M., Hirsch E., Hantraye P., Deglon N. and Brouillet E. (2006) Involvement of mitochondrial complex II defects in neuronal death produced by N-terminus fragment of mutated huntingtin. *Mol. Biol. Cell* 17, 1652-1663. ISSN: 1059-1524 (Print); ISSN: 1059-1524 (Linking)

Benn C. L., Sun T., Sadri-Vakili G., McFarland K. N., DiRocco D. P., Yohrling G. J., Clark T. W., Bouzou B. and Cha J. H. (2008) Huntingtin modulates transcription, occupies gene promoters in vivo, and binds directly to DNA in a polyglutamine-dependent manner. *J. Neurosci.* 28, 10720-10733. ISSN: 1529-2401 (Electronic); ISSN: 0270-6474 (Linking)

Bito H., Deisseroth K. and Tsien R. W. (1996) CREB phosphorylation and dephosphorylation: a Ca(2+)- and stimulus duration-dependent switch for hippocampal gene expression. *Cell* 87, 1203-1214. ISSN: 0092-8674 (Print); ISSN: 0092-8674 (Linking)

Bizat N., Hermel J. M., Boyer F., Jacquard C., Creminon C., Ouary S., Escartin C., Hantraye P., Kajewski S. and Brouillet E. (2003) Calpain is a major cell death effector in selective striatal degeneration induced in vivo by 3-nitropropionate: implications for Huntington's disease. *J. Neurosci.* 23, 5020-5030. ISSN: 1529-2401 (Electronic); ISSN: 0270-6474 (Linking)

Bogdanov M. B., Andreassen O. A., Dedeoglu A., Ferrante R. J. and Beal M. F. (2001) Increased oxidative damage to DNA in a transgenic mouse model of Huntington's disease. *J. Neurochem.* 79, 1246-1249. ISSN: 0022-3042 (Print); ISSN: 0022-3042 (Linking)

Bossy-Wetzel E., Petrilli A. and Knott A. B. (2008) Mutant huntingtin and mitochondrial dysfunction. *Trends Neurosci.* 31, 609-616. ISSN: 0166-2236 (Print); ISSN: 0166-2236 (Linking)

Brouillet E., Conde F., Beal M. F. and Hantraye P. (1999) Replicating Huntington's disease phenotype in experimental animals. *Prog. Neurobiol.* 59, 427-468. ISSN: 0301-0082 (Print); ISSN: 0301-0082 (Linking)

Brouillet E., Jacquard C., Bizat N. and Blum D. (2005) 3-Nitropropionic acid: a mitochondrial toxin to uncover physiopathological mechanisms underlying striatal degeneration in Huntington's disease. *J. Neurochem.* 95, 1521-1540. ISSN: 0022-3042 (Print); ISSN: 0022-3042 (Linking)

Brouillet E., Jenkins B. G., Hyman B. T., Ferrante R. J., Kowall N. W., Srivastava R., Roy D. S., Rosen B. R. and Beal M. F. (1993) Age-dependent vulnerability of the striatum to the mitochondrial toxin 3-nitropropionic acid. *J. Neurochem.* 60, 356-359. ISSN: 0022-3042 (Print); ISSN: 0022-3042 (Linking)

Browne S. E., Bowling A. C., MacGarvey U., Baik M. J., Berger S. C., Muqit M. M., Bird E. D. and Beal M. F. (1997) Oxidative damage and metabolic dysfunction in Huntington's disease: selective vulnerability of the basal ganglia. *Ann. Neurol.* 41, 646-653. ISSN: 0364-5134 (Print); ISSN: 0364-5134 (Linking)

Browne S. E., Ferrante R. J. and Beal M. F. (1999) Oxidative stress in Huntington's disease. *Brain Pathol.* 9, 147-163. ISSN: 1015-6305 (Print): ISSN: 1015-6305 (Linking)

Brustovetsky N., Brustovetsky T., Purl K. J., Capano M., Crompton M. and Dubinsky J. M. (2003) Increased susceptibility of striatal mitochondria to calcium-induced permeability transition. *J. Neurosci.* 23, 4858-4867. ISSN: 1529-2401 (Electronic); ISSN: 0270-6474 (Linking)

Butterworth J., Yates C. M. and Reynolds G. P. (1985) Distribution of phosphate-activated glutaminase, succinic dehydrogenase, pyruvate dehydrogenase and gamma-glutamyl transpeptidase in post-mortem brain from Huntington's disease and agonal cases. *J. Neurol. Sci.* 67, 161-171. ISSN: 0022-510X (Print); ISSN: 0022-510X (Linking)

Cereghetti G. M., Costa V. and Scorrano L. (2010) Inhibition of Drp1-dependent mitochondrial fragmentation and apoptosis by a polypeptide antagonist of calcineurin. *Cell Death. Differ.* 17, 1785-1794. ISSN: 1476-5403 (Electronic); ISSN: 1350-9047 (Linking)

Chang D. T., Rintoul G. L., Pandipati S. and Reynolds I. J. (2006) Mutant huntingtin aggregates impair mitochondrial movement and trafficking in cortical neurons. *Neurobiol. Dis.* 22, 388-400. ISSN: 0969-9961 (Print); ISSN: 0969-9961 (Linking)

Chaturvedi R. K., Adhihetty P., Shukla S., Hennessy T., Calingasan N., Yang L., Starkov A., Kiaei M., Cannella M., Sassone J., Ciammola A., Squitieri F. and Beal M. F. (2009) Impaired PGC-1alpha function in muscle in Huntington's disease. *Hum. Mol. Genet.* 18, 3048-3065. ISSN: 1460-2083 (Electronic); ISSN: 0964-6906 (Linking)

Chen C. M., Wu Y. R., Cheng M. L., Liu J. L., Lee Y. M., Lee P. W., Soong B. W. and Chiu D. T. (2007) Increased oxidative damage and mitochondrial abnormalities in the peripheral blood of Huntington's disease patients. *Biochem. Biophys. Res. Commun.* 359, 335-340. ISSN: 0006-291X (Print); ISSN: 0006-291X (Linking)

Chen H. and Chan D. C. (2009) Mitochondrial dynamics--fusion, fission, movement, and mitophagy--in neurodegenerative diseases. *Hum. Mol. Genet.* 18, R169-R176. ISSN: 1460-2083 (Electronic); ISSN: 0964-6906 (Linking)

Chen-Plotkin A. S., Sadri-Vakili G., Yohrling G. J., Braveman M. W., Benn C. L., Glajch K. E., DiRocco D. P., Farrell L. A., Krainc D., Gines S., MacDonald M. E. and Cha J. H. (2006) Decreased association of the transcription factor Sp1 with genes downregulated in Huntington's disease. *Neurobiol. Dis.* 22, 233-241. ISSN: 0969-9961 (Print); ISSN: 0969-9961 (Linking)

Chiang M. C., Chern Y. and Huang R. N. (2011) PPARgamma rescue of the mitochondrial dysfunction in Huntington's disease. *Neurobiol. Dis.* ISSN: 1095-953X (Electronic); ISSN: 0969-9961 (Linking)

Choo Y. S., Johnson G. V., MacDonald M., Detloff P. J. and Lesort M. (2004) Mutant huntingtin directly increases susceptibility of mitochondria to the calcium-induced permeability transition and cytochrome c release. *Hum. Mol. Genet.* 13, 1407-1420. ISSN: 0964-6906 (Print); ISSN: 0964-6906 (Linking)

Ciammola A., Sassone J., Alberti L., Meola G., Mancinelli E., Russo M. A., Squitieri F. and Silani V. (2006) Increased apoptosis, Huntingtin inclusions and altered differentiation in muscle cell cultures from Huntington's disease subjects. *Cell Death. Differ.* 13, 2068-2078. ISSN: 1350-9047 (Print); ISSN: 1350-9047 (Linking)

Connor B. and Dragunow M. (1998) The role of neuronal growth factors in neurodegenerative disorders of the human brain. *Brain Res. Brain Res. Rev.* 27, 1-39. ISSN: 0165-0173

Cornett J., Smith L., Friedman M., Shin J. Y., Li X. J. and Li S. H. (2006) Context-dependent dysregulation of transcription by mutant huntingtin. *J. Biol. Chem.* 281, 36198-36204. ISSN: 0021-9258 (Print); ISSN: 0021-9258 (Linking)

Costa V., Giacomello M., Hudec R., Lopreiato R., Ermak G., Lim D., Malorni W., Davies K. J., Carafoli E. and Scorrano L. (2010) Mitochondrial fission and cristae disruption increase the response of cell models of Huntington's disease to apoptotic stimuli. *EMBO Mol. Med.* 2, 490-503. ISSN: 1757-4684 (Electronic); ISSN: 1757-4676 (Linking)

Cui L., Jeong H., Borovecki F., Parkhurst C. N., Tanese N. and Krainc D. (2006) Transcriptional repression of PGC-1alpha by mutant huntingtin leads to mitochondrial dysfunction and neurodegeneration. *Cell* 127, 59-69. ISSN: 0092-8674 (Print); ISSN: 0092-8674 (Linking)

Damiano M., Galvan L., Deglon N. and Brouillet E. (2010) Mitochondria in Huntington's disease. *Biochim. Biophys. Acta* 1802, 52-61. ISSN: 0006-3002 (Print); ISSN: 0006-3002 (Linking)

De Souza E. B. (1995) Corticotropin-releasing factor receptors: physiology, pharmacology, biochemistry and role in central nervous system and immune disorders. *Psychoneuroendocrinology* 20, 789-819. ISSN: 0306-4530 (Print); ISSN: 0306-4530 (Linking)

del Hoyo P., Garcia-Redondo A., de B. F., Molina J. A., Sayed Y., Alonso-Navarro H., Caballero L., Arenas J. and Jimenez-Jimenez F. J. (2006) Oxidative stress in skin fibroblasts cultures of patients with Huntington's disease. *Neurochem. Res.* 31, 1103-1109. ISSN: 0364-3190 (Print); ISSN: 0364-3190 (Linking)

Du K. and Montminy M. (1998) CREB is a regulatory target for the protein kinase Akt/PKB. *J. Biol. Chem.* 273, 32377-32379. ISSN: 0021-9258 (Print); ISSN: 0021-9258 (Linking)

Dunah A. W., Jeong H., Griffin A., Kim Y. M., Standaert D. G., Hersch S. M., Mouradian M. M., Young A. B., Tanese N. and Krainc D. (2002) Sp1 and TAFII130 transcriptional activity disrupted in early Huntington's disease. *Science* 296, 2238-2243. ISSN: 1095-9203 (Electronic); ISSN: 0036-8075 (Linking)

Ferreira I. L., Cunha-Oliveira T., Nascimento M. V., Ribeiro M., Proenca M. T., Januario C., Oliveira C. R. and Rego A. C. (2011) Bioenergetic dysfunction in Huntington's disease human cybrids. *Exp. Neurol.* 231, 127-134. ISSN: 1090-2430 (Electronic); ISSN: 0014-4886 (Linking)

Ferreira I. L., Nascimento M. V., Ribeiro M., Almeida S., Cardoso S. M., Grazina M., Pratas J., Santos M. J., Januario C., Oliveira C. R. and Rego A. C. (2010) Mitochondrial-dependent apoptosis in Huntington's disease human cybrids. *Exp. Neurol.* 222, 243-255. ISSN: 1090-2430 (Electronic); ISSN: 0014-4886 (Linking)

Ferrer I., Blanco R., Cutillas B. and Ambrosio S. (2000) Fas and Fas-L expression in Huntington's disease and Parkinson's disease. *Neuropathol. Appl. Neurobiol.* 26, 424-433. ISSN: 0305-1846 (Print); ISSN: 0305-1846 (Linking)

Frim D. M., Simpson J., Uhler T. A., Short M. P., Bossi S. R., Breakefield X. O. and Isacson O. (1993) Striatal degeneration induced by mitochondrial blockade is prevented by biologically delivered NGF. *J. Neurosci. Res.* 35, 452-458. ISSN: 0360-4012 (Print); ISSN: 0360-4012 (Linking)

Gafni J. and Ellerby L. M. (2002) Calpain activation in Huntington's disease. *J. Neurosci.* 22, 4842-4849. ISSN: 1529-2401 (Electronic); ISSN: 0270-6474 (Linking)

Gauthier L. R., Charrin B. C., Borrell-Pages M., Dompierre J. P., Rangone H., Cordelieres F. P., De M. J., MacDonald M. E., Lessmann V., Humbert S. and Saudou F. (2004) Huntingtin controls neurotrophic support and survival of neurons by enhancing BDNF vesicular transport along microtubules. *Cell* 118, 127-138. ISSN: 0092-8674 (Print); ISSN: 0092-8674 (Linking)

Gil J. M. and Rego A. C. (2008) Mechanisms of neurodegeneration in Huntington's disease. *Eur. J. Neurosci.* 27, 2803-2820. ISSN: 1460-9568 (Electronic); ISSN: 0953-816X (Linking)

Gines S., Seong I. S., Fossale E., Ivanova E., Trettel F., Gusella J. F., Wheeler V. C., Persichetti F. and MacDonald M. E. (2003) Specific progressive cAMP reduction implicates energy deficit in presymptomatic Huntington's disease knock-in mice. *Hum. Mol. Genet.* 12, 497-508. ISSN: 0964-6906 (Print); ISSN: 0964-6906 (Linking)

Goebel H. H., Heipertz R., Scholz W., Iqbal K. and Tellez-Nagel I. (1978) Juvenile Huntington chorea: clinical, ultrastructural, and biochemical studies. *Neurology* 28, 23-31. ISSN: 0028-3878 (Print); ISSN: 0028-3878 (Linking)

Graham R. K., Deng Y., Carroll J., Vaid K., Cowan C., Pouladi M. A., Metzler M., Bissada N., Wang L., Faull R. L., Gray M., Yang X. W., Raymond L. A. and Hayden M. R. (2010) Cleavage at the 586 amino acid caspase-6 site in mutant huntingtin influences caspase-6 activation in vivo. *J. Neurosci.* 30, 15019-15029. ISSN: 1529-2401 (Electronic); ISSN: 0270-6474 (Linking)

Griffith J. P., Kim J. L., Kim E. E., Sintchak M. D., Thomson J. A., Fitzgibbon M. J., Fleming M. A., Caron P. R., Hsiao K. and Navia M. A. (1995) X-ray structure of calcineurin inhibited by the immunophilin-immunosuppressant FKBP12-FK506 complex. *Cell* 82, 507-522. ISSN: 0092-8674 (Print); ISSN: 0092-8674 (Linking)

Gu M., Gash M. T., Mann V. M., Javoy-Agid F., Cooper J. M. and Schapira A. H. (1996) Mitochondrial defect in Huntington's disease caudate nucleus. *Ann. Neurol.* 39, 385-389. ISSN: 0364-5134 (Print); ISSN: 0364-5134 (Linking)

Hansson O., Petersen A., Leist M., Nicotera P., Castilho R. F. and Brundin P. (1999) Transgenic mice expressing a Huntington's disease mutation are resistant to quinolinic acid-induced striatal excitotoxicity. *Proc. Natl. Acad. Sci. U. S. A* 96, 8727-8732. ISSN: 0027-8424 (Print); ISSN: 0027-8424 (Linking)

Hernandez-Espinosa D. and Morton A. J. (2006) Calcineurin inhibitors cause an acceleration of the neurological phenotype in a mouse transgenic for the human Huntington's disease mutation. *Brain Res. Bull.* 69, 669-679. ISSN: 0361-9230 (Print); ISSN: 0361-9230 (Linking)

Hersch S. M., Gevorkian S., Marder K., Moskowitz C., Feigin A., Cox M., Como P., Zimmerman C., Lin M., Zhang L., Ulug A. M., Beal M. F., Matson W., Bogdanov M., Ebbel E., Zaleta A., Kaneko Y., Jenkins B., Hevelone N., Zhang H., Yu H., Schoenfeld D., Ferrante R. and Rosas H. D. (2006) Creatine in Huntington disease is safe, tolerable, bioavailable in brain and reduces serum 8OH2'dG. *Neurology* 66, 250-252. ISSN: 1526-632X (Electronic); ISSN: 0028-3878 (Linking)

Horton T. M., Graham B. H., Corral-Debrinski M., Shoffner J. M., Kaufman A. E., Beal M. F. and Wallace D. C. (1995) Marked increase in mitochondrial DNA deletion levels in the cerebral cortex of Huntington's disease patients. *Neurology* 45, 1879-1883. ISSN: 0028-3878 (Print); ISSN: 0028-3878 (Linking)

Huang E. J. and Reichardt L. F. (2003) Trk receptors: roles in neuronal signal transduction. *Annu. Rev. Biochem.* 72, 609-642. ISSN: 0066-4154 (Print); ISSN: 0066-4154 (Linking)

Illuzzi J. L., Vickers C. A. and Kmiec E. B. (2011) Modifications of p53 and the DNA Damage Response in Cells Expressing Mutant Form of the Protein Huntingtin. *J. Mol. Neurosci.* 45, 256-268. ISSN: 1559-1166 (Electronic); ISSN: 0895-8696 (Linking)

Impey S., Obrietan K., Wong S. T., Poser S., Yano S., Wayman G., Deloulme J. C., Chan G. and Storm D. R. (1998) Cross talk between ERK and PKA is required for Ca2+ stimulation of CREB-dependent transcription and ERK nuclear translocation. *Neuron* 21, 869-883. ISSN: 0896-6273 (Print); ISSN: 0896-6273 (Linking)

Jenkins B. G., Koroshetz W. J., Beal M. F. and Rosen B. R. (1993) Evidence for impairment of energy metabolism in vivo in Huntington's disease using localized 1H NMR spectroscopy. *Neurology* 43, 2689-2695. ISSN: 0028-3878 (Print); ISSN: 0028-3878 (Linking)

Jin Y. N. and Johnson G. V. (2010) The interrelationship between mitochondrial dysfunction and transcriptional dysregulation in Huntington disease. *J. Bioenerg. Biomembr.* 42, 199-205. ISSN: 1573-6881 (Electronic); ISSN: 0145-479X (Linking)

Kasraie S., Houshmand M., Banoei M. M., Ahari S. E., Panahi M. S., Shariati P., Bahar M. and Moin M. (2008) Investigation of tRNA(Leu/Lys) and ATPase 6 genes mutations in Huntington's disease. *Cell Mol. Neurobiol.* 28, 933-938. ISSN: 1573-6830 (Electronic); ISSN: 0272-4340 (Linking)

Kaufman B. A., Durisic N., Mativetsky J. M., Costantino S., Hancock M. A., Grutter P. and Shoubridge E. A. (2007) The mitochondrial transcription factor TFAM coordinates the assembly of multiple DNA molecules into nucleoid-like structures. *Mol. Biol. Cell* 18, 3225-3236. ISSN: 1059-1524 (Print): ISSN: 1059-1524 (Linking)

Kells A. P., Fong D. M., Dragunow M., During M. J., Young D. and Connor B. (2004) AAV-mediated gene delivery of BDNF or GDNF is neuroprotective in a model of Huntington disease. *Mol. Ther.* 9, 682-688. ISSN: 1525-0016 (Print); ISSN: 1525-0016 (Linking)

Kelly D. P. and Scarpulla R. C. (2004) Transcriptional regulatory circuits controlling mitochondrial biogenesis and function. *Genes Dev.* 18, 357-368. ISSN: 0890-9369 (Print); ISSN: 0890-9369 (Linking)

Kiechle T., Dedeoglu A., Kubilus J., Kowall N. W., Beal M. F., Friedlander R. M., Hersch S. M. and Ferrante R. J. (2002) Cytochrome C and caspase-9 expression in Huntington's disease. *Neuromolecular. Med.* 1, 183-195. ISSN: 1535-1084 (Print); ISSN: 1535-1084 (Linking)

Kim G. W., Gasche Y., Grzeschik S., Copin J. C., Maier C. M. and Chan P. H. (2003) Neurodegeneration in striatum induced by the mitochondrial toxin 3-nitropropionic acid: role of matrix metalloproteinase-9 in early blood-brain barrier disruption? *J. Neurosci.* 23, 8733-8742. ISSN: 1529-2401 (Electronic); ISSN: 0270-6474 (Linking)

Kim J., Moody J. P., Edgerly C. K., Bordiuk O. L., Cormier K., Smith K., Beal M. F. and Ferrante R. J. (2010) Mitochondrial loss, dysfunction and altered dynamics in Huntington's disease. *Hum. Mol. Genet.* 19, 3919-3935. ISSN: 1460-2083 (Electronic); ISSN: 0964-6906 (Linking)

Kim Y. J., Yi Y., Sapp E., Wang Y., Cuiffo B., Kegel K. B., Qin Z. H., Aronin N. and DiFiglia M. (2001) Caspase 3-cleaved N-terminal fragments of wild-type and mutant huntingtin are present in normal and Huntington's disease brains, associate with membranes, and undergo calpain-dependent proteolysis. *Proc. Natl. Acad. Sci. U. S. A* 98, 12784-12789. ISSN: 0027-8424 (Print); ISSN: 0027-8424 (Linking)

King M. P. and Attardi G. (1989) Human cells lacking mtDNA: repopulation with exogenous mitochondria by complementation. *Science* 246, 500-503. ISSN: 0036-8075 (Print); ISSN: 0036-8075 (Linking)

Klivenyi P., Ferrante R. J., Gardian G., Browne S., Chabrier P. E. and Beal M. F. (2003) Increased survival and neuroprotective effects of BN82451 in a transgenic mouse model of Huntington's disease. *J. Neurochem.* 86, 267-272. ISSN: 0022-3042 (Print); ISSN: 0022-3042 (Linking)

Koroshetz W. J., Jenkins B. G., Rosen B. R. and Beal M. F. (1997) Energy metabolism defects in Huntington's disease and effects of coenzyme Q10. *Ann. Neurol.* 41, 160-165. ISSN: 0364-5134 (Print); ISSN: 0364-5134 (Linking)

Kroemer G. and Reed J. C. (2000) Mitochondrial control of cell death. *Nat. Med.* 6, 513-519. ISSN: 1078-8956 (Print); ISSN: 1078-8956 (Linking)

Kuhl D. E., Phelps M. E., Markham C. H., Metter E. J., Riege W. H. and Winter J. (1982) Cerebral metabolism and atrophy in Huntington's disease determined by 18FDG and computed tomographic scan. *Ann. Neurol.* 12, 425-434. ISSN: 0364-5134 (Print); ISSN: 0364-5134 (Linking)

Kumar P. and Kumar A. (2009) Neuroprotective effect of cyclosporine and FK506 against 3-nitropropionic acid induced cognitive dysfunction and glutathione redox in rat: possible role of nitric oxide. *Neurosci. Res.* 63, 302-314. ISSN: 0168-0102 (Print); ISSN: 0168-0102 (Linking)

Kuwert T., Lange H. W., Langen K. J., Herzog H., Aulich A. and Feinendegen L. E. (1990) Cortical and subcortical glucose consumption measured by PET in patients with Huntington's disease. *Brain* 113 (Pt 5), 1405-1423. ISSN: 0006-8950 (Print); ISSN: 0006-8950 (Linking)

Lee J., Kim C. H., Simon D. K., Aminova L. R., Andreyev A. Y., Kushnareva Y. E., Murphy A. N., Lonze B. E., Kim K. S., Ginty D. D., Ferrante R. J., Ryu H. and Ratan R. R. (2005) Mitochondrial cyclic AMP response element-binding protein (CREB) mediates mitochondrial gene expression and neuronal survival. *J. Biol. Chem.* 280, 40398-40401. ISSN: 0021-9258 (Print); ISSN: 0021-9258 (Linking)

Ley R., Balmanno K., Hadfield K., Weston C. and Cook S. J. (2003) Activation of the ERK1/2 signaling pathway promotes phosphorylation and proteasome-dependent degradation of the BH3-only protein, Bim. *J. Biol. Chem.* 278, 18811-18816. ISSN: 0021-9258 (Print); ISSN: 0021-9258 (Linking)

Li S. H., Cheng A. L., Zhou H., Lam S., Rao M., Li H. and Li X. J. (2002) Interaction of Huntington disease protein with transcriptional activator Sp1. *Mol. Cell Biol.* 22, 1277-1287. ISSN: 0270-7306 (Print); ISSN: 0270-7306 (Linking)

Lin J., Wu P. H., Tarr P. T., Lindenberg K. S., St-Pierre J., Zhang C. Y., Mootha V. K., Jager S., Vianna C. R., Reznick R. M., Cui L., Manieri M., Donovan M. X., Wu Z., Cooper M. P., Fan M. C., Rohas L. M., Zavacki A. M., Cinti S., Shulman G. I., Lowell B. B., Krainc D. and Spiegelman B. M. (2004) Defects in adaptive energy metabolism with CNS-linked hyperactivity in PGC-1alpha null mice. *Cell* 119, 121-135. ISSN: 0092-8674 (Print); ISSN: 0092-8674 (Linking)

Lin J., Yang R., Tarr P. T., Wu P. H., Handschin C., Li S., Yang W., Pei L., Uldry M., Tontonoz P., Newgard C. B. and Spiegelman B. M. (2005) Hyperlipidemic effects of dietary saturated fats mediated through PGC-1beta coactivation of SREBP. *Cell* 120, 261-273. ISSN: 0092-8674 (Print); ISSN: 0092-8674 (Linking)

Lodi R., Schapira A. H., Manners D., Styles P., Wood N. W., Taylor D. J. and Warner T. T. (2000) Abnormal in vivo skeletal muscle energy metabolism in Huntington's disease and dentatorubropallidoluysian atrophy. *Ann. Neurol.* 48, 72-76. ISSN: 0364-5134 (Print); ISSN: 0364-5134 (Linking)

Luciano F., Jacquel A., Colosetti P., Herrant M., Cagnol S., Pages G. and Auberger P. (2003) Phosphorylation of Bim-EL by Erk1/2 on serine 69 promotes its degradation via the proteasome pathway and regulates its proapoptotic function. *Oncogene* 22, 6785-6793. ISSN: 0950-9232 (Print); ISSN: 0950-9232 (Linking)

Luthi-Carter R., Hanson S. A., Strand A. D., Bergstrom D. A., Chun W., Peters N. L., Woods A. M., Chan E. Y., Kooperberg C., Krainc D., Young A. B., Tapscott S. J. and Olson J. M. (2002) Dysregulation of gene expression in the R6/2 model of polyglutamine disease: parallel changes in muscle and brain. *Hum. Mol. Genet.* 11, 1911-1926. ISSN: 0964-6906 (Print); ISSN: 0964-6906 (Linking)

Martin E., Betuing S., Pages C., Cambon K., Auregan G., Deglon N., Roze E. and Caboche J. (2011) Mitogen- and stress-activated protein kinase 1-induced neuroprotection in Huntington's disease: role on chromatin remodeling at the PGC-1-alpha promoter. *Hum. Mol. Genet.* 20, 2422-2434. ISSN: 1460-2083 (Electronic); ISSN: 0964-6906 (Linking)

Masters S. C., Yang H., Datta S. R., Greenberg M. E. and Fu H. (2001) 14-3-3 inhibits Bad-induced cell death through interaction with serine-136. *Mol. Pharmacol.* 60, 1325-1331. ISSN: 0026-895X (Print); ISSN: 0026-895X (Linking)

Matthews R. P., Guthrie C. R., Wailes L. M., Zhao X., Means A. R. and McKnight G. S. (1994) Calcium/calmodulin-dependent protein kinase types II and IV differentially regulate CREB-dependent gene expression. *Mol. Cell Biol.* 14, 6107-6116. ISSN: 0270-7306 (Print); ISSN: 0270-7306 (Linking)

Mayr B. and Montminy M. (2001) Transcriptional regulation by the phosphorylation-dependent factor CREB. *Nat. Rev. Mol. Cell Biol.* 2, 599-609. ISSN: 1471-0072 (Print); ISSN: 1471-0072 (Linking)

Mochel F. and Haller R. G. (2011) Energy deficit in Huntington disease: why it matters. *J. Clin. Invest* 121, 493-499. ISSN: 1932-6203 (Electronic); ISSN: 1932-6203 (Linking)

Morimoto N., Nagano I., Deguchi K., Murakami T., Fushimi S., Shoji M. and Abe K. (2004) Leber hereditary optic neuropathy with chorea and dementia resembling Huntington disease. *Neurology* 63, 2451-2452. ISSN: 1526-632X (Electronic); ISSN: 0028-3878 (Linking)

Napolitano M., Centonze D., Gubellini P., Rossi S., Spiezia S., Bernardi G., Gulino A. and Calabresi P. (2004) Inhibition of mitochondrial complex II alters striatal expression of genes involved in glutamatergic and dopaminergic signaling: possible implications for Huntington's disease. *Neurobiol. Dis.* 15, 407-414. ISSN: 0969-9961 (Print); ISSN: 0969-9961 (Linking)

Nucifora F. C., Jr., Sasaki M., Peters M. F., Huang H., Cooper J. K., Yamada M., Takahashi H., Tsuji S., Troncoso J., Dawson V. L., Dawson T. M. and Ross C. A. (2001) Interference by huntingtin and atrophin-1 with cbp-mediated transcription leading to cellular toxicity. *Science* 291, 2423-2428. ISSN: 0036-8075 (Print); ISSN: 0036-8075 (Linking)

Olah J., Klivenyi P., Gardian G., Vecsei L., Orosz F., Kovacs G. G., Westerhoff H. V. and Ovadi J. (2008) Increased glucose metabolism and ATP level in brain tissue of Huntington's disease transgenic mice. *FEBS J.* 275, 4740-4755. ISSN: 1742-464X (Print); ISSN: 1742-464X (Linking)

Oliveira J. M. (2010) Nature and cause of mitochondrial dysfunction in Huntington's disease: focusing on huntingtin and the striatum. *J. Neurochem.* 114, 1-12. ISSN: 1471-4159 (Electronic); ISSN: 0022-3042 (Linking)

Oliveira J. M., Chen S., Almeida S., Riley R., Goncalves J., Oliveira C. R., Hayden M. R., Nicholls D. G., Ellerby L. M. and Rego A. C. (2006) Mitochondrial-dependent Ca2+ handling in Huntington's disease striatal cells: effect of histone deacetylase inhibitors. *J. Neurosci.* 26, 11174-11186. ISSN: 1529-2401 (Electronic); ISSN: 0270-6474 (Linking)

Oliveira J. M. and Goncalves J. (2009) In situ mitochondrial Ca2+ buffering differences of intact neurons and astrocytes from cortex and striatum. *J. Biol. Chem.* 284, 5010-5020. ISSN: 0021-9258 (Print); ISSN: 0021-9258 (Linking)

Oliveira J. M., Jekabsons M. B., Chen S., Lin A., Rego A. C., Goncalves J., Ellerby L. M. and Nicholls D. G. (2007) Mitochondrial dysfunction in Huntington's disease: the bioenergetics of isolated and in situ mitochondria from transgenic mice. *J. Neurochem.* 101, 241-249. ISSN: 0022-3042 (Print); ISSN: 0022-3042 (Linking)

Ona V. O., Li M., Vonsattel J. P., Andrews L. J., Khan S. Q., Chung W. M., Frey A. S., Menon A. S., Li X. J., Stieg P. E., Yuan J., Penney J. B., Young A. B., Cha J. H. and Friedlander R. M. (1999) Inhibition of caspase-1 slows disease progression in a mouse model of Huntington's disease. *Nature* 399, 263-267. ISSN: 0028-0836 (Print); ISSN: 0028-0836 (Linking)

Orr A. L., Li S., Wang C. E., Li H., Wang J., Rong J., Xu X., Mastroberardino P. G., Greenamyre J. T. and Li X. J. (2008) N-terminal mutant huntingtin associates with mitochondria and impairs mitochondrial trafficking. *J. Neurosci.* 28, 2783-2792. ISSN: 1529-2401 (Electronic); ISSN: 0270-6474 (Linking)

Pandey M., Mohanakumar K. P. and Usha R. (2010) Mitochondrial functional alterations in relation to pathophysiology of Huntington's disease. *J. Bioenerg. Biomembr.* 42, 217-226. ISSN: 1573-6881 (Electronic); ISSN: 0145-479X (Linking)

Pang Z. and Geddes J. W. (1997) Mechanisms of cell death induced by the mitochondrial toxin 3-nitropropionic acid: acute excitotoxic necrosis and delayed apoptosis. *J. Neurosci.* 17, 3064-3073. ISSN: 0270-6474 (Print); ISSN: 0270-6474 (Linking)

Panov A. V., Gutekunst C. A., Leavitt B. R., Hayden M. R., Burke J. R., Strittmatter W. J. and Greenamyre J. T. (2002) Early mitochondrial calcium defects in Huntington's disease are a direct effect of polyglutamines. *Nat. Neurosci.* 5, 731-736. ISSN: 1097-6256 (Print); ISSN: 1097-6256 (Linking)

Pardo R., Colin E., Regulier E., Aebischer P., Deglon N., Humbert S. and Saudou F. (2006) Inhibition of calcineurin by FK506 protects against polyglutamine-huntingtin toxicity through an increase of huntingtin phosphorylation at S421. *J. Neurosci.* 26, 1635-1645. ISSN: 1529-2401 (Electronic); ISSN: 0270-6474 (Linking)

Parker W. D., Jr., Boyson S. J., Luder A. S. and Parks J. K. (1990) Evidence for a defect in NADH: ubiquinone oxidoreductase (complex I) in Huntington's disease. *Neurology* 40, 1231-1234. ISSN: 0028-3878 (Print); ISSN: 0028-3878 (Linking)

Perez-Navarro E., Canudas A. M., Akerund P., Alberch J. and Arenas E. (2000) Brain-derived neurotrophic factor, neurotrophin-3, and neurotrophin-4/5 prevent the death of striatal projection neurons in a rodent model of Huntington's disease. *J. Neurochem.* 75, 2190-2199. ISSN: 0022-3042 (Print); ISSN: 0022-3042 (Linking)

Perez-Severiano F., Rios C. and Segovia J. (2000) Striatal oxidative damage parallels the expression of a neurological phenotype in mice transgenic for the mutation of Huntington's disease. *Brain Res.* 862, 234-237. ISSN: 0006-8993 (Print); ISSN: 0006-8993 (Linking)

Perez-Severiano F., Santamaria A., Pedraza-Chaverri J., Medina-Campos O. N., Rios C. and Segovia J. (2004) Increased formation of reactive oxygen species, but no changes in glutathione peroxidase activity, in striata of mice transgenic for the Huntington's disease mutation. *Neurochem. Res.* 29, 729-733. ISSN: 0364-3190 (Print); ISSN: 0364-3190 (Linking)

Perkinton M. S., Ip J. K., Wood G. L., Crossthwaite A. J. and Williams R. J. (2002) Phosphatidylinositol 3-kinase is a central mediator of NMDA receptor signalling to MAP kinase (Erk1/2), Akt/PKB and CREB in striatal neurones. *J. Neurochem.* 80, 239-254. ISSN: 0022-3042 (Print); ISSN: 0022-3042 (Linking)

Perluigi M., Poon H. F., Maragos W., Pierce W. M., Klein J. B., Calabrese V., Cini C., De M. C. and Butterfield D. A. (2005) Proteomic analysis of protein expression and oxidative modification in r6/2 transgenic mice: a model of Huntington disease. *Mol. Cell Proteomics.* 4, 1849-1861. ISSN: 1535-9476 (Print); ISSN: 1535-9476 (Linking)

Pineda J. R., Pardo R., Zala D., Yu H., Humbert S. and Saudou F. (2009) Genetic and pharmacological inhibition of calcineurin corrects the BDNF transport defect in Huntington's disease. *Mol. Brain* 2, 33. ISSN: 1756-6606 (Electronic); ISSN: 1756-6606 (Linking)

Polidori M. C., Mecocci P., Browne S. E., Senin U. and Beal M. F. (1999) Oxidative damage to mitochondrial DNA in Huntington's disease parietal cortex. *Neurosci. Lett.* 272, 53-56. ISSN: 0304-3940 (Print); ISSN: 0304-3940 (Linking)

Powers W. J., Haas R. H., Le T., Videen T. O., Hershey T., McGee-Minnich L. and Perlmutter J. S. (2007a) Normal platelet mitochondrial complex I activity in Huntington's disease. *Neurobiol. Dis.* 27, 99-101. ISSN: 0969-9961 (Print); ISSN: 0969-9961 (Linking)

Powers W. J., Videen T. O., Markham J., McGee-Minnich L., Antenor-Dorsey J. V., Hershey T. and Perlmutter J. S. (2007b) Selective defect of in vivo glycolysis in early Huntington's disease striatum. *Proc. Natl. Acad. Sci. U. S. A* 104, 2945-2949. ISSN: 0027-8424 (Print); ISSN: 0027-8424 (Linking)

Pugazhenthi S., Nesterova A., Sable C., Heidenreich K. A., Boxer L. M., Heasley L. E. and Reusch J. E. (2000) Akt/protein kinase B up-regulates Bcl-2 expression through cAMP-response element-binding protein. *J. Biol. Chem.* 275, 10761-10766. ISSN: 0021-9258 (Print); ISSN: 0021-9258 (Linking)

Quintanilla R. A. and Johnson G. V. (2009) Role of mitochondrial dysfunction in the pathogenesis of Huntington's disease. *Brain Res. Bull.* 80, 242-247. ISSN: 1873-2747 (Electronic); ISSN: 0361-9230 (Linking)

Rigamonti D., Bauer J. H., De-Fraja C., Conti L., Sipione S., Sciorati C., Clementi E., Hackam A., Hayden M. R., Li Y., Cooper J. K., Ross C. A., Govoni S., Vincenz C. and Cattaneo E. (2000) Wild-type huntingtin protects from apoptosis upstream of caspase-3. *J. Neurosci.* 20, 3705-3713. ISSN: 1529-2401 (Electronic); ISSN: 0270-6474 (Linking)

Rigamonti D., Sipione S., Goffredo D., Zuccato C., Fossale E. and Cattaneo E. (2001) Huntingtin's neuroprotective activity occurs via inhibition of procaspase-9 processing. *J. Biol. Chem.* 276, 14545-14548. ISSN: 0021-9258 (Print); ISSN: 0021-9258 (Linking)

Rosenstock T. R., de Brito O. M., Lombardi V., Louros S., Ribeiro M., Almeida S., Ferreira I. L., Oliveira C. R. and Rego A. C. (2011) FK506 ameliorates cell death features in Huntington's disease striatal cell models. *Neurochem. Int.* ISSN: 1872-9754 (Electronic); ISSN: 0197-0186 (Linking)

Rosenstock T. R., Duarte A. I. and Rego A. C. (2010) Mitochondrial-associated metabolic changes and neurodegeneration in Huntington's disease - from clinical features to the bench. *Curr. Drug Targets.* 11, 1218-1236. ISSN: 1873-5592 (Electronic); ISSN: 1389-4501 (Linking)

Rouaux C., Jokic N., Mbebi C., Boutillier S., Loeffler J. P. and Boutillier A. L. (2003) Critical loss of CBP/p300 histone acetylase activity by caspase-6 during neurodegeneration. *EMBO J.* 22, 6537-6549. ISSN: 0261-4189 (Print); ISSN: 0261-4189 (Linking)

Ryu J. K., Kim J., Cho S. J., Hatori K., Nagai A., Choi H. B., Lee M. C., McLarnon J. G. and Kim S. U. (2004) Proactive transplantation of human neural stem cells prevents degeneration of striatal neurons in a rat model of Huntington disease. *Neurobiol. Dis.* 16, 68-77. ISSN: 0969-9961 (Print); ISSN: 0969-9961 (Linking)

Saft C., Zange J., Andrich J., Muller K., Lindenberg K., Landwehrmeyer B., Vorgerd M., Kraus P. H., Przuntek H. and Schols L. (2005) Mitochondrial impairment in patients and asymptomatic mutation carriers of Huntington's disease. *Mov Disord.* 20, 674-679. ISSN: 0885-3185 (Print); ISSN: 0885-3185 (Linking)

Saha R. N., Liu X. and Pahan K. (2006) Up-regulation of BDNF in astrocytes by TNF-alpha: a case for the neuroprotective role of cytokine. *J. Neuroimmune. Pharmacol.* 1, 212-222. ISSN: 1557-1904 (Electronic); ISSN: 1557-1890 (Linking)

Sanchez I., Xu C. J., Juo P., Kakizaka A., Blenis J. and Yuan J. (1999) Caspase-8 is required for cell death induced by expanded polyglutamine repeats. *Neuron* 22, 623-633. ISSN: 0896-6273 (Print); ISSN: 0896-6273 (Linking)

Santamaria A., Perez-Severiano F., Rodriguez-Martinez E., Maldonado P. D., Pedraza-Chaverri J., Rios C. and Segovia J. (2001) Comparative analysis of superoxide dismutase activity between acute pharmacological models and a transgenic mouse model of Huntington's disease. *Neurochem. Res.* 26, 419-424. ISSN: 0364-3190 (Print); ISSN: 0364-3190 (Linking)

Saudou F., Finkbeiner S., Devys D. and Greenberg M. E. (1998) Huntingtin acts in the nucleus to induce apoptosis but death does not correlate with the formation of intranuclear inclusions. *Cell* 95, 55-66. ISSN: 0092-8674 (Print); ISSN: 0092-8674 (Linking)

Sawa A., Wiegand G. W., Cooper J., Margolis R. L., Sharp A. H., Lawler J. F., Jr., Greenamyre J. T., Snyder S. H. and Ross C. A. (1999) Increased apoptosis of Huntington disease lymphoblasts associated with repeat length-dependent mitochondrial depolarization. *Nat. Med.* 5, 1194-1198. ISSN: 1078-8956 (Print); ISSN: 1078-8956 (Linking)

Scarpulla R. C. (2002) Nuclear activators and coactivators in mammalian mitochondrial biogenesis. *Biochim. Biophys. Acta* 1576, 1-14. ISSN: 0006-3002 (Print); ISSN: 0006-3002 (Linking)

Scarpulla R. C. (2011) Metabolic control of mitochondrial biogenesis through the PGC-1 family regulatory network. *Biochim. Biophys. Acta* 1813, 1269-1278. ISSN: 0006-3002 (Print); ISSN: 0006-3002 (Linking)

Scheid M. P., Schubert K. M. and Duronio V. (1999) Regulation of bad phosphorylation and association with Bcl-x(L) by the MAPK/Erk kinase. *J. Biol. Chem.* 274, 31108-31113. ISSN: 0021-9258 (Print); ISSN: 0021-9258 (Linking)

Shih A. Y., Imbeault S., Barakauskas V., Erb H., Jiang L., Li P. and Murphy T. H. (2005) Induction of the Nrf2-driven antioxidant response confers neuroprotection during mitochondrial stress in vivo. *J. Biol. Chem.* 280, 22925-22936. ISSN: 0021-9258 (Print); ISSN: 0021-9258 (Linking)

Shimohata T., Nakajima T., Yamada M., Uchida C., Onodera O., Naruse S., Kimura T., Koide R., Nozaki K., Sano Y., Ishiguro H., Sakoe K., Ooshima T., Sato A., Ikeuchi T., Oyake M., Sato T., Aoyagi Y., Hozumi I., Nagatsu T., Takiyama Y., Nishizawa M., Goto J., Kanazawa I., Davidson I., Tanese N., Takahashi H. and Tsuji S. (2000) Expanded polyglutamine stretches interact with TAFII130, interfering with CREB-dependent transcription. *Nat. Genet.* 26, 29-36. ISSN: 1061-4036 (Print); ISSN: 1061-4036 (Linking)

Shirendeb U., Reddy A. P., Manczak M., Calkins M. J., Mao P., Tagle D. A. and Reddy P. H. (2011) Abnormal mitochondrial dynamics, mitochondrial loss and mutant huntingtin oligomers in Huntington's disease: implications for selective neuronal damage. *Hum. Mol. Genet.* 20, 1438-1455. ISSN: 1460-2083 (Electronic); ISSN: 0964-6906 (Linking)

Solans A., Zambrano A., Rodriguez M. and Barrientos A. (2006) Cytotoxicity of a mutant huntingtin fragment in yeast involves early alterations in mitochondrial OXPHOS complexes II and III. *Hum. Mol. Genet.* 15, 3063-3081. ISSN: 0964-6906 (Print); ISSN: 0964-6906 (Linking)

Song W., Chen J., Petrilli A., Liot G., Klinglmayr E., Zhou Y., Poquiz P., Tjong J., Pouladi M. A., Hayden M. R., Masliah E., Ellisman M., Rouiller I., Schwarzenbacher R., Bossy B., Perkins G. and Bossy-Wetzel E. (2011) Mutant huntingtin binds the mitochondrial fission GTPase dynamin-related protein-1 and increases its enzymatic activity. *Nat. Med.* 17, 377-382. ISSN: 1546-170X (Electronic); ISSN: 1078-8956 (Linking)

Sorbi S., Bird E. D. and Blass J. P. (1983) Decreased pyruvate dehydrogenase complex activity in Huntington and Alzheimer brain. *Ann. Neurol.* 13, 72-78. ISSN: 0364-5134 (Print); ISSN: 0364-5134 (Linking)

Sorolla M. A., Rodriguez-Colman M. J., Tamarit J., Ortega Z., Lucas J. J., Ferrer I., Ros J. and Cabiscol E. (2010) Protein oxidation in Huntington disease affects energy production and vitamin B6 metabolism. *Free Radic. Biol. Med.* 49, 612-621. ISSN: 1873-4596 (Electronic); ISSN: 0891-5849 (Linking)

Squitieri F., Maglione V., Orobello S. and Fornai F. (2011) Genotype-, aging-dependent abnormal caspase activity in Huntington disease blood cells. *J. Neural Transm.* ISSN: 1435-1463 (Electronic); ISSN: 0300-9564 (Linking)

St-Pierre J., Drori S., Uldry M., Silvaggi J. M., Rhee J., Jager S., Handschin C., Zheng K., Lin J., Yang W., Simon D. K., Bachoo R. and Spiegelman B. M. (2006) Suppression of reactive oxygen species and neurodegeneration by the PGC-1 transcriptional coactivators. *Cell* 127, 397-408. ISSN: 0092-8674 (Print); ISSN: 0092-8674 (Linking)

Stahl W. L. and Swanson P. D. (1974) Biochemical abnormalities in Huntington's chorea brains. *Neurology* 24, 813-819. ISSN: 0028-3878 (Print); ISSN: 0028-3878 (Linking)

Steffan J. S., Bodai L., Pallos J., Poelman M., McCampbell A., Apostol B. L., Kazantsev A., Schmidt E., Zhu Y. Z., Greenwald M., Kurokawa R., Housman D. E., Jackson G. R., Marsh J. L. and Thompson L. M. (2001) Histone deacetylase inhibitors arrest polyglutamine-dependent neurodegeneration in Drosophila. *Nature* 413, 739-743. ISSN: 0028-0836 (Print); ISSN: 0028-0836 (Linking)

Steffan J. S., Kazantsev A., Spasic-Boskovic O., Greenwald M., Zhu Y. Z., Gohler H., Wanker E. E., Bates G. P., Housman D. E. and Thompson L. M. (2000) The Huntington's disease protein interacts with p53 and CREB-binding protein and represses transcription. *Proc. Natl. Acad. Sci. U. S. A* 97, 6763-6768. ISSN: 0027-8424 (Print); ISSN: 0027-8424 (Linking)

Stoy N., Mackay G. M., Forrest C. M., Christofides J., Egerton M., Stone T. W. and Darlington L. G. (2005) Tryptophan metabolism and oxidative stress in patients with Huntington's disease. *J. Neurochem.* 93, 611-623. ISSN: 0022-3042 (Print); ISSN: 0022-3042 (Linking)

Strand A. D., Baquet Z. C., Aragaki A. K., Holmans P., Yang L., Cleren C., Beal M. F., Jones L., Kooperberg C., Olson J. M. and Jones K. R. (2007) Expression profiling of Huntington's disease models suggests that brain-derived neurotrophic factor depletion plays a major role in striatal degeneration. *J. Neurosci.* 27, 11758-11768. ISSN: 1529-2401 (Electronic); ISSN: 0270-6474 (Linking)

Sugars K. L. and Rubinsztein D. C. (2003) Transcriptional abnormalities in Huntington disease. *Trends Genet.* 19, 233-238. ISSN: 0168-9525 (Print); ISSN: 0168-9525 (Linking)

Swerdlow R. H., Parks J. K., Cassarino D. S., Shilling A. T., Bennett J. P., Jr., Harrison M. B. and Parker W. D., Jr. (1999) Characterization of cybrid cell lines containing mtDNA from Huntington's disease patients. *Biochem. Biophys. Res. Commun.* 261, 701-704. ISSN: 0006-291X (Print); ISSN: 0006-291X (Linking)

Tabrizi S. J., Workman J., Hart P. E., Mangiarini L., Mahal A., Bates G., Cooper J. M. and Schapira A. H. (2000) Mitochondrial dysfunction and free radical damage in the Huntington R6/2 transgenic mouse. *Ann. Neurol.* 47, 80-86. ISSN: 0364-5134 (Print); ISSN: 0364-5134 (Linking)

Taherzadeh-Fard E., Saft C., Akkad D. A., Wieczorek S., Haghikia A., Chan A., Epplen J. T. and Arning L. (2011) PGC-1alpha downstream transcription factors NRF-1 and TFAM are genetic modifiers of Huntington disease. *Mol. Neurodegener.* 6, 32. ISSN: 1750-1326 (Electronic); ISSN: 1750-1326 (Linking)

Tellez-Nagel I., Johnson A. B. and Terry R. D. (1974) Studies on brain biopsies of patients with Huntington's chorea. *J. Neuropathol. Exp. Neurol.* 33, 308-332. ISSN: 0022-3069 (Print); ISSN: 0022-3069 (Linking)

Trushina E., Dyer R. B., Badger J. D., Ure D., Eide L., Tran D. D., Vrieze B. T., Legendre-Guillemin V., McPherson P. S., Mandavilli B. S., Van H. B., Zeitlin S., McNiven M., Aebersold R., Hayden M., Parisi J. E., Seeberg E., Dragatsis I., Doyle K., Bender A., Chacko C. and McMurray C. T. (2004) Mutant huntingtin impairs axonal trafficking in mammalian neurons in vivo and in vitro. *Mol. Cell Biol.* 24, 8195-8209. ISSN: 0270-7306 (Print); ISSN: 0270-7306 (Linking)

Turner C., Cooper J. M. and Schapira A. H. (2007) Clinical correlates of mitochondrial function in Huntington's disease muscle. *Mov Disord.* 22, 1715-1721. ISSN: 0885-3185 (Print); ISSN: 0885-3185 (Linking)

Vis J. C., Schipper E., de Boer-van Huizen RT, Verbeek M. M., de Waal R. M., Wesseling P., ten Donkelaar H. J. and Kremer B. (2005) Expression pattern of apoptosis-related markers in Huntington's disease. *Acta Neuropathol.* 109, 321-328. ISSN: 0001-6322 (Print); ISSN: 0001-6322 (Linking)

Wang H., Lim P. J., Karbowski M. and Monteiro M. J. (2009) Effects of overexpression of huntingtin proteins on mitochondrial integrity. *Hum. Mol. Genet.* 18, 737-752. ISSN: 1460-2083 (Electronic); ISSN: 0964-6906 (Linking)

Wang H. G., Pathan N., Ethell I. M., Krajewski S., Yamaguchi Y., Shibasaki F., McKeon F., Bobo T., Franke T. F. and Reed J. C. (1999) Ca2+-induced apoptosis through calcineurin dephosphorylation of BAD. *Science* 284, 339-343. ISSN: 0036-8075 (Print); ISSN: 0036-8075 (Linking)

Wellington C. L., Ellerby L. M., Hackam A. S., Margolis R. L., Trifiro M. A., Singaraja R., McCutcheon K., Salvesen G. S., Propp S. S., Bromm M., Rowland K. J., Zhang T., Rasper D., Roy S., Thornberry N., Pinsky L., Kakizuka A., Ross C. A., Nicholson D. W., Bredesen D. E. and Hayden M. R. (1998) Caspase cleavage of gene products associated with triplet expansion disorders generates truncated fragments containing the polyglutamine tract. *J. Biol. Chem.* 273, 9158-9167. ISSN: 0021-9258 (Print); ISSN: 0021-9258 (Linking)

Weydt P., Pineda V. V., Torrence A. E., Libby R. T., Satterfield T. F., Lazarowski E. R., Gilbert M. L., Morton G. J., Bammler T. K., Strand A. D., Cui L., Beyer R. P., Easley C. N., Smith A. C., Krainc D., Luquet S., Sweet I. R., Schwartz M. W. and La Spada A. R. (2006) Thermoregulatory and metabolic defects in Huntington's disease transgenic mice implicate PGC-1alpha in Huntington's disease neurodegeneration. *Cell Metab* 4, 349-362. ISSN: 1550-4131 (Print); ISSN: 1550-4131 (Linking)

Weydt P., Soyal S. M., Gellera C., Didonato S., Weidinger C., Oberkofler H., Landwehrmeyer G. B. and Patsch W. (2009) The gene coding for PGC-1alpha modifies age at onset in Huntington's Disease. *Mol. Neurodegener.* 4, 3.ISSN: 1750-1326 (Electronic); ISSN: 1750-1326 (Linking)

Xifro X., Garcia-Martinez J. M., Del T. D., Alberch J. and Perez-Navarro E. (2008) Calcineurin is involved in the early activation of NMDA-mediated cell death in mutant huntingtin knock-in striatal cells. *J. Neurochem.* 105, 1596-1612. ISSN: 1471-4159 (Electronic); ISSN: 0022-3042 (Linking)

Xifro X., Giralt A., Saavedra A., Garcia-Martinez J. M., Diaz-Hernandez M., Lucas J. J., Alberch J. and Perez-Navarro E. (2009) Reduced calcineurin protein levels and activity in exon-1 mouse models of Huntington's disease: role in excitotoxicity. *Neurobiol. Dis.* 36, 461-469. ISSN: 1095-953X (Electronic); ISSN: 0969-9961 (Linking)

Yamamoto K. K., Gonzalez G. A., Biggs W. H., III and Montminy M. R. (1988) Phosphorylation-induced binding and transcriptional efficacy of nuclear factor CREB. *Nature* 334, 494-498. ISSN: 0028-0836 (Print); ISSN: 0028-0836 (Linking)

Zhai W., Jeong H., Cui L., Krainc D. and Tjian R. (2005) In vitro analysis of huntingtin-mediated transcriptional repression reveals multiple transcription factor targets. *Cell* 123, 1241-1253. ISSN: 0092-8674 (Print); ISSN: 0092-8674 (Linking)

Zhang X. D., Wang Y., Wang Y., Zhang X., Han R., Wu J. C., Liang Z. Q., Gu Z. L., Han F., Fukunaga K. and Qin Z. H. (2009a) p53 mediates mitochondria dysfunction-triggered autophagy activation and cell death in rat striatum. *Autophagy.* 5, 339-350. ISSN: 1554-8635 (Electronic); ISSN: 1554-8627 (Linking)

Zhang X. D., Wang Y., Wu J. C., Lin F., Han R., Han F., Fukunaga K. and Qin Z. H. (2009b) Down-regulation of Bcl-2 enhances autophagy activation and cell death induced by mitochondrial dysfunction in rat striatum. *J. Neurosci. Res.* 87, 3600-3610. ISSN: 1097-4547 (Electronic); ISSN: 0360-4012 (Linking)

Zuccato C., Ciammola A., Rigamonti D., Leavitt B. R., Goffredo D., Conti L., MacDonald M. E., Friedlander R. M., Silani V., Hayden M. R., Timmusk T., Sipione S. and Cattaneo E. (2001) Loss of huntingtin-mediated BDNF gene transcription in Huntington's disease. *Science* 293, 493-498. ISSN: 0036-8075 (Print); ISSN: 0036-8075 (Linking)

Zuccato C., Liber D., Ramos C., Tarditi A., Rigamonti D., Tartari M., Valenza M. and Cattaneo E. (2005) Progressive loss of BDNF in a mouse model of Huntington's disease and rescue by BDNF delivery. *Pharmacol. Res.* 52, 133-139. ISSN: 1043-6618 (Print); ISSN: 1043-6618 (Linking)

Zuccato C., Tartari M., Crotti A., Goffredo D., Valenza M., Conti L., Cataudella T., Leavitt B. R., Hayden M. R., Timmusk T., Rigamonti D. and Cattaneo E. (2003) Huntingtin interacts with REST/NRSF to modulate the transcription of NRSE-controlled neuronal genes. *Nat. Genet.* 35, 76-83. ISSN: 1061-4036 (Print); ISSN: 1061-4036 (Linking)

Part 2

Therapeutic Targets in Huntington's Disease

5

Cellular Therapies for Huntington's Disease

C. M. Kelly and A. E. Rosser

Brain Repair Group, School of Biosciences, Cardiff
UK

1. Introduction

Huntington's Disease is an autosomal dominant neurodegenerative disorder with an incidence of 5 to 10 per 100,000 in the Caucasian community. The clinical symptoms of HD are chorea, parkinsonism, dystonia, intellectual impairment, emotional and psychiatric disturbances as well as dysphasia, dysarthria, rigidity and gait disturbances. The depression that is associated with HD is thought to be secondary to the motor abnormalities, given that it develops prior to the appearance of any other symptoms (Folstein, 1989). To date symptomatic treatments are the only available treatments for HD as there are no disease-modifying therapies.

The pathology of HD is characterised by a loss of medium spiny projection neurons in the head of the caudate and putamen of the striatum (Ross and Margolis, 2001) which form part of a complex circuitry comprising parallel feedback loops involving discrete areas of cortex and subcortical structures. As a result of the neuronal loss there is eventually significant atrophy of these structures, with a compensatory expansion of the lateral ventricles. With disease progression the overall brain weight decreases by 25-30%, which reflects additional atrophy of other brain areas such as the cerebral cortex. Gliosis is also seen in the pathology alongside the marked neuronal loss. Neuronal loss in the cortex is found to be layer specific with the greatest loss seen in layer VI and significant amounts of loss seen in layers III and V (Reddy et al., 1999, Ross and Margolis, 2001). The relatively focal loss of medium spiny GABAergic projection neurons in the striatum presents an opportunity to explore neural transplantation as a strategy for cell replacement and circuit reconstruction. For neural transplantation to be successful it is dependant on the cells surviving the transplantation procedure and being able to integrate into the host brain (striatum) and become physiologically active (Lindvall and Hagell, 2002).

2. Clinical trials for neural transplantation

Much of the ground breaking clinical research on neural transplants was done for Parkinson's Disease (PD), beginning in the late 1980s. These trials used primary human foetal mesencephalic tissue as the donor tissue and transplanted it into the host striatum, which is the normal target area of these cells. The mesencephalic tissue contains fate-committed dopaminergic neuroblasts, which have the capacity to differentiate into fully mature dopaminergic neurons following transplantation. For this to be successful certain criteria need to be adhered to, these include harvesting tissue between specific gestational ages and the optimisation of tissue preparation methodologies. If one considers the PD trials in which these principles are taken into account and which use good longitudinal assessment, then results to date in the PD trials have demonstrated improvements in a range of motor skills and many, but not all, of the patients have been able to reduce or even eliminate their daily intake of L-dopa (Hagell et al., 2002, Mendez et al., 2008, Olanow et al., 1996). However, there is variability in the success of this approach, which may be a direct result of variations in transplant methodology as well as differences in patient selection criteria (Freed et al., 2001, Freeman et al., 2000, Kordower et al., 2008, Li et al., 2008, Lindvall et al., 1990). Some of these trials have also highlighted the possibility of dyskinetic side effects in a proportion of patients (Freed et al., 2001), and the reasons for these is currently a topic of active investigation (Hagell et al., 2002, Carta et al., 2010, Lane et al., 2009a, Lane et al., 2009b, Politis et al., 2011, Politis et al., 2010, Steece-Collier et al., 2009). Following several years of round table discussions about how to move forward, a new multicentre European trial has been initiated and it is expected that patients will begin to be transplanted in 2012. This trial has taken all of the new data and the experiences learned from the past to ensure that the best possible protocols are adhered to in all centres, with the aim that the patients receive the best possible tissue transplant.

Parallel clinical trials of neural transplantation in HD are at a much earlier stage than the PD trials and are currently underway in a small number of centres around the world (Bachoud-Levi et al., 2000a, Freeman et al., 2000, Hauser et al., 2002, Kopyov et al., 1998a, Kopyov et al., 1998b, Rosser et al., 2002, Reuter et al., 2008, Philpott et al., 1997, Cicchetti et al., 2009). The French trial, based in Créteil, was the first to provide efficacy data, based on systematic long-term evaluation of their patients. Three of the five patients, having received bilateral striatal implants, were reported to show substantial improvement over several years (Bachoud-Levi et al., 2006, Bachoud-Levi et al., 2000c). More recently there has been an expansion of the French trial to include other French-speaking regions in Europe and a total of 40 patients will eventually receive transplants and will undergo follow-up, although no efficacy data is available as yet. In another study in Florida, 6 of 7 patients appeared to show improvement but one declined significantly, so that the overall group changes were not significant (Hauser et al., 2002). One patient died after 18 months due to cardiovascular disease and post mortem analysis of this patient's brain showed surviving graft tissue that was not affected by the underlying disease progression, at least at this time point (Freeman et al., 2000). The graft tissue was positive for striatal markers such as acetylcholinesterase, calbindin, calretinin, dopamine and tyrosine hydroxylase. Moreover, there was no sign of immune rejection in the graft region (Freeman et al., 2000). In the same study 3 patients developed subdural haemorrhages and 2 required surgical drainage (Hauser et al., 2002). These events may have been related to the stage of disease, which was rather more advanced than for the patients in the French or UK studies, in that more advanced cases of HD tend to have more cerebral atrophy with an accompanying increased risk of intracranial bleeding peri-operatively. Small numbers of patients have received grafts in several other centres with reports of safety (Kopyov et al., 1998a, Rosser et al., 2002), and although efficacy studies are underway in these centres, systematic reports have not yet been published. More recently it has been reported following post mortem analysis 10 years after transplantation in the Florida study, that the grafted cells had themselves been subjected to the disease process (Cicchetti et al., 2009). This raises issues about the long-term viability of transplantation as a therapy for HD, however, as this is only a report of 3 patients caution has to be taken not to misrepresent the field as a whole.

The UK trial (Rosser et al., 2002) is currently on hold due to EU regulations on tissue handling for transplantation, which now requires that all tissue be treated under good manufacturing practice (GMP). The French trial is not limited by such regulations due to their use of tissue pieces grafts as apposed to the cell suspension grafts used in the UK. There is little clear evidence to date stating that one method is better than the other (Watts et al., 2000) however, from the data that is available there is a suggestion that tissue pieces induce a more intense immune response post transplantation (Cooper et al., 2009). It is the belief in the UK that cell suspensions allow for greater integration of the cells into the host brain.

The initial studies of cell transplantation in HD are providing accumulating evidence of the conditions for safety, and preliminary evidence for efficacy. However, the limited availability of foetal tissue and the difficulty in ensuring the high degree of standardisation and quality control when a continuous source of fresh donor tissue is required from elective surgical abortion limits the widespread use of neural transplantation as a practical therapy. It has recently been shown that foetal tissue obtained from medical terminations of pregnancy is a viable source of tissue for transplant studies (Kelly et al., 2011). The use of medically sourced tissue will circumvent some of the logistical issues that were envisaged using surgical tissue due to the limited supply. Despite this new source of fresh foetal tissue there is still ethical and legislative concerns about abortion and the large number of donors required to support each operation, that restrict the number of patients that can receive grafts to a few specialist centres in a restricted number of countries. These issues have stimulated the search for alternative sources of donor cells or tissue that circumvent the problems associated with primary foetal tissue collection.

3. Alternative cell sources

The ability to generate a large stable population of cells to circumvent the supply issue and also to allow regular characterisation to ensure stability of the quality and character of the tissue, without the need for separate characterisation of each and every collection as is the case with primary tissue transplants is the ideal characteristic of an alternative cell source. Also, tissue storage methods need to be refined and validated so that the cells can be delivered on demand, to advance optimal clinical management of the recipient, rather than the surgeon and patient being constrained to surgery around an erratic schedule of tissue availability. The trials using primary foetal tissue thus provide a 'proof of concept' of the cell transplantation strategy as the basis for developing a practical therapy using a standardised, quality-controlled source of cells available to any appropriately equipped neurosurgical facility on demand. Several options are now being investigated as potential sources of donor tissue.

Stem cells are a possible source of cells for neural transplantation in HD and have attracted much attention in the last decade. Stem cells undergo self-renewal by symmetric division and can also undergo asymmetric division to produce another stem cell and a more differentiated progeny (Morrison et al., 1997, Watt and Hogan, 2000). Some multipotential cells may persist into adulthood, either by remaining quiescent in specific regions of the CNS parenchyma or by continued self-renewal (Morrison et al., 1997). Such cells are now referred to as "tissue specific stem cells" (Fuchs and Segre, 2000, Watt and Hogan, 2000). Embryonic stem (ES) cells have the potential to differentiate into all cell types under the correct conditions. Stem cells from a range of sources have potential as donor cells for neural transplantation. However, whatever the source, therapeutic application will require that cells can be directed to differentiate into the precise phenotype required to replace the cells lost to the disease process, and specifically medium spiny neurons for HD. We describe here stem cell sources under consideration as potential donor cells in this context, and the extent to which directed differentiation has been achieved. This list is not exhaustive but covers at least the main categories of stem cells that are currently being explored as alternative cell sources for neural transplantation in HD as well as a number of other neurodegenerative disorders.

3.1 Adult neural stem cells (ANSCs)

ANSCs are tissue-specific stem cell and are derived from the mature brain. Altman and colleagues provided the first clear evidence, using 3H-thymidine autoradiography, that a low level of neurogenesis is ongoing in the dentate gyrus of adult rats (Altman and Das, 1965). ANSCs have since been confirmed in two main regions of the CNS: the sub granular layers of the dentate gyrus, from where the newly-formed neurons repopulate the dentate gyrus (Gage et al., 1995); and the subventricular zone (SVZ) of the lateral ventricles (Alvarez-Buylla et al., 2002), from where the newly formed neurons migrate via the rostral migratory stream to the olfactory bulb (Lois and Alvarez-Buylla, 1994). It has also been reported that neural stem cells may also reside in other regions of the brain, albeit at an even lower concentration, including cortex (Gould et al., 1999, Rietze et al., 2000) and the medial-rostral part of the substantia nigra pars compacta in the lining of the cerebroventricular system of the midbrain (Zhao et al., 2003), although these reports remain controversial (Frielingsdorf et al., 2004).

The attraction of ANSCs as a donor supply for neural transplantation would be the possibility of autologous transplants, thus bypassing the immunological issues of graft rejection, which can be severe in the case of xenografts and not entirely benign even for allografts. Furthermore, it may eventually be possible to recruit such cells for endogenous repair without a requirement for their isolation and re-implantation. That is, it might be possible to stimulate the resident population of ANSCs to migrate to the site of degeneration. However, adult neural stem cells remain difficult to isolate and grow in culture and the factors that would be required to enhance the proliferation of these cells and their differentiation into the particular phenotypes relevant to the site of degeneration remains unknown. Therefore, these cells are less likely to be of beneficial clinical use for transplantation in Huntington's Disease patients.

3.2 Neural stem (NS) cells

Neural stem (NS) cells are those cells that are derived from the developing or adult brain but which are already committed to a neural fate. These cells can be expanded in culture where they undergo asymmetrical division and have been shown to have the potential to differentiate into all cell types of the nervous system, neurons, astrocytes and oligodendrocytes. NS cells can be isolated from the developing brain and in the presence of specific growth factors such as EGF and FGF-2 these cells will form free floating spheres of cells "neurospheres". Animal experiments using these cells have been carried out using tissue from E14 (embryonic day14) mouse striatal tissue and it was verified that the spheres formed from these cells are multipotential (Reynolds and Weiss, 1996). Clonal analysis in the presence of FGF-2 has shown it to be mitogenic for NS cells (Drago et al., 1991, Gensburger et al., 1987, Ray and Gage, 1994, Ray et al., 1993, Richards et al., 1992, Vicario-Abejon et al., 1995).

Several growth factors have the potential to enhance the neuronal differentiation of these cells down particular lineages, including nerve growth factor (NGF), insulin-like growth factor (IGF) and tumour necrosis factor (TNFα) (Arsenijevic et al., 2001, Cattaneo and McKay, 1990, Santa-Olla and Covarrubias, 1995, Tropepe et al., 1997). Identifying an appropriate growth factor cocktail appropriate to the phenotype associated with each particular application may be a necessary prelude to using these cells for transplantation.

It has been found with molecular characterisation of foetal NS cells in vitro that they retain a degree of their site-specific identity when environmental cues are absent but when co-cultured with cells of different origin they can adopt a new fate (Fricker et al., 1999, Parmar et al., 2002). IsletI and Er81 are genes associated with striatal development and their expression is found to be maintained over time in culture, but with neuronal differentiation, expression of striatal specific neuronal markers such as DARPP-32 and Islet1 are lost, although they do express homeobox transcription factors Dlx and MEIS2, which are associated with ventral forebrain development (Parmar et al., 2002, Skogh et al., 2003). Thus, it appears that expansion of NS cells in culture may restrict the differentiation potential of the cells. Further evidence for this has been demonstrated in disease models where these NS cells can survive post-transplantation following a short period of expansion; but that this is compromised by longer expansion times (Zietlow et al., 2005). One interpretation of these findings is that positional information is lost with continued expansion so that when long-term expanded cells are placed in an environment such as the adult CNS, they are not exposed to the developmental signals that they would see in the developing brain and are thus unable to differentiate into neurons appropriate to the site from which they were derived (for example medium spiny neurons from striatally-derived NS cells). However, when grafted to the neonatal brain, similar cells appear to respond to developmental signals and regional determinants by differentiating in a site-specific manner (Englund et al., 2002a, Englund et al., 2002b, Rosser et al., 2000) suggesting that they retain the capacity to respond to developmental signals if they are present.

From these and many other studies it is clear that NS cells may have the potential for neural transplantation. However, for this to become successful it is imperative that we first optimise the conditions in which these cells are expanded so as to increase the frequency at which these cells differentiate into the appropriate phenotype. It may be that we are now at a point where we can take what has been learnt from the directed differentiation of stem cells (as described below) and developmental biology and apply it to NS cells. Such factors as sonic hedgehog and dikkopf to mention but a few, which have been identified as important in striatal development and for directing the differentiation of stem cells, may be of benefit to maintaining the positional identity of the NS cells as well as directing the undifferentiated cells within this culture system that have not yet gone through their terminal differentiation, given the heterogeneic nature of the cells in question (El-Akabawy et al., 2011). The immunogenicity of these cells is another factor that needs to be taken into consideration for neural transplantation. Several studies have looked at the immunogenicity of these cells (Akesson et al., 2009, Al Nimer et al., 2004, Hori et al., 2007, Odeberg et al.,

2005, Ubiali et al., 2007, Laguna Goya et al., 2011) and it has been shown that these cells when expanded in culture become more immunogenic, and so patients receiving these cells would need to be immunosuppressed to prevent graft rejection taking place.

3.3 ES cells

Embryonic stem (ES) cells are generated from the inner cell mass (ICM) of the blastocyst passing the first step of cell differentiation and giving rise to trophectoderm (Evans and Kaufman, 1981, Martin, 1981). ES cells have the ability to extensively proliferate and self-renew whilst maintaining their pluripotentcy. ES cells are able to differentiate into all cell types of the three germ layers—ectoderm, mesoderm, and endoderm, and when transplanted are capable of germline transmission to generate chimeric animals which is in contrast to embryonic carcinoma cells (EC) cells (Bradley et al., 1984). Thus, ES cells can be used to generate models of disease and to understand developmental pathways by introducing modifications into the mouse germline. Human ES (hES) cells were first derived in 1998 (Thomson et al., 1998) and also have the potential to differentiate into cells of all three germ layers (Amit et al., 2000). However, the conditions used for culturing mouse and hES cells are different in that hES cells do not survive in leukemia inhibitory factor (LIF) containing media, a prerequisite for mouse ES cell culture (Daheron et al, 2004; Humphrey et al., 2004). They are pluripotent and can be propagated in culture for long periods of time in an undifferentiated state (Blau et al., 2001, Odorico et al., 2001, Schuldiner et al., 2001).

The ability of these cells to divide in culture over long periods of time highlights their potential for cell transplantation in that they would alleviate the logistical issues associated with primary tissue transplants. However, despite this, the important step of directing the differentiation of these cells into specific cell types is proving difficult. Whilst the default differentiation pathway appears to be that of a neural lineage, the specificity of the neuronal differentiation is limited. In the Parkinson's Disease model where large numbers of dopamine (DA) neurons are required there has been significant developments in directing the differentiation of ES cells into the required phenotype using factors such as retinoic acid and sonic hedghog (shh). In the case of HD where a population of medium spiny DARPP-32 positive neurons are required there is a very limited literature. Bouton and Kato (Bouhon et al., 2006, Kato et al., 2004) have reported on their ability to direct the differentiation of mouse ES cells into a ventral lineage where the cells maintained the expression of ventral markers that are typical of striatal neurons over a short time in culture. In the case of human ES cells, to date there is only one report of DARPP-32 positive neurons (Aubry et al., 2008). In this study the authors report that the DARPP-32 positive cells generated in culture had the ability to differentiate into such mature neurons in vivo following xenotransplantation into the lesioned rat brain model of HD. However, this is the only study reporting such data and to date there is no further evidence of a working protocol generating large populations of these neurons from stem cells. As part of a European consortium to address this issue several groups have come together to facilitate this issue and it is anticipated that new data will come to the fore in the not too distant future.

There have been significant ethical disputes associated with the derivation and use of human ES cells, including concerns over the use of human embryos, and fears related to their potential for human cloning (McHugh, 2004, Sandel, 2004). As a result of these ethical issues many countries have restricted or banned human ES cell research. Nevertheless, other countries have actively supported the development of human ES cell research because of the perceived potential for therapeutic benefit in a wide range of diseases. Some, including the UK, allow cloning of human embryos for therapeutic purposes, while imposing tight regulations to preclude their use for reproductive cloning.

However, despite the great potential of these cells one major caveat is their potential to form tumours. It is crucial that a method be developed for eliminating any possible ES cells from the differentiated population as one single ES cell could have devastating affects if transplanted into the host brain.

3.4 Induced pluripotent stem (iPS) cells

Induced pluripotent stem cells were first described in 2006 (Takahashi and Yamanaka, 2006). Introducing four exogenous transcription factors to differentiated cells and nurturing those cells in an embryonic environment the authors were able to directly reprogramme the cells as pluripotent like cells. Yamanaka and Takahashi in 2006 after much work and many different combinations of factors concluded that the four factors-Oct4, Sox2, c-Myc, and Klf4, which are present at high levels in ES cells are sufficient to transform mouse fibroblasts into cells that mimic ES cells (Figure 1). Subsequently, there have been many reports strengthening this finding (Brambrink et al., 2008, Kaji et al., 2009, Maherali et al., 2007, Meissner et al., 2007, Nakagawa et al., 2008, Stadtfeld et al., 2008, Takahashi et al., 2007, Wernig et al., 2007, Yamanaka, 2008, Yu et al., 2007, Okita et al., 2007, Wernig et al., 2008). iPS cells morphologically look identical to ES cells and as a result more detailed epigenetic characterisation is required to confirm the presence of iPS cell colonies in culture (Figure 2).

Following from this initial work, there have been many refinements to the initial viral based protocol using various methods from a non viral approach to small molecules to generate similar cells and using different factors (Haase et al., 2009, Kim et al., 2009, Sidhu, 2011, Soldner et al., 2009, Yu et al., 2009, Kaji et al., 2009, Okita et al., 2008, Park et al., 2008b, Stadtfeld et al., 2008, Woltjen et al., 2009) with each reporting positive generation of iPS cells with different levels of efficiency. In 2008 the first human iPS cells were described (Park et al., 2008a, Park et al., 2008b) and as with mouse iPS cells there has since been several reports of iPS cell generation from human tissues including; human fetal tissue, adult neural cells, adult fibroblasts, foreskin and disease specific sources, thus highlighting the potential usefulness of these cells both from a scientific and clinical perspective.

The molecular mechanisms of somatic cells reprogramming are still unclear. The wide range of time points to recognise the iPS colonies were reported from numerous studies; the epigenetic events during the reprogramming process and the up or down regulation of involving pluripotent genes are still a mystery. It is not known whether the reprogramming of somatic cells to pluripotent cells is a timed sequential process or if it's a random process, but what is important is that more studies are needed in order to understand the molecular function and use these cells before they are to be used in any clinical research.

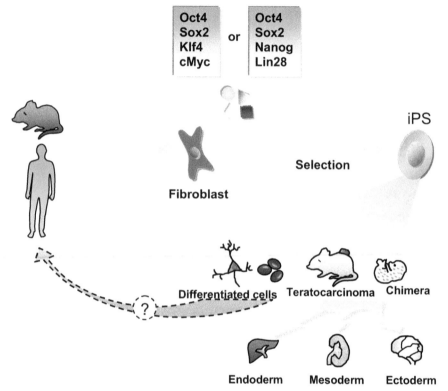

Fig. 1. Schematic drawing demonstrates direct reprogramming mouse and human fibroblasts to iPS cells with four defined factors Oct4, Sox2, Klf4, c-Myc, and Lin28. After selection, iPS cells are derived. These cells could differentiate into all cell types within three germ layers as assayed by teratoma formation and developmental contribution. (Adapted from (Welstead et al., 2008)

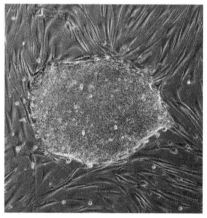

Fig. 2. A colony of pluripotent stem cells derived under non viral conditions.

3.5 Therapeutic potential of iPS cells

The ultimate goal of iPS cell derivation for degenerative diseases is to provide transplantable patient-specific cell sources that overcome ethical and immune rejection difficulties as found with other donor cell sources. Hematopoietic progenitors (HPs) derived from iPS cells were the first to be reported to successfully rescue and improve all pathological conditions in a mouse sickle cell anemia model (Hanna et al., 2007). This early study is a promising step forward in the quest to generate a suitable cell source for transplantation studies.

Interestingly, one year later, Wernig reported the functional benefits and behavioral improvements using iPS cell derived NSCs transplanted into a PD rat model (Wernig et al., 2008). Wernig claimed that in vitro NSCs generated from an iPS cell line were able to differentiate into all neural cell types (β-III tubulin, GFAP, O4 positive staining) including dopaminergic neurons after patterning factors had been added to the culture (FGF8 and sonic hedgehog) (Wernig et al., 2008). In addition, migration of NSCs from iPS cells was observed in various brain regions such as the striatum, midbrain, and hypothalamus after injection to the lateral ventricle of mouse embryos (E13.5-14.5). Furthermore, functional restoration and behavioral improvement were confirmed by action potential initiation, synaptophysin expression, and bias movement reduction from reprogramming somatic cells derived neurons (Wernig et al., 2008).

These studies provide evidence that iPS cells have high potential as an alternative donor cell source for cell replacement in regenerative medicine. To date there is no literature pertaining to the differentiation of DARPP-32 positive medium spiny neurons from iPS cells however, given the fast pace of this ever evolving field it is anticipated that such data will become available in the not too distant future.

However, as with ES cells and NSCs there is an associated risk of tumour formation. In comparison to the other cell sources, iPS cells have the potential to be generated on a patient specific basis and so may overcome this issue to some extent. The need to go through the ES like state is problematic as it renders the cells tumorigenic in nature and so makes them less attractive than initially envisaged.

Recently there have been reports about the possibility of generating functional neurons from fibroblast cells without having to go through the stem cell state (Parmar and Jakobsson, 2011, Pfisterer et al., 2011). As with iPS cells this is a viral based protocol using a combination of three different factors, namely; Ascl1, Brn2 and Myt1l (Forsberg et al., 2010, Ieda et al., 2010). This exciting development circumvents the issue of tumorgenicity that is associated with current ES and iPS protocols but is limited in that large numbers of cells cannot be generated. Therefore whilst this approach currently is optimistic, there are issues that will need to be overcome if this is to become a viable option for cell therapy.

3.6 Trans-differentiation of other tissue-specific stem cell populations

Another approach is to attain trans-differentiation of a non-neural tissue-specific stem cell population, the classic one being bone-marrow-derived stem cells. This population have the advantage of being more easily harvested than either foetal or adult neural stem cells, but the disadvantage that they do not by default produce neurally differentiated cells.

There is some evidence that trans-differentiation can be achieved, although this remains an area of dispute. Mesenchymal stem cells (MSCs) which are derived from the bone marrow and under normal conditions give rise to chondrocytes, adipocytes and cells of the blood lineage have been reported to trans-differentiate to ectodermal and endodermal cell fates (Zhao et al., 2002). In vitro, MSCs have also been shown to differentiate to form neurons and astrocytes. MSCs transplanted into the rat brain survive and express markers of neuroectodermal cells as well as having a functional effect (Deng et al., 2006, Bertani et al., 2005). This ability to trans-differentiate is not unique to MSCs, as neural stem cells have also been shown to have this ability, where they were seen to differentiate into muscle (Galli et al., 2000). However, evidence suggests that this plasticity may be a result of cell fusion based on studies that have looked at the potential of MSCs to differentiate into hepatocytes (Vassilopoulos et al., 2003, Wang et al., 2003), the increasing body of evidence for MSC trans-differentiation would suggest that this may in fact be true. This issue will need to be clarified for these cells to be serious contenders for neural transplantation.

The best characterised of the tissue-specific stem cells are the Hematopoietic stem cells (HSCs), which are also derived from the bone marrow, and reconstitute the blood. Two classes of HSC have been identified in mouse, those that survive for around 2 months, (the short term, ST-HSC), and those that survive for greater than 6 months, (the long term, LT-HSC) (Blau et al., 2001). Fluorescence-activated cell sorting (FACS) has been used to positively select cells based on the expression of specific cell surface markers. HSCs can be highly enriched up to 10,000 fold and then transplanted into the bone marrow of patients (Lagasse et al., 2001) for the treatment of oncogenic blood diseases. In an animal model of spinal cord injury, HSCs have been shown to survive for 5 weeks after transplantation, differentiate into astrocytes, oligodendrocytes and neuronal precursors and show improvement in functional behaviour using hindlimb motor function (Koshizuka et al., 2004), although no mature neurons were identified.

Human umbilical cord blood is easily retrieved following labour without the risk of harm to the mother or child and has been reported to contain multipotential progenitor cells that apparently have the ability to trans-differentiate into neuronal and glial cells (Sanchez-Ramos et al., 2001). Transplantation of these cells into the neonatal and adult brain have shown potential to survive and differentiate into neurons and glia (Li et al., 2004, Nan et al., 2005, Sanberg et al., 2005, Willing et al., 2003, Zigova et al., 2002). It may be that intravenous delivery rather than neural transplantation will be a more advantageous method of administering these cells for therapeutic benefit, based on a study by Willing et al (2003) where there was significant improvement in certain behavioural tasks when compared to animals receiving neural transplants of cells directly to the striatum. However, further studies are necessary to validate the potential of these cells and again, the issue of cell fusion needs to be addressed in this context.

3.7 Xenogenic tissue

Xenotransplantation offers the opportunity of breeding animals for foetal striatal tissue donation under conditions where the supply can be regulated according to demand; where the breeding stock is inbred, well characterised and controlled for pathogens; and where tissue collection and preparation can be undertaken under standardised sterile good manufacturing practice (GMP) conditions. The most likely donor candidate is porcine tissue, the advantages being: the extensive experience of animal husbandry within this farm species; the reliability of breeding; the large size of the litters; the possibility of sterile collection under standardised conditions; the comparable size and time course of development of the pig and human brain; and the potential application of transgenic technology to porcine tissue, which would open up the possibility of genetic manipulation, for example to modify the immunogenicity of transplanted tissue.

Transplantation of xenogeneic tissues into the immunosuppressed host CNS has been performed using a number of species, for example human to rat, pig to rat, rat to mouse and vice versa (Armstrong et al., 2002, Deacon et al., 1999, Galpern et al., 1996, Garcia et al., 1995, Isacson et al., 2001, Svendsen et al., 1997). Both primary and expanded tissue graft experiments have been reported using xenogenic tissue. The grafted tissue has been found to survive transplantation, axonal and glial fibre projections from the grafts, and make synapses with the host brain.

Clinical studies of CNS xenotransplantation are limited. Primary porcine embryonic striatal tissue has been transplanted into the caudate and putamen of 12 immunosuppressed PD patients with some clinical improvements reported, although there was little convincing evidence of graft survival (Isacson et al., 2001). The immune response from these grafts was more vigorous than that seen in human to rodent models. One patient died 7 months post-operatively for reasons unrelated to the graft, and was found to have very small numbers of surviving neurons in the graft region, raising the possibility that the majority had been rejected. In the same series, 12 HD patients received porcine striatal grafts but, again, there was little evidence of graft survival or functional effect. Twelve months of post-operative analysis of these patients demonstrated no change in the mean total functional capacity score (Fink et al., 2000).

Two key issues need to be resolved for xenografts to progress to practical therapeutic trials. The first relates to the fact, as illustrated by the first pilot clinical trial reported above, that xenografted tissue is largely rejected in the absence of effective immune protection. Two alternative strategies were adopted in the Diacrin trial – daily treatment with CsA or treatment with an antibody against major histocompatability complex 1 (MHC 1) to block the host T cell response (Fink et al., 2000). There is no clear evidence that either strategy proved effective for yielding good cell survival in patients, and it is surprising that the study had progressed on the basis that preliminary reports of the same strategies in primates were equally ineffective. Combination immunoprotection strategies to promote xenograft survival are an area of active research (Armstrong et al., 2001, Harrower and Barker, 2004). We described a new method that would allow long term xenograft survival of human fetal tissue in the rat brain (Kelly et al., 2009). In this method we took advantage of the naïve state of the neonatal rat pup immune system and induced what we describe as desensitisation to xenogenic tissue. Subsequent neural transplants into the adult rat brain resulted in good graft survival up to 40 weeks post transplantation without any immunosuppression. This method now allows long-term evaluation of xenogenic cells both anatomically and more importantly functionally in animal models of disease. Another approach that has been described to block the immune response to ES and iPS derived cells is to use an antibody response against the co-stimulatory molecules involved in the T cell response (Pearl et al., 2011). This method has only been reported for short-term graft survival and as yet no long-term efficacy data is available for functional evaluation of xenogenic cells using this approach.

The second key issue that requires resolution relates to safety of xenografted tissues. In the light of the recent spread of bovine spongiform encephalopathy to man in the form of new variant Creutzfeld-Jacob Disease, and the difficulty in controlling the spread of animal pathogens, as exemplified by the recent UK foot-and-mouth epidemic, there is widespread concern world-wide about the difficulties of eliminating the possibility of transmitting animal diseases to man. This may be particularly risky in the context of transplantation of tissues directly into the immunosuppressed CNS. The concern is not just for the recipient but, in the case of porcine endogenous retrovirus (PERVs), whether direct transfer into the brain might provide a route of transmission that allows virus mutation into new forms of viruses that give rise to unpredicted new diseases in man, even giving rise to de novo epidemics. Although the chances of such mutation are recognised to be very low, the cost of occurrence could be devastatingly high. Moreover, the risk of generating a new disease by an unknown mechanism is one that it is impossible to absolutely exclude by any known safety screen. The regulatory climate is consequently such that any novel xenograft approach is unlikely to gain approval for trial in the foreseeable future, at least in Europe. In the absence of having suffered the same major BSE, CJD and FMD epidemics, US regulations, although strict, are somewhat more permissive, with the result that most academic and commercial research of developing xenotransplantation as a therapeutic strategy for the CNS has moved westwards across the Atlantic over the last 10 years.

3.8 Genetically engineered cells

A variety of cells may be engineered in vitro either for the purpose of producing molecules of potential importance for CNS release (for example, in the form of polymer encapsulated cells, as below), or to alter the properties of a cell to render it potentially useful for circuit reconstruction. Of course, these strategies are not necessarily mutually exclusive - trophic factor support may be crucial for transplanted cells to survive and integrate in the host brain, and genetically engineering cells to release trophic factors in the graft region is one potential method for optimising graft survival.

The herpes simplex viral vector was the first virus to be tested as a method of introducing genes into the adult CNS (During et al., 1994, Fraefel et al., 1996, Song et al., 1997). More recently, other viral vectors have been introduced, including adenovirus, the recombinant adeno-associated virus (rAAV), lentivirus and pseudotyped vectors. The rAAV vector is more efficient than the HSV in that it is possible to achieve much higher levels of expression. The use of such vectors has allowed genes to be transferred to a specific group of cells in the CNS (Janson et al., 2001), and has provided support for the efficacy of factors such as GDNF for PD (Eslamboli et al., 2003, Kirik et al., 2000, Mandel et al., 1999, Mandel et al., 1997) and CNTF for HD (Emerich, 2004, Kahn et al., 1996, Mittoux et al., 2002, Regulier et al., 2002).

Polymer capsules have been considered as a system for trophic factor delivery to the CNS as they have the advantages of being relatively cheap to produce and can also be removed from the CNS as required, but the major drawback is that the effect is not long lasting

(Emerich et al., 1994). Where a limited amount of a protein is required for relatively short periods of time, polymer microspheres are an attractive alternative as they are biodegradable and subsequent surgical procedures are not required for retrieval (Date et al., 2001). However, improvements in the duration of release have been obtained by the use of encapsulated cells engineered to produce the desired molecules (Emerich, 1999, Emerich et al., 1997). Here, cells engineered to secrete specific substances such as neurotrophic factors are protected from the host immune system by a semi-permeable selective biocompatible outer membrane (Emerich, 1999, Emerich, 2004, Emerich et al., 1998, Emerich et al., 1997, Emerich et al., 1996). The outer membrane allows the entry of nutrients to the cells whilst also allowing the exit of neuroactive molecules. The advantage of this strategy is that it allows for the implantation of xenogeneic cells, which may be much easier to obtain or engineer than human cells. This approach has been used for delivery of factors such as GDNF in animal models of PD (Date et al., 2001, Sautter et al., 1998) and CNTF in animal models of HD (Emerich et al., 1997).

In the case of HD there have been several studies using polymer encapsulated cells for the delivery of CNTF. Baby hamster fibroblasts have been genetically modified to produce hCNTF and incorporated into polymer capsules (Anderson et al., 1996, Emerich et al., 1996). Both rodent and primate studies have been carried out incorporating this method (Anderson et al., 1996; Emerich et al., 1996; Emerich et al., 1997; Emerich and Winn, 2004; Kordower et al., 2000; Mittoux et al., 2000). These animal studies suggested that CNTF can protect striatal neurons against subsequent damage from an excitotoxic lesion. As well as protecting specific populations of striatal neurons from lesion-induced cell death, behavioural improvement was observed on skilled motor and cognitive tasks when compared to control animals. Encapsulated CNTF released by BHK cells were used in a clinical trial in France (Bachoud-Levi et al., 2000b), however, it was subsequently found that on removal of the capsule the cells failed to release sufficient amount of CNTF. The trial has reported safety and feasibility of this approach but further work is required to optimise the capsule for release of CNTF (Bloch et al., 2004). Nevertheless, the use of encapsulated cells for the delivery of growth factors and neurotrophic factors is an attractive alternative and may be required in combination with neural transplantation as a means of providing trophic support to the grafted cells.

Another potential cell source is immortalised cell lines, the neurally committed lines, such as the Ntera2 cell line, RN33B and Hib5. Functional benefit has been reported using these cells in various animal models (Catapano et al., 1999, Lundberg et al., 1996, Miyazono et al., 1995, Saporta et al., 2001). The Ntera2 cell line has been the most widely used. These cells are derived from human embryonal carcinomas and are terminally differentiated in vitro with retinoic acid. They have been found to respond to environmental cues when transplanted into the excitotoxically lesioned striatum (Saporta et al., 2001; Miyazono et al., 1995), sending out target-specific projections as well as expressing a site-specific phenotype. Grafting Ntera2 cells into the excitotoxic lesioned striatum resulted in neuronal differentiation, and a preliminary study reported rather dramatic functional effects (Hurlbert et al., 1999). However, on more detailed analysis the cells did not express any striatal-specific markers and there was no sustained improvement on skilled paw reaching and cylinder placing (Fricker-Gates et al., 2004). Transplantation of the RN33B cell line to the lesioned and non-lesioned striatum of rats has demonstrated their potential to differentiate into neurons in a site-specific way and form connections with target areas such as the globus pallidus (Lundberg et al., 1996), although only a proportion of the cells showed this differentiation potential. A major disadvantage of using such cell lines is the genotypic variability that arises from the immortalization process (Renfranz et al., 1991), and the risk that cells continue to proliferate to form tumours after transplantation.

4. Good manufacturing practice (GMP)

One of the major stumbling blocks for clinical trials of cell transplantation in Europe has been the introduction of the human tissue directive. This directive stipulates that all tissues used for human patients must be handled under clean room conditions. As a result many trials have been stopped to allow time to implement these new conditions. Each member state of the EU has taken their own interpretation of the directive and in the UK this is regulated by the human tissue authority (HTA). It is a requirement that any facility used to manipulate the cells/tissue used for transplantation into patients be licenced and governed by a strict set of guidelines. As a result in the case of the UK trial (NEST-UK) no patients have been transplanted in the last decade.

5. Conclusion

For HD, Cell transplantation is a promising therapy based on the current data from clinical trials. However, it is limited by the availability of a reliable source of cells that can replace the lost cells and reform the connections required for functional benefit. The proof of principle data from human fetal tissue studies highlights the effectiveness of the approach and the need for an alternative cell source. This chapter has highlighted some of the possible alternatives available and the potential of each one. Whilst the focus is very much on stem cells it is important that other cells also be considered as each has its own caveats. Which cell source is likely to make it to the clinical is not certain at this time and it is clear that much work is required before this can happen. Whilst much is known about cell sources and their potential for PD it is clear that the HD field is a long way behind. It is important that we as scientist stay focused on the goal and work together to move the field forward. As well as the issues of differentiation, tumour formation and cell number we also need to be mindful of the regulatory issues when devising such protocols and how they will adapt to GMP conditions. There is increasing emphasis on the use of GMP grade products for such studies, which are widely available. HD is a devastating disease and we are driven by the need for a therapy that works to make the lives of these patients less distressful.

6. References

Akesson, E., Wolmer-Solberg, N., Cederarv, M., Falci, S. & Odeberg, J. 2009. Human neural stem cells and astrocytes, but not neurons, suppress an allogeneic lymphocyte response. *Stem Cell Res*, 2, 56-67.

Al Nimer, F., Wennersten, A., Holmin, S., Meijer, X., Wahlberg, L. & Mathiesen, T. 2004. MHC expression after human neural stem cell transplantation to brain contused rats. *NeuroReport*, 15, 1871-5.

Altman, J. & Das, G. D. 1965. Autoradiographic and histological evidence of postnatal hippocampal neurogenesis in rats. *J Comp Neurol.*, 124, 319-335.

Alvarez-Buylla, A., Seri, B. & Doetsch, F. 2002. Identification of neural stem cells in the adult vertebrate brain. *Brain Research Bulletin,* 57, 751-758.

Amit, M., Carpenter, M. K., Inokuma, M. S., Chiu, C. P., Harris, C. P., Waknitz, M. A., Itskovitz-Eldor, J. & Thomson, J. A. 2000. Clonally derived human embryonic stem cell lines maintain pluripotency and proliferative potential for prolonged periods of culture. *Developmental Biology,* 227, 271-8.

Anderson, K. D., Panayotatos, N., Corcoran, T. L., Lindsay, R. M. & Wiegand, S. J. 1996. Ciliary neurotrophic factor protects striatal output neurons in an animal model of Huntington's Disease. *Proceedings of the National Academy of Sciences,* 93, 7346-7351.

Armstrong, R. J., Harrower, T. P., Hurelbrink, C. B., Mclaughin, M., Ratcliffe, E. L., Tyers, P., Richards, A., Dunnett, S. B., Rosser, A. E. & Barker, R. A. 2001. Porcine neural xenografts in the immunocompetent rat: immune response following grafting of expanded neural precursor cells. *Neuroscience,* 106, 201-216.

Armstrong, R. J., Hurelbrink, C. B., Tyers, P., Ratcliffe, E. L., Richards, A., Dunnett, S. B., Rosser, A. E. & Barker, R. A. 2002. The potential for circuit reconstruction by expanded neural precursor cells explored through porcine xenografts in a rat model of Parkinson's Disease. *Exp Neurol,* 175, 98-111.

Arsenijevic, Y., Weiss, S., Schneider, B. & Aebischer, P. 2001. Insulin-Like Growth Factor-1 Is Necessary for Neural Stem Cell Prolferation and Demonstartes Distinct Actions of Epidermal Growth Factor and Fibroblast Growth Factor-2. *Journal of Neuroscience,* 27(18), 7194-7202.

Aubry, L., Bugi, A., Lefort, N., Rousseau, F., Peschanski, M. & Perrier, A. L. 2008. Striatal progenitors derived from human ES cells mature into DARPP32 neurons in vitro and in quinolinic acid-lesioned rats. *Proc Natl Acad Sci U S A,* 105, 16707-12.

Bachoud-Levi, A., Bourdet, C., Brugieres, P., Nguyen, J. P., Grandmougin, T., Haddad, B., Jeny, R., Bartolomeo, P., Boisse, M. F., Barba, G. D., Degos, J. D., Ergis, A. M., Lefaucheur, J. P., Lisovoski, F., Pailhous, E., Remy, P., Palfi, S., Defer, G. L., Cesaro, P., Hantraye, P. & Peschanski, M. 2000a. Safety and tolerability assessment of intrastriatal neural allografts in five patients with Huntington's Disease. *Exp Neurol,* 161, 194-202.

Bachoud-Levi, A. C., Deglon, N., Nguyen, J. P., Bloch, J., Bourdet, C., Winkel, L., Remy, P., Goddard, M., Lefaucheur, J. P., Brugieres, P., Baudic, S., Cesaro, P., Peschanski, M. & Aebischer, P. 2000b. Neuroprotective gene therapy for Huntington's Disease using a polymer encapsulated BHK cell line engineered to secrete human CNTF. *Hum.Gene Ther.,* 11, 1723-1729.

Bachoud-Levi, A. C., Gaura, V., Brugieres, P., Lefaucheur, J. P., Boisse, M. F., Maison, P., Baudic, S., Ribeiro, M. J., Bourdet, C., Remy, P., Cesaro, P., Hantraye, P. & Peschanski, M. 2006. Effect of fetal neural transplants in patients with Huntington's Disease 6 years after surgery: a long-term follow-up study. *Lancet Neurol,* 5, 303-9.

Bachoud-Levi, A. C., Remy, P., Nguyen, J. P., Brugieres, P., Lefaucheur, J. P., Bourdet, C., Baudic, S., Gaura, V., Maison, P., Haddad, B., Boisse, M. F., Grandmougin, T., Jeny, R., Bartolomeo, P., Dalla Barba, G., Degos, J. D., Lisovoski, F., Ergis, A. M., Pailhous, E., Cesaro, P., Hantraye, P. & Peschanski, M. 2000c. Motor and cognitive improvements in patients with Huntington's Disease after neural transplantation. *Lancet,* 356, 1975-9.

Bertani, N., Malatesta, P., Volpi, G., Sonego, P. & Perris, R. 2005. Neurogenic potential of human mesenchymal stem cells revisited: analysis by immunostaining, time-lapse video and microarray. *Journal of cell science*, 118, 3925-36.

Blau, H. M., Brazelton, T. R. & Weimann, J. M. 2001. The evolving concept of a stem cell: Entity or function? *Cell*, 105, 829-841.

Bloch, J., Bachoud-Levi, A. C., Deglon, N., Lefaucheur, J. P., Winkel, L., Palfi, S., Nguyen, J. P., Bourdet, C., Gaura, V., Remy, P., Brugieres, P., Boisse, M. F., Baudic, S., Cesaro, P., Hantraye, P., Aebischer, P. & Peschanski, M. 2004. Neuroprotective gene therapy for Huntington's Disease, using polymer-encapsulated cells engineered to secrete human ciliary neurotrophic factor: results of a phase I study. *Hum.Gene Ther.*, 15, 968-975.

Bouhon, I. A., Joannides, A., Kato, H., Chandran, S. & Allen, N. D. 2006. Embryonic stem cell-derived neural progenitors display temporal restriction to neural patterning. *Stem Cells*, 24, 1908-13.

Bradley, A., Evans, M., Kaufman, M. H. & Robertson, E. 1984. Formation of germ-line chimaeras from embryo-derived teratocarcinoma cell lines. *Nature*, 309, 255-6.

Brambrink, T., Foreman, R., Welstead, G. G., Lengner, C. J., Wernig, M., Suh, H. & Jaenisch, R. 2008. Sequential expression of pluripotency markers during direct reprogramming of mouse somatic cells. *Cell Stem Cell*, 2, 151-9.

Carta, M., Carlsson, T., Munoz, A., Kirik, D. & Bjorklund, A. 2010. Role of serotonin neurons in the induction of levodopa- and graft-induced dyskinesias in Parkinson's Disease. *Mov Disord*, 25 Suppl 1, S174-9.

Catapano, L. A., Sheen, V. L., Leavitt, B. R. & Macklis, J. D. 1999. Differentiation of transplanted neural precursors varies regionally in adults striatum. *NeuroReport*, 10, 3971-3977.

Cattaneo, E. & Mckay, R. 1990. Proliferation and differentiation of neuronal stem cells regulated by nerve growth factor. *Nature*, 347, 762-765.

Cicchetti, F., Saporta, S., Hauser, R. A., Parent, M., Saint-Pierre, M., Sanberg, P. R., Li, X. J., Parker, J. R., Chu, Y., Mufson, E. J., Kordower, J. H. & Freeman, T. B. 2009. Neural transplants in patients with Huntington's Disease undergo disease-like neuronal degeneration. *Proceedings of the National Academy of Sciences of the United States of America*, 106, 12483-8.

Cooper, O., Astradsson, A., Hallett, P., Robertson, H., Mendez, I. & Isacson, O. 2009. Lack of functional relevance of isolated cell damage in transplants of Parkinson's Disease patients. *J Neurol*, 256 Suppl 3, 310-6.

Date, I., Shingo, T., Yoshida, H., Fujiwara, K., Kobayashi, K., Takeuchi, A. & Ohmoto, T. 2001. Grafting of encapsulated genetically modified cells secreting GDNF into the striatum of parkinsonian model rats. *Cell Transplantation*, 10, 397-401.

Deacon, T., Whatley, B., Leblanc, C., Lin, L. & Isacson, O. 1999. Pig Fetal Septal Neurons Implanted Into the Hippocampus of Aged or Cholinergic Deafferented Rats Grow Axons and Form Cross-Species Synapses in Appropriate Target Regions. *Cell Transplantation*, 8, 111-129.

Deng, J., Petersen, B. E., Steindler, D. A., Jorgensen, M. L. & Laywell, E. D. 2006. Mesenchymal stem cells spontaneously express neural proteins in culture and are neurogenic after transplantation. *Stem Cells*, 24, 1054-64.

Drago, J., Murphy, M., Carroll, S. M., Harvey, P. P. & Bartlett, P. F. 1991. Fibroblast growth factor-mediated proliferation of central nervous system precursors depends on endogenous production of insulin-like growth factor 1. *Proc.Natl.Acad.Sci.USA*, 88, 2199-2203.

During, M. J., Naegele, J. R., O'malley, K. L. & Geller, A. I. 1994. Long-term behavioral recovery in parkinsonian rats by an HSV vector expressing tyrosine hydroxylase. *Science*, 266, 1399-1403.

El-Akabawy, G., Medina, L. M., Jeffries, A., Price, J. & Modo, M. 2011. Purmorphamine Increases DARPP-32 Differentiation in Human Striatal Neural Stem Cells Through the Hedgehog Pathway. *Stem Cells Dev.*

Emerich, D. F. 1999. Encapsulated CNTF-producing cells for Huntington's Disease. *Cell Transplant.*, 8, 581-582.

Emerich, D. F. 2004. Sertoli cell grafts for Huntington's disease. An opinion. *Neurotox Res*, 5, 567.

Emerich, D. F., Bruhn, S., Chu, Y. & Kordower, J. H. 1998. Cellular delivery of CNTF but not NT-4/5 prevents degeneration of striatal neurons in a rodent model of Huntington's Disease. *Cell Transplant.*, 7, 213-225.

Emerich, D. F., Cain, C. K., Greco, C., Saydoff, J. A., Hu, Z. Y., Liu, H. J. & Lindner, M. D. 1997. Cellular delivery of human CNTF prevents motor and cognitive dysfunction in a rodent model of Huntington's disease. *Cell Transplantation*, 6, 249-266.

Emerich, D. F., Hammang, J. P., Baetge, E. E. & Winn, S. R. 1994. Implantation of polymer-encapsulated human nerve growth factor-secreting fibroblasts attenuates the behavioral and neuropathological consequences of quinolinic acid injections into rodent striatum. *Exp.Neurol.*, 130, 141-150.

Emerich, D. F., Lindner, M. D., Winn, S. R., Chen, E. Y., Frydel, B. R. & Kordower, J. H. 1996. Implants of encapsulated human CNTF-producing fibroblasts prevent behavioral deficits and striatal degeneration in a rodent model of Huntington's Disease. *Journal of Neuroscience*, 16, 5168-5181.

Englund, U., Bjorklund, A., Wictorin, K., Lindvall, O. & Kokaia, M. 2002a. Grafted neural stem cells develop into functional pyramidal neurons and integrate into host cortical circuitry. *Proceedings of the National Academy of Sciences*, 99, 17089.

Englund, U., Fricker-Gates, R. A., Lundberg, C., Bjorklund, A. & Wictorin, K. 2002b. Transplantation of human neural progenitor cells into the neonatal rat brain: Extensive migration and differentiation with long-distance axonal projections. *Experimental Neurology*, 173, 1-21.

Eslamboli, A., Cummings, R. M., Ridley, R. M., Baker, H. F., Muzyczka, N., Burger, C., Mandel, R. J., Kirik, D. & Annett, L. E. 2003. Recombinant adeno-associated viral vector (rAAV) delivery of GDNF provides protection against 6-OHDA lesion in the common marmoset monkey (Callithrix jacchus). *Exp.Neurol.*, 184, 536-548.

Evans, M. J. & Kaufman, M. H. 1981. Establishment in culture of pluripotential cells from mouse embryos. *Nature*, 292, 154-6.

Fink, J. S., Schumacher, J. M., Ellias, S. L., Palmer, E. P., Saint-Hilaire, M., Shannon, K., Penn, R., Starr, P., Vanhorne, C., Kott, H. S., Dempsey, P. K., Fischman, A. J., Raineri, R., Manhart, C., Dinsmore, J. & Isacson, O. 2000. Porcine xenografts in Parkinson's Disease and Huntington's Disease patients: preliminary results. *Cell Transplant.*, 9, 273-278.

Folstein, S. E. 1989. The Psychopathology of Huntingtons-Disease. *Journal of Nervous and Mental Disease,* 177, 645-645.

Forsberg, M., Carlen, M., Meletis, K., Yeung, M. S., Barnabe-Heider, F., Persson, M. A., Aarum, J. & Frisen, J. 2010. Efficient reprogramming of adult neural stem cells to monocytes by ectopic expression of a single gene. *Proceedings of the National Academy of Sciences of the United States of America,* 107, 14657-61.

Fraefel, C., Song, S., Lim, F., Lang, P., Yu, L., Wang, Y., Wild, P. & Geller, A. I. 1996. Helper virus-free transfer of herpes simplex virus type 1 plasmid vectors into neural cells. *J.Virol.,* 70, 7190-7197.

Freed, C. R., Greene, P. E., Breeze, R. E., Tsai, W. Y., Dumouchiel, W., Kao, R., Dillon, S., Winfield, H., Culver, S., Trojanowski, J. Q., Eidelberg, D. & Fahn, S. 2001. Transplantation of embryonic dopamine neurons for severe Parkinson's Disease. *The New England Journal of Medicine,* 344, 710-719.

Freeman, T. B., Cicchetti, F., Hauser, R. A., Deacon, T. W., Li, X. J., Hersch, S. M., Nauert, G. M., Sanberg, P. R., Kordower, J. H., Saporta, S. & Isacson, O. 2000. Transplanted fetal striatum in Huntington's Disease: Phenotypic development and lack of pathology. *Proceedings of the National Academy of Sciences,* 97, 13877-13882.

Fricker, R. A., Carpenter, M. K., Winkler, C., Greco, C., Gates, M. & Bjorklund, A. 1999. Site-Specific Migration and Neuroanl Differentition of Human Neural Progenitor Cells after Transplantation in the Adult Rat Brain. *The Jouranl of Neuroscience,* 19, 5990-6005.

Fricker-Gates, R. A., White, A., Gates, M. A. & Dunnett, S. B. 2004. Striatal neurons in striatal grafts are derived from both post-mitotic cells and dividing progenitors. *European Journal of Neuroscience,* 19, 513-520.

Frielingsdorf, H., Schwarz, K., Brundin, P. & Mohapel, P. 2004. No evidence for new dopaminergic neurons in the adult mammalian substantia nigra. *Proc.Natl.Acad.Sci.U.S.A,* 101, 10177-10182.

Fuchs, E. & Segre, J. A. 2000. Stem cells: a new lease on life. *Cell,* 100, 143-155.

Gage, F. H., Ray, J. & Fisher, L. J. 1995. Isolation, characterization, and use of stem cells from the CNS. *Annual Reiew of Neuroscience,* 18, 159-192.

Galli, R., Borello, U., Gritti, A., Giulia Minasi, M., Bjornson, C., Coletta, M., Mora, M., De Angelis, M. G. C., Fiocco, R., Cossu, G. & Vescovi, A. L. 2000. Skeletal myogenic potential of human and mouse neural stem cells. *Nature,* 3, 986-991.

Galpern, W. R., Burns, L. H., Deacon, T. W., Dismore, J. & Isacson, O. 1996. Xenotransplantation of Porcine Fetal Ventral Mesencephalon in a Rat Model of Parkinson's Disease: Functional Recovery and Graft Morphology. *Experimental Neurology,* 140, 1-13.

Garcia, A. R., Deacon, T. W., Dinsmore, J. & Isacson, O. 1995. Extensive Axonal and Glial Fiber Growth from Fetal Porcine Cortical Xenografts in the Adult Rat Cortex. *Cell Transplantation,* 4, 515-527.

Gensburger, C., Labourdette, G. & Sensenbrenner, M. 1987. Brain basic fibroblast growth factor stimulates the proliferation of rat neuronal precursor cells in vitro. *FEBS Letters,* 217, 1-5.

Gould, E., Reeves, A. J., Graziano, M. S. A. & Gross, C. G. 1999. Neurogenesis in the neocortex of adult primates. *Science,* 286, 548-552.

Haase, A., Olmer, R., Schwanke, K., Wunderlich, S., Merkert, S., Hess, C., Zweigerdt, R., Gruh, I., Meyer, J., Wagner, S., Maier, L. S., Han, D. W., Glage, S., Miller, K., Fischer, P., Scholer, H. R. & Martin, U. 2009. Generation of induced pluripotent stem cells from human cord blood. *Cell Stem Cell,* 5, 434-41.

Hagell, P., Piccine, P., Bjâ≠◊Rklund, A., Brundin, P., Rehncrona, S., Widner, H., Crabb, L., Pavese, N., Oertel, W. H., Quinn, N., Brooks, D. J. & Lindvall, O. 2002. Dyskinesias following neural transplantation in Parkinson's Disease. *Nature Neuroscience,* 5, 627-628.

Harrower, T. P. & Barker, R. A. 2004. The emerging technologies of neural xenografting and stem cell transplantation for treating neurodegenerative disorders. *Drugs Today (Barc),* 40, 171-89.

Hauser, R. A., Furtado, S., Cimino, C. R., Delgado, H., Eichler, S., Schwartz, S., Scott, D., Nauert, G. M., Soety, E., Sossi, V., Holt, D. A., Sanberg, P. R., Stoessl, A. J. & Freeman, T. B. 2002. Bilateral human fetal striatal transplantation in Huntington's Disease. *Neurology,* 58, 687-95.

Hori, J., Ng, T. F., Shatos, M., Klassen, H., Streilein, J. W. & Young, M. J. 2007. Neural progenitor cells lack immunogenicity and resist destruction as allografts. 2003. *Ocul Immunol Inflamm,* 15, 261-73.

Humphrey, R. K., Beattie, G. M., Lopez, A. D., Bucay, N., King, C. C., Firpo, M. T., Rose-John, S. & Hayek, A. 2004. Maintenance of pluripotency in human embryonic stem cells is STAT3 independent. *Stem Cells,* 22, 522-30.

Hurlbert, M. S., Gianani, R. I., Hutt, C., Freed, C. R. & Kaddis, F. G. 1999. Neural transplantation of hNT neurons for Huntington's Disease. *Cell Transplant.,* 8, 143-151.

Ieda, M., Fu, J. D., Delgado-Olguin, P., Vedantham, V., Hayashi, Y., Bruneau, B. G. & Srivastava, D. 2010. Direct reprogramming of fibroblasts into functional cardiomyocytes by defined factors. *Cell,* 142, 375-86.

Isacson, O., Costantini, J. M., Cicchetti, F., Chung, S. & Kim, K. S. 2001. Cell implantation therapies for Parkinson's Disease using neural stem, transgenic or xenogenic donor, cells. *Parkinsonism and Related Disorders,* 7, 205-212.

Janson, C. G., Mcphee, S. W. J., Leone, P., Freese, A. & During, M. J. 2001. Viral-based gene transfer to the mammalian CNS for functional genome studies. *Trends in Neuroscience,* 24, 706-712.

Kahn, A., Haase, G., Akli, S. & Guidotti, J. E. 1996. [Gene therapy of neurological diseases]. *C.R.Seances Soc.Biol.Fil.,* 190, 9-11.

Kaji, K., Norrby, K., Paca, A., Mileikovsky, M., Mohseni, P. & Woltjen, K. 2009. Virus-free induction of pluripotency and subsequent excision of reprogramming factors. *Nature,* 458, 771-5.

Kato, H., Bouhon, I. A., Chandran, S. & Allen, N. D. 2004. Critical factors influencing fate determination and developmental plasticity of embryonic stem cells derived neural precursor cells. *Submitted.*

Kelly, C. M., Precious, S. V., Scherf, C., Penketh, R., Amso, N. N., Battersby, A., Allen, N. D., Dunnett, S. B. & Rosser, A. E. 2009. Neonatal desensitization allows long-term survival of neural xenotransplants without immunosuppression. *Nat Methods,* 6, 271-3.

Kelly, C. M., Precious, S. V., Torres, E. M., Harrison, A., Williams, D., Scherf, C., Weyrauch, U. M., Lane, E. L., Allen, N. D., Penketh, R., Amso, N., Kemp, P., Dunnett, S. B. & Rosser, A. E. 2011. Medical terminations of pregnancy: a viable source of tissue for cell replacement therapy for neurodegenerative disorders. *Cell Transplantation*.

Kim, D., Kim, C. H., Moon, J. I., Chung, Y. G., Chang, M. Y., Han, B. S., Ko, S., Yang, E., Cha, K. Y., Lanza, R. & Kim, K. S. 2009. Generation of human induced pluripotent stem cells by direct delivery of reprogramming proteins. *Cell Stem Cell*, 4, 472-6.

Kirik, D., Rosenblad, C., Bjorklund, A. & Mandel, R. J. 2000. Long-term rAAV-mediated gene transfer of GDNF in the rat Parkinson's model: intrastriatal but not intranigral transduction promotes functional regeneration in the lesioned nigrostriatal system. *Journal of Neuroscience*, 20, 4686-4700.

Kopyov, O. V., Jacques, S. & Eagle, K. S. 1998a. Fetal transplantation for the treatment of neurodegenerative diseases - Current status and future potential. *Cns Drugs*, 9, 77-83.

Kopyov, O. V., Jacques, S., Lieberman, A., Duma, C. M. & Eagle, K. S. 1998b. Safety of intrastriatal neurotransplantation for Huntington's Disease patients. *Experimental Neurology*, 149, 97-108.

Kordower, J. H., Chu, Y., Hauser, R. A., Freeman, T. B. & Olanow, C. W. 2008. Lewy body-like pathology in long-term embryonic nigral transplants in Parkinson's Disease. *Nat Med*, 14, 504-6.

Koshizuka, S., Okada, S., Okawa, A., Koda, M., Murasawa, M., Hashimoto, M., Kamada, T., Yoshinaga, K., Murakami, M., Moriya, H. & Yamazaki, M. 2004. Transplanted hematopoietic stem cells from bone marrow differentiate into neural lineage cells and promote functional recovery after spinal cord injury in mice. *J Neuropathol.Exp.Neurol.*, 63, 64-72.

Lagasse, E., Shizuru, J. A., Uchida, N., Tsukamoto, A. & Weissman, I. L. 2001. Toward regenerative medicine. *Immunity*, 14, 425-436.

Laguna Goya, R., Busch, R., Mathur, R., Coles, A. J. & Barker, R. A. 2011. Human fetal neural precursor cells can up-regulate MHC class I and class II expression and elicit CD4 and CD8 T cell proliferation. *Neurobiol Dis*, 41, 407-14.

Lane, E. L., Brundin, P. & Cenci, M. A. 2009a. Amphetamine-induced abnormal movements occur independently of both transplant- and host-derived serotonin innervation following neural grafting in a rat model of Parkinson's Disease. *Neurobiol Dis*, 35, 42-51.

Lane, E. L., Vercammen, L., Cenci, M. A. & Brundin, P. 2009b. Priming for L-DOPA-induced abnormal involuntary movements increases the severity of amphetamine-induced dyskinesia in grafted rats. *Exp Neurol*, 219, 355-8.

Li, H. J., Liu, H. Y., Zhao, Z. M., Lu, S. H., Yang, R. C., Zhu, H. F., Cai, Y. L., Zhang, Q. J. & Han, Z. C. 2004. [Transplantation of human umbilical cord stem cells improves neurological function recovery after spinal cord injury in rats]. *Zhongguo Yi.Xue.Ke.Xue.Yuan Xue.Bao.*, 26 38-42.

Li, J. Y., Englund, E., Holton, J. L., Soulet, D., Hagell, P., Lees, A. J., Lashley, T., Quinn, N. P., Rehncrona, S., Bjorklund, A., Widner, H., Revesz, T., Lindvall, O. & Brundin, P. 2008. Lewy bodies in grafted neurons in subjects with Parkinson's Disease suggest host-to-graft disease propagation. *Nat Med*, 14, 501-3.

Lindvall, O., Brundin, P., Widner, H., Rehncrona, S., Gustavii, B., Frackowiak, R., Leenders, K. L., Sawle, G., Rothwell, J. C., Marsden, D. & Bjâ≠0Rklund, A. 1990. Grafts of fetal dopamine neurons survive and improve motor function in Parkinson's Disease. *Science,* 247, 574-577.

Lindvall, O. & Hagell, P. 2002. Cell replacement therapy in human neurodegenerative disorders. *Clinical Neuroscience Research,* 2 86-92.

Lois, C. & Alvarez-Buylla, A. 1994. Long-distance neuronal migration in the adult mammalian brain. *Science,* 264, 1145-1148.

Lundberg, C., Winkler, C., Whittemore, S. R. & Bjorklund, A. 1996. Conditionally immortalized neural progenitor cells grafted to the striatum exhibit site-specific neuronal differentiation and establish connections with the host globus pallidus. *Neurobiol.Dis.,* 3, 33-50.

Maherali, N., Sridharan, R., Xie, W., Utikal, J., Eminli, S., Arnold, K., Stadtfeld, M., Yachechko, R., Tchieu, J., Jaenisch, R., Plath, K. & Hochedlinger, K. 2007. Directly reprogrammed fibroblasts show global epigenetic remodeling and widespread tissue contribution. *Cell Stem Cell,* 1, 55-70.

Mandel, R. J., Snyder, R. O. & Leff, S. E. 1999. Recombinant adeno-associated viral vector-mediated glial cell line-derived neurotrophic factor gene transfer protects nigral dopamine neurons after onset of progressive degeneration in a rat model of Parkinson's Disease. *Exp.Neurol.,* 160, 205-214.

Mandel, R. J., Spratt, S. K., Snyder, R. O. & Leff, S. E. 1997. Midbrain injection of recombinant adeno-associated virus encoding rat glial cell line-derived neurotrophic factor protects nigral neurons in a progressive 6-hydroxydopamine-induced degeneration model of Parkinson's Disease in rats. *Proc.Natl.Acad.Sci.U.S.A,* 94, 14083-14088.

Martin, G. R. 1981. Isolation of a pluripotent cell line from early mouse embryos cultured in medium conditioned by teratocarcinoma stem cells. *Proceedings of the National Academy of Sciences of the United States of America,* 78, 7634-8.

Mchugh, P. R. 2004. Zygote and "clonote"--the ethical use of embryonic stem cells. *N.Engl.J.Med.,* 351, 209-211.

Meissner, A., Wernig, M. & Jaenisch, R. 2007. Direct reprogramming of genetically unmodified fibroblasts into pluripotent stem cells. *Nat Biotechnol,* 25, 1177-81.

Mendez, I., Vinuela, A., Astradsson, A., Mukhida, K., Hallett, P., Robertson, H., Tierney, T., Holness, R., Dagher, A., Trojanowski, J. Q. & Isacson, O. 2008. Dopamine neurons implanted into people with Parkinson's Disease survive without pathology for 14 years. *Nat Med,* 14, 507-9.

Mittoux, V., Ouary, S., Monville, C., Lisovoski, F., Poyot, T., Conde, F., Escartin, C., Robichon, R., Brouillet, E., Peschanski, M. & Hantraye, P. 2002. Corticostriatopallidal Neuroprotection by Adenovirus-Mediated Ciliary Neurotrophic Factor Gene Transfer in a Rat Model of Progressive Striatal Degeneration. *Journal of Neuroscience,* 22, 4478-4486.

Miyazono, M., Lee, V. M. & Trojanowski, J. Q. 1995. Proliferation, cell death, and neuronal differentiation in transplanted human embryonal carcinoma (NTera2) cells depend on the graft site in nude and severe combined immunodeficient mice. *Lab Invest,* 73, 273-283.

Morrison, S. J., Ahah, N. M. & Anderson, D. J. 1997. Regulatory mechanisms in stem cell biology. *Cell,* 88, 287-298.

Nakagawa, M., Koyanagi, M., Tanabe, K., Takahashi, K., Ichisaka, T., Aoi, T., Okita, K., Mochiduki, Y., Takizawa, N. & Yamanaka, S. 2008. Generation of induced pluripotent stem cells without Myc from mouse and human fibroblasts. *Nat Biotechnol,* 26, 101-6.

Nan, Z., Grande, A., Sanberg, C. D., Sanberg, P. R. & Low, W. C. 2005. Infusion of human umbilical cord blood ameliorates neurologic deficits in rats with hemorrhagic brain injury. *Ann.N.Y.Acad.Sci.,* 1049, 84-96.

Odeberg, J., Piao, J. H., Samuelsson, E. B., Falci, S. & Akesson, E. 2005. Low immunogenicity of in vitro-expanded human neural cells despite high MHC expression. *J Neuroimmunol,* 161, 1-11.

Odorico, J. S., Kaufman, D. S. & Thomson, J. A. 2001. Multilineage differentiation from Human Embryonic Stem Cell Lines. *Stem Cells,* 19, 193-204.

Okita, K., Ichisaka, T. & Yamanaka, S. 2007. Generation of germline-competent induced pluripotent stem cells. *Nature,* 448, 313-7.

Okita, K., Nakagawa, M., Hyenjong, H., Ichisaka, T. & Yamanaka, S. 2008. Generation of mouse induced pluripotent stem cells without viral vectors. *Science,* 322, 949-53.

Olanow, C. W., Kordower, J. H. & Freeman, T. B. 1996. Fetal nigral transplantation as a therapy for Parkinson's Disease. *Trends in Neurosciences,* 19, 102-109.

Park, I. H., Lerou, P. H., Zhao, R., Huo, H. & Daley, G. Q. 2008a. Generation of human-induced pluripotent stem cells. *Nat Protoc,* 3, 1180-6.

Park, I. H., Zhao, R., West, J. A., Yabuuchi, A., Huo, H., Ince, T. A., Lerou, P. H., Lensch, M. W. & Daley, G. Q. 2008b. Reprogramming of human somatic cells to pluripotency with defined factors. *Nature,* 451, 141-6.

Parmar, M. & Jakobsson, J. 2011. Turning skin into dopamine neurons. *Cell Res.*

Parmar, M., Skogh, C., Bjorklund, A. & Campbell, K. 2002. Regional specification of neurosphere cultures derived from subregions of the embryonic telencephalon. *Mol.Cell Neurosci,* 21 645-656.

Pearl, J. I., Lee, A. S., Leveson-Gower, D. B., Sun, N., Ghosh, Z., Lan, F., Ransohoff, J., Negrin, R. S., Davis, M. M. & Wu, J. C. 2011. Short-term immunosuppression promotes engraftment of embryonic and induced pluripotent stem cells. *Cell Stem Cell,* 8, 309-17.

Pfisterer, U., Kirkeby, A., Torper, O., Wood, J., Nelander, J., Dufour, A., Bjorklund, A., Lindvall, O., Jakobsson, J. & Parmar, M. 2011. Direct conversion of human fibroblasts to dopaminergic neurons. *Proc Natl Acad Sci U S A,* 108, 10343-8.

Philpott, L. M., Kopyov, O. V., Lee, A. J., Jacques, S., Duma, C. M., Caine, S., Yang, M. & Eagle, K. S. 1997. Neuropsychological functioning following fetal striatal transplantation in Huntington's chorea: three case presentations. *Cell Transplantation,* 6, 203-12.

Politis, M., Oertel, W. H., Wu, K., Quinn, N. P., Pogarell, O., Brooks, D. J., Bjorklund, A., Lindvall, O. & Piccini, P. 2011. Graft-induced dyskinesias in Parkinson's Disease: High striatal serotonin/dopamine transporter ratio. *Mov Disord.*

Politis, M., Wu, K., Loane, C., Quinn, N. P., Brooks, D. J., Rehncrona, S., Bjorklund, A., Lindvall, O. & Piccini, P. 2010. Serotonergic neurons mediate dyskinesia side effects in Parkinson's patients with neural transplants. *Sci Transl Med,* 2, 38ra46.

Ray, J. & Gage, F. H. 1994. Spinal Cord Neuroblasts Proliferate in Response to Basic Fibroblast Growth Factor. *The Jouranl of Neuroscience,* 14, 3548-3564.

Ray, J., Peterson, M., Schinstine, M. & Gage, F. H. 1993. Proliferation,differentiation, and long-term culture of primary hippocampal neurons. *Neurobiology,* 90, 3602-3606.

Reddy, P. H., Williams, M. & Tagle, D. A. 1999. Recent advances in understanding the pathogenesis of Huntington's Disease. *Trends in Neuroscience,* 22, 248-254.

Regulier, E., Pereira, D. A., Sommer, B., Aebischer, P. & Deglon, N. 2002. Dose-dependent neuroprotective effect of ciliary neurotrophic factor delivered via tetracycline-regulated lentiviral vectors in the quinolinic acid rat model of Huntington's Disease. *Hum.Gene Ther.,* 13 1981-1990.

Renfranz, P. J., Cunningham, M. G. & Mckay, R. D. 1991. Region-specific differentiation of the hippocampal stem cell line HiB5 upon implantation into the developing mammalian brain. *Cell,* 66 713-729.

Reuter, I., Tai, Y. F., Pavese, N., Chaudhuri, K. R., Mason, S., Polkey, C. E., Clough, C., Brooks, D. J., Barker, R. A. & Piccini, P. 2008. Long-term clinical and positron emission tomography outcome of fetal striatal transplantation in Huntington's Disease. *Journal of neurology, neurosurgery, and psychiatry,* 79, 948-51.

Reynolds, B. A. & Weiss, S. 1996. Clonal and Population Analyses Demonstrate That an EGF-Responsive Mammalian Embryonic CNS Precursor Is a Stem Cell. *Developmental Biology,* 175, 1-13.

Richards, L. J., Kilpatrick, T. J. & Bartlett, P. F. 1992. De novo generation of neuroanl cells from the adult mouse brain. *Proc.Natl.Acad.Sci.USA,* 89, 8591-8595.

Rietze, R., Poulin, P. & Weiss, S. 2000. Mitotically active cells that generate neurons and astrocytes are present in multiple regions of the adult mouse hippocampus. *Journal of Comparative Neurology,* 424, 397-408.

Ross, C. A. & Margolis, R. L. 2001. Huntington's Disease. *Clinical Neuroscience Research,* 1, 142-152.

Rosser, A. E., Barker, R. A., Harrower, T., Watts, C., Farrington, M., Ho, A. K., Burnstein, R. M., Menon, D. K., Gillard, J. H., Pickard, J. & Dunnett, S. B. 2002. Unilateral transplantation of human primary fetal tissue in four patients with Huntington's Disease: NEST-UK safety report ISRCTN no 36485475. *J Neurol Neurosurg Psychiatry,* 73, 678-85.

Rosser, A. E., Tyers, P. & Dunnett, S. B. 2000. The morphological development of neurons derived from EGF- and FGF-2-driven human CNS precursors depends on their site of integration in the neonatal rat brain. *Eur J Neurosci,* 12, 2405-13.

Sanberg, P. R., Willing, A. E., Garbuzova-Davis, S., Saporta, S., Liu, G., Sanberg, C. D., Bickford, P. C., Klasko, S. K. & El Badri, N. S. 2005. Umbilical cord blood-derived stem cells and brain repair. *Ann.N.Y.Acad.Sci.,* 1049 67-83.

Sanchez-Ramos, J., Song, S., Kamath, S. G., Zigova, T., Willing, A., Cardozo-Pelaez, F., Stedford, T., Chopp, M. & Sanberg, P. R. 2001. Expression of neural markers in human umbilical cord blood. *Experimental Neurology,* 171, 109-115.

Sandel, M. J. 2004. Embryo ethics--the moral logic of stem-cell research. *N.Engl.J.Med.,* 351, 207-209.

Santa-Olla, J. & Covarrubias, L. 1995. Epidermal Growth Factor (EGF), Transforming Growth Factor-Ã (T GF-Ã), and Basic Fibroblast Growth Factor (bFGF) Differentially Influence Neural Precursor Cells of Mouse Embryonic Mesencephalon. *Journal of Neuroscience Research,* 42, 172-183.

Saporta, S., Willing, A. E., Zigova, T., Daadi, M. M. & Sanberg, P. R. 2001. Comparison of calcium-binding proteins expressed in cultured hNT neurons and hNT neurons transplanted into the rat striatum. *Exp.Neurol.,* 167, 252-259.

Sautter, J., Tseng, J. L., Braguglia, D., Aebischer, P., Spenger, C., Seiler, R. W., Widmer, H. R. & Zurn, A. D. 1998. Implants of polymer-encapsulated genetically modified cells releasing glial cell line-derived neurotrophic factor improve survival, growth, and function of fetal dopaminergic grafts. *Experimental Neurology,* 149 230-236.

Schuldiner, M., Eiges, R., Eden, A., Yanuka, O., Itskovitz-Eldor, J., Goldstein, R. S. & Benvenisty, N. 2001. Induced neuronal differentiation of human embryonic stem cells. *Brain Research,* 913, 201-205.

Sidhu, K. S. 2011. New approaches for the generation of induced pluripotent stem cells. *Expert Opin Biol Ther,* 11, 569-79.

Skogh, C., Parmar, M. & Campbell, K. 2003. The differentiation potential of precursor cells from the mouse lateral ganglionic eminence is restricted by in vitro expansion. *Neuroscience,* 120, 379-385.

Soldner, F., Hockemeyer, D., Beard, C., Gao, Q., Bell, G. W., Cook, E. G., Hargus, G., Blak, A., Cooper, O., Mitalipova, M., Isacson, O. & Jaenisch, R. 2009. Parkinson's Disease patient-derived induced pluripotent stem cells free of viral reprogramming factors. *Cell,* 136, 964-77.

Song, S., Wang, Y., Bak, S. Y., Lang, P., Ullrey, D., Neve, R. L., O'malley, K. L. & Geller, A. I. 1997. An HSV-1 vector containing the rat tyrosine hydroxylase promoter enhances both long-term and cell type-specific expression in the midbrain. *J.Neurochem.,* 68 1792-1803.

Stadtfeld, M., Nagaya, M., Utikal, J., Weir, G. & Hochedlinger, K. 2008. Induced pluripotent stem cells generated without viral integration. *Science,* 322, 945-9.

Steece-Collier, K., Soderstrom, K. E., Collier, T. J., Sortwell, C. E. & Maries-Lad, E. 2009. Effect of levodopa priming on dopamine neuron transplant efficacy and induction of abnormal involuntary movements in parkinsonian rats. *J Comp Neurol,* 515, 15-30.

Svendsen, C. N., Caldwell, M. A., Shen, J., Ter Borg, M. G., Rosser, A. E., Tyres, P., Karmiol, S. & Dunnett, S. B. 1997. Long-Term Survival of Human Central Nervous System Progenitor Cells Transplanted into a Rat Model of Parkinson's Disease. *Experimental Neurology,* 148, 135-146.

Takahashi, K., Tanabe, K., Ohnuki, M., Narita, M., Ichisaka, T., Tomoda, K. & Yamanaka, S. 2007. Induction of pluripotent stem cells from adult human fibroblasts by defined factors. *Cell,* 131, 861-72.

Takahashi, K. & Yamanaka, S. 2006. Induction of pluripotent stem cells from mouse embryonic and adult fibroblast cultures by defined factors. *Cell,* 126, 663-76.

Thomson, J. A., Itskovitz-Eldor, J., Shapiro, S. S., Waknitz, M. A., Swiergiel, J. J., Marshall, V. S. & Jones, J. M. 1998. Embryonic stem cell lines derived from human blastocysts. *Science,* 282, 1145-7.

Tropepe, V., Craig, C. G., Morshead, C. M. & Van Der Kooy, D. 1997. Transforming Growth Factor-a Null and Senescent Mice Show Decreased Neural Progenitor Cell Proliferation in the Forebrain Subependyma. *The Jouranl of Neuroscience,* 17, 7850-7859.

Ubiali, F., Nava, S., Nessi, V., Frigerio, S., Parati, E., Bernasconi, P., Mantegazza, R. & Baggi, F. 2007. Allorecognition of human neural stem cells by peripheral blood lymphocytes despite low expression of MHC molecules: role of TGF-beta in modulating proliferation. *Int Immunol,* 19, 1063-74.

Vassilopoulos, G., Wang, P. R. & Russell, D. W. 2003. Transplanted bone marrow regenerates liver by cell fusion. *Nature,* 422, 901-904.

Vicario-Abejon, C., Johe, K. K., Hazel, T. G., Collazo, D. & Mckay, R. D. 1995. Functions of basic fibroblast growth factor and neurotrophins in the differentiation of hippocampal neurons. *Neuron,* 15, 105-114.

Wang, X., Willenbring, H., Akkari, Y., Torimaru, Y., Foster, M., Al Dhalimy, M., Lagasse, E., Finegold, M., Olson, S. & Grompe, M. 2003. Cell fusion is the principal source of bone-marrow-derived hepatocytes. *Nature,* 422, 897-901.

Watt, F. M. & Hogan, B. L. M. 2000. Out of eden:Stem cells and their niches. *Science,* 287, 1427-1430.

Watts, C., Brasted, P. J. & Dunnett, S. B. 2000. The Morphology, Integration, and Functional Efficacy of Striatal Grafts Differ Between Cell Suspensions and Tissue Pieces. *Cell Transplantation,* 9 395-407.

Welstead, G. G., Schorderet, P. & Boyer, L. A. 2008. The reprogramming language of pluripotency. *Curr Opin Genet Dev,* 18, 123-9.

Wernig, M., Lengner, C. J., Hanna, J., Lodato, M. A., Steine, E., Foreman, R., Staerk, J., Markoulaki, S. & Jaenisch, R. 2008. A drug-inducible transgenic system for direct reprogramming of multiple somatic cell types. *Nat Biotechnol,* 26, 916-24.

Wernig, M., Meissner, A., Foreman, R., Brambrink, T., Ku, M., Hochedlinger, K., Bernstein, B. E. & Jaenisch, R. 2007. In vitro reprogramming of fibroblasts into a pluripotent ES-cell-like state. *Nature,* 448, 318-24.

Willing, A. E., Lixian, J., Milliken, M., Poulos, S., Zigova, T., Song, S., Hart, C., Sanchez-Ramos, J. & Sanberg, P. R. 2003. Intravenous versus intrastriatal cord blood administration in a rodent model of stroke. *J Neurosci Res.,* 73, 296-307.

Woltjen, K., Michael, I. P., Mohseni, P., Desai, R., Mileikovsky, M., Hamalainen, R., Cowling, R., Wang, W., Liu, P., Gertsenstein, M., Kaji, K., Sung, H. K. & Nagy, A. 2009. piggyBac transposition reprograms fibroblasts to induced pluripotent stem cells. *Nature,* 458, 766-70.

Yamanaka, S. 2008. Induction of pluripotent stem cells from mouse fibroblasts by four transcription factors. *Cell Prolif,* 41 Suppl 1, 51-6.

Yu, J., Hu, K., Smuga-Otto, K., Tian, S., Stewart, R., Slukvin, Ii & Thomson, J. A. 2009. Human induced pluripotent stem cells free of vector and transgene sequences. *Science,* 324, 797-801.

Yu, J., Vodyanik, M. A., Smuga-Otto, K., Antosiewicz-Bourget, J., Frane, J. L., Tian, S., Nie, J., Jonsdottir, G. A., Ruotti, V., Stewart, R., Slukvin, Ii & Thomson, J. A. 2007. Induced pluripotent stem cell lines derived from human somatic cells. *Science,* 318, 1917-20.

Zhao, L.-R., Duan, W.-M., Reyes, M., Keene, C. D., Verfaillie, C. M. & Low, W. C. 2002. Human Bone Marrow Stem Cells Exhibit Neural Phenotypes and Ameliorate Neurological Deficits after Grafting into the Ischemic Brain of Rats. *Experimental Neurology,* 174, 11-20.

Zhao, M., Momma, S., Delfani, K., Carlen, M., Cassidy, R. M., Johansson, C. B., Brismar, H., Shupliakov, O., Frisen, J. & Janson, A. M. 2003. Evidence for neurogenesis in the adult mammalian substantia nigra. *Proceedings of the National Academy of Sciences,* 100, 7925.
Zietlow, R., Pekarik, V., Armstrong, R. J., Tyers, P., Dunnett, S. B. & Rosser, A. E. 2005. The survival of neural precursor cell grafts is influenced by in vitro expansion. *Journal of anatomy,* 207, 227-40.
Zigova, T., Song, S., Willing, A. E., Hudson, J. E., Newman, M. B., Saporta, S., Sanchez-Ramos, J. & Sanberg, P. R. 2002. Human umbilical cord blood cells express neural antigens after transplantation into the developing rat brain. *Cell Transplant.,* 11, 265-274.

6

Ameliorating Huntington's Disease by Targeting Huntingtin mRNA

Melvin M. Evers[1], Rinkse Vlamings[2,3],
Yasin Temel[2,3] and Willeke M. C. van Roon-Mom[1]
*[1]Center for Human and Clinical Genetics,
Leiden University Medical Center, Leiden,
[2]Departments of Neuroscience and Neurosurgery,
Maastricht University Medical Center, Maastricht,
[3]European Graduate School of Neuroscience (EURON),
The Netherlands*

1. Introduction

To date there are 9 known neurological diseases caused by an expanded polyglutamine (polyQ) repeat, with the most prevalent being Huntington's Disease (HD) (Cummings & Zoghbi, 2000). HD is a progressive autosomal dominant disorder. It is caused by a CAG repeat expansion in the *HTT* gene, which results in an expansion of a polyQ stretch at the N-terminal end of the huntingtin (htt) protein. This polyQ expansion plays a central role in the disease and results in the accumulation of cytoplasmic and nuclear aggregates. In this chapter we will discuss wild-type htt function and the gain of toxic function of mutant htt in HD. Currently no treatment is available to delay onset or slow disease progression. However, recently developed RNA modulating therapies have great potential to lower mutant htt levels in HD. Already promising results in animal and human studies for other neurodegenerative disorders have been obtained, from which HD research can learn.

2. Huntington's Disease

HD is an autosomal dominantly inherited neurodegenerative disorder. HD is rare, but more common in Western countries. The prevalence of HD in America is approximately 5 in 100,000 (Shoulson & Young, 2011) and in Europe, the prevalence of HD may be even higher with estimates in England and Wales as high as 12 in 100,000 individuals (Rawlins, 2010).

Post-mortem studies show that there is a 10-20 percent weight reduction in HD brains (Vonsattel et al., 1985). Neurodegeneration occurs throughout the forebrain with the GABAergic medium spiny neurons of the striatum as its first prominent victim, and to a lesser extent neurons in the cerebral cortex (Levesque et al., 2003). Severe cell loss in the striatal complex, the caudate nucleus and putamen results in striatal atrophy. This is accompanied by an enlargement of the lateral ventricles. The medium spiny projection neurons, containing enkephalin, are more susceptive to degeneration than substance P containing neurons while interneurons seem to be spared (Walker, 2007). With disease progression, degeneration expands throughout the HD brain and other structures become affected (Vonsattel et al., 1985). Cortical atrophy is characterized by thinning of the cerebral cortex and the underlying white matter. Neuronal loss is abundant in cortical layers III, V and VI (Rosas et al., 2008) but is also prominent in the CA1 region of the hippocampus, with a reduction of about 9 percent (Rosas et al., 2003).

Disease onset usually occurs around midlife and is clinically characterized by a combination of symptoms: cognitive impairments, movement abnormalities, and emotional disturbances. Motor symptoms of HD include chorea and occasionally bradykinesia and dystonia (Tabrizi et al., 2009). Choreic movements, recognized as involuntary and unwanted movements, start in the distal extremities. During the course of HD these movements become more profound and eventually all other muscles of the body are affected. These symptoms can initially appear as lack of concentration or nervousness and unsteady gait (Kremer et al., 1992). Psychiatric symptoms often precede the onset of motor symptoms. Irritability is commonly one of the first signs and occurs throughout the course of the disease. Other psychiatric symptoms involve anxiety, obsessive and compulsive behavior while apathy and psychosis can appear in advanced stages. However, the most frequent psychiatric symptom is depression (Craufurd et al., 2001). Like psychiatric symptoms, cognitive symptoms can be present prior to the onset of the motor symptoms. The cognitive symptoms comprise mainly impairment in executive functions, including abstract thinking, problem solving, and attention (Snowden et al., 2002). Furthermore, the ability to learn new skills is affected (Paulsen et al., 2001). Altogether these symptoms substantially impede social and professional functioning. Eventually patients are incapable to adequately perform daily activities finally leading to progressive disability, requiring full-time care, followed by death (Simpson, 2007). Death generally occurs 15 to 20 years post diagnosis due to complications such as pneumonia, falls, dysphagia, heart disease or suicide.

The disease is caused by a CAG trinucleotide repeat expansion within the coding region of the *HTT* gene. The *HTT* gene was the first autosomal disease locus to be mapped by genetic linkage analysis in 1983 (Gusella et al., 1983) on the short arm of chromosome 4 (4p16.3). The huntingtin protein (htt) was found to be ubiquitously expressed throughout the body, with highest expression in testis and brain (Strong et al., 1993), however, cells in the brain are specifically vulnerable to the toxic function of mutant htt. The CAG repeat expansion in the *HTT* gene results in an expanded polyQ repeat in the htt protein (The Huntington's Disease Collaborative Research Group, 1993). When the number of CAG repeats exceeds 39, the gene encodes a mutated form of the htt protein that is prone to aggregation. Alleles ranging 36 to 39 repeats, lead to an incomplete and variable penetrance of the disease or to a very late onset (McNeil et al., 1997). Repeat numbers exceeding 55-60 result in clinical manifestation of the disease before the age of 20, known as Juvenile Huntington's Disease (JHD) (Andresen et al., 2007) and both sexes are affected with the same frequency (Walker, 2007). Intergenerational CAG changes are extremely rare on normal chromosomes but on expanded chromosomes changes in CAG size take place in approximately 70 percent of meioses and expansion is more likely via the paternal line (Kremer et al., 1995).

There is a strong inverse correlation between repeat numbers and the age of onset of the disease. The repeat length accounts for approximately 70 percent of the variance in age of onset (Roos, 2010). However, no correlation with repeat size is apparent for the progression and duration of the disease. Furthermore, neuropathological changes, such as atrophy and inclusion load are clearly correlated with the CAG repeat number.

For patients, only symptomatic treatment is available and a treatment to slow down the progression or delay the onset of the disease remains elusive.

2.1 Huntingtin protein

When the *HTT* gene was discovered in 1993, the htt protein had an unknown function. Since then, enormous research efforts have revealed many functions of the wild-type protein (discussed in the present paragraph) and many toxic gain of functions of the mutant protein (discussed in the next paragraph).

Wild-type htt is mainly localized in the cytoplasm, although a small proportion is present in the nucleus (de Rooij et al., 1996; Kegel et al., 2002). The protein is known to be associated with microtubules, the plasma membrane, Golgi complex, the endoplasmic reticulum, and mitochondria. Furthermore htt is associated with vesicular structures, such as clathrin-coated and non-coated vesicles, autophagic vesicles, endosomal compartments or caveolae (Kegel et al., 2005; Strehlow et al., 2007; Rockabrand et al., 2007; Atwal et al., 2007; Caviston et al., 2011).

Three of the first 17 amino acids at the amino terminus of htt are lysines, which are targets for post translational modifications that regulate htt half-life and are proposed to be involved in targeting htt to various intracellular membrane-associated organelles (Kalchman et al., 1996; Steffan et al., 2004; Kegel et al., 2005; Atwal et al., 2007; Rockabrand et al., 2007). The first 17 amino acids of htt have also been suggested to act as nuclear export signal (NES) by interaction with the nuclear pore protein translocated promoter region (Tpr) that then transports N-terminal htt fragments out of the nucleus (Cornett et al., 2005). The polyQ repeat starts at the 18th amino acid and is thought to form a polar zipper structure, which has been implicated in the interaction between different polyQ-containing transcription factors (Perutz et al., 1994; Harjes & Wanker, 2003). The polyQ stretch is followed by a polyproline repeat, which is thought to be involved in keeping the protein soluble (Steffan et al., 2004). Additionally, three main HEAT (htt, elongation factor 3, protein phosphatase 2A, and the yeast PI3-kinase TOR1) repeat motifs are identified which are known to form superhelical structures and are involved in protein-protein interactions (Takano & Gusella, 2002; Li et al., 2006). Htt is palmitoylated at the cysteine residue 214 by htt interacting protein (Hip) 14, which is thought to be involved in htt trafficking (Huang et al., 2004). Htt has various proteolytic cleavage motifs, with a hotspot between amino acid 500 and 600, which are recognized by various proteases, such as caspases 1, 3, 6, 7 and 8 and calpain (Gafni & Ellerby, 2002; Wellington et al., 2002; Kim et al., 2006). In contrast to mutant htt, the significance of wild-type htt cleavage is not completely clear.

2.2 Mutant htt gain of toxic function in HD

Expanded polyQ proteins are known to undergo conformational changes, which result in the hallmark of polyQ disorders, protein aggregates. The aggregates can already be found before the onset of the first symptoms (Weiss et al., 2008). Remarkably, there is growing evidence suggesting that these aggregates are not good indicators for disease onset and progression (Wanker, 2000; van Roon-Mom et al., 2006). The rate of aggregate formation is correlated to the length of the polyQ repeat (Legleiter et al., 2010). Whether accumulation of these aggregates is neurotoxic or neuroprotective is still under debate since evidence also suggests that soluble mutant htt is the main toxic component (Davies et al., 1997; Saudou et al., 1998; Arrasate et al., 2004). While the expanded polyQ repeat displays pathogenic properties it is probably not essential for normal function (Clabough & Zeitlin, 2006). Mutant htt is more disposed to proteolysis and it was shown that small N-terminal htt fragments are more toxic than full length mutant htt (Cooper et al., 1998). Proteolytic cleavage of mutant htt results in nuclear localization of toxic N-terminal mutant htt fragments. These N-terminal mutant htt fragments are important in the pathological process. Mutant htt fragments within the striatum of HD brains clearly differ from those of control brains, suggesting cleavage is disease specific (Mende-Mueller et al., 2001) and htt caspase-6 resistant HD mice did not show neuronal dysfunction (Graham et al., 2006).

Various transcription factors have been found to co-localize with htt aggregates, such as TATA box binding protein (TBP), CREB binding protein (CBP) and p53 (Steffan et al., 2000; van Roon-Mom et al., 2002). These co-aggregated proteins can no longer assert their normal function and could thereby contribute to HD pathology (Nucifora, Jr. et al., 2001)

Mutant htt is also suggested to act as pro-apoptotic factor triggering cell death. Htt is found to bind to the pro-apoptotic factor p53. Interestingly, p53 deficient HD mice displayed increased striatal inclusion body formation (Ryan et al., 2006). Expression of mutant htt in p53 deficient mice improved the lifespan probably by increased apoptosis initiated by mutant htt (Ryan & Scrable, 2008).

In HD the fusion machinery and axonal transport are impaired. Accumulated N-terminal fragments block the axonal machinery, resulting in transport defects (Gunawardena et al., 2003). Endocytosis is thought to be impaired since the synaptic vesicle protein PACSIN1 has an altered subcellular location in early stage HD patients (Modregger et al., 2002). Finally, various proteins involved in exocytosis are known to have decreased expression levels in HD patients. Proteins involved in docking and fusion of vesicles show reduced transcript expression, suggesting a defect in the neurotransmitter release machinery in HD patients (Smith et al., 2007).

N-terminal mutant htt fragments are found to be associated with the surface of mitochondria in transgenic and knock-in HD mice (Panov et al., 2002; Orr et al., 2008). The accumulation of mutant htt on mitochondria is increasing with age and correlates with disease progression. This impaired mitochondrial trafficking by N-terminal mutant htt could lead to decreased ATP supply in nerve terminals (Orr et al., 2008). Mutant htt is also suggested to be involved mitochondrial energy metabolism defects. Metabolic energy defects could be the result of mutant htt's capability to induce mitochondrial permeability transition pore opening. This leads to low mitochondrial membrane potential and high glutamate transmission, resulting in overactive glutamate NMDA receptors (excitotoxicity) (Choo et al., 2004). Abnormal mitochondrial respiratory chain function leads to reduced ATP levels and subsequent partially depolarized membrane. This voltage change leads to chronic calcium influx and activation of proteases, causing more reactive oxygen species (ROS) production. Further, increased ROS production gives rise to oxidative stress and could contribute to the vicious circle (Browne & Beal, 2006).

2.3 Loss of wild-type function in HD

As described above, the main cause of HD is a gain of toxic mutant htt function. Since various functions and post-translational modifications of htt are altered in HD, loss of wild-type htt function could also be involved. Htt expression is important for normal cellular function since knock-out of the homologous htt mouse gene was found to be early embryonic lethal (Zeitlin et al., 1995). Previous studies have shown that approximately 50% of htt protein level is required to maintain cell functionality (Dragatsis et al., 2000). Next to embryonic development, htt is also involved in regulation of apoptosis, transcription, intracellular transport and BDNF transcription (Zuccato et al., 2001; Imarisio et al., 2008).

Wild-type htt is reported to act as protector of the brain cells from apoptotic stimuli (Rigamonti et al., 2000). Reduced wild-type htt expression in transgenic HD mice resulted in worsening of the behavioural deficits and survival. In addition, no severe striatal abnormalities were visible in those HD mice, which could mean that the striatal phenotype is mainly caused by mutant htt toxicity (Zhang et al., 2003). Furthermore, overexpression of wild-type htt protected these mice against neurodegeneration. Removal of endogenous htt in a *Drosophila melanogaster (D. melanogaster)* HD model was found to exacerbate the neurodegenerative phenotype associated, suggesting that loss of normal htt function might also contribute to HD pathogenesis (Zhang et al., 2009).

3. HTT RNA

Although the main toxic component is the htt protein, recent evidence suggests that also HTT RNA could have toxic properties. There is also recent evidence for antisense transcription through the *HTT* locus. In this paragraph we will review the importance of these findings.

3.1 Htt RNA gain of function in HD

Trinucleotide expansion disorders occur either in untranslated genomic regions (UTRs) resulting in a toxic RNA gain of function or loss of gene function, or in coding regions resulting in a gain of toxic protein function (Orr & Zoghbi, 2007). Until recently, it was believed that HD is solely caused by a toxic gain of function of the polyQ protein and to a lesser extent, loss of wild-type function. However, recent evidence suggests that the mutant CAG repeats of the HTT RNA transcript could also have toxic properties (Fig. 1). This RNA toxicity is caused by the long hairpin structures of the expanded RNA that result in abnormal interactions with double stranded RNA-binding proteins.

The CAG repeat hairpin in the HTT transcript was found to be stabilized by the flanking (CCG)n repeat (de Mezer et al., 2011). The resulting double stranded CAG RNA hairpin formed intranuclear foci that co-localized with the muscleblind-like 1 (MBNL1) splicing factor (Jiang et al., 2004). Altered MBNL1 function is implicated in RNA toxicity of CUG repeat expansion disorders such as myotonic dystrophy type 1 (DM1) (Kanadia et al., 2003). DM1 is caused by a CTG repeat expansion at the 3′ UTR of the *DMPK* gene. The CTG repeats are known to form stable hairpin structures that are toxic by causing abnormal alternative splicing by MBNL1 binding and sequestering in nuclear foci (Fardaei et al., 2001; Kanadia et al., 2003). Similar to expanded CUG repeats in DM1, synthesized expanded CAG repeats also resulted in abnormal alternative splicing in both transiently transfected and patient-derived cells (Mykowska et al., 2011). The RNA toxicity modifier MBNL1 was also found to be involved in another polyQ disease, namely spinocerebellar ataxia 3 (SCA3). MBNL1 was found to be up-regulated in a *D. melanogaster* model of SCA3. The neurodegenerative disorder SCA3 is caused by a CAG repeat expansion in the *ATXN3* gene, which results in the expression of a polyQ containing ataxin-3 protein. Upregulation of the *D. melanogaster* homolog of MBNL1 (*mbl*) was found to enhance pathogenic ataxin-3 protein induced toxicity, as well as pathogenic mutant htt protein induced toxicity (Li et al., 2008).

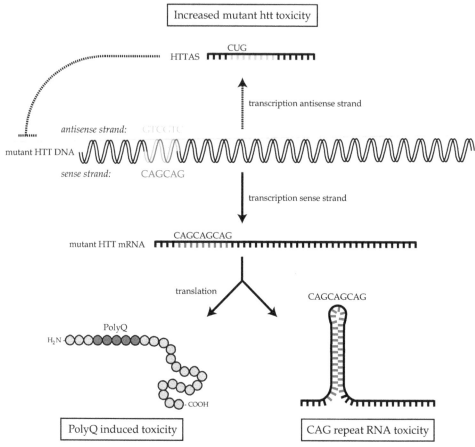

Fig. 1. Schematic representation of modes of huntingtin toxicity in HD. Mutant htt transcription results in mutant HTT mRNA which can form double stranded hairpins through the expanded CAG repeat and adjacent CCG repeat. The CAG hairpin is involved in MBNL1 induced alternative splicing and toxicity. The main pathological process in HD involves the translation of expanded CAG repeat-containing mRNA into a toxic polyQ protein. Antisense transcription through the *HTT* gene results in a HTT antisense transcript (HTTAS). This HTTAS regulates HTT sense levels. In HD there is lower expression of HTTAS, resulting in increased levels of the HTT sense transcript and increased mutant htt toxicity.

HD and SCA3 transgenes with a CAG repeat interrupted by CAA codons (expressing an identical polyQ protein as compared to a pure CAG repeat) showed only a mild phenotype, indicating the importance of the expanded pure CAG repeat for the toxic phenotype. Interestingly, both full CAG repeats and CAA interrupted CAG repeats showed similar levels of protein inclusions, indicating that the phenotype severity does not correlate with the number of inclusions (Li et al., 2008).

Recently, transgenic mice expressing a GFP construct with 200 CAGs in the 3' UTR resulted in reduced GFP levels as compared to animals with 23 CAG repeats in their 3' UTR of the GFP construct (Hsu et al., 2011). Furthermore, these CAG_{200} mice showed nuclear RNA foci and a reduced breeding efficiency, which supports the gain of RNA toxicity hypothesis.

Transgenic *Caenorhabditis elegans* (*C. elegans*) expressing various CAG repeat lengths in the 3' UTR of a GFP gene showed a length-dependent toxicity. Worms with an 83 CAG repeat did not show any phenotype, whereas *C. elegans* expressing 200 CAGs died within a few days. Both 125 CUGs and 125 CAGs co-localized in nuclear foci with *C. elegans* MBNL1 homolog CeMBL and overexpression of CeMBL partly reversed the CAG 125 induced phenotype (Wang et al., 2011).

In contrast to the above studies, there is also evidence that the CAG repeat RNA is not toxic. Expression of a cDNA construct with 79 CAG repeats in the 3' UTR did not induce cell death, whereas a construct expressing 79 CAGs in the coding region did induce cell death (Ikeda et al., 1996). This was also found in two other polyQ disorders, spinocerebellar ataxia 1 (SCA1) and spinobulbar muscular atrophy (SBMA). A SCA1 mouse model with impaired nuclear localization signal in ataxin-1 did not show nuclear inclusion bodies and did not display the disease phenotype (Klement et al., 1998). Furthermore, impairing nuclear localization of the androgen receptor (AR) in SBMA by castration showed marked improvements of disease pathology, also suggesting that the pathology is mainly caused by gain of toxic protein and not RNA (Katsuno et al., 2002). A *D. melanogaster* model of CAG toxicity expressing a repeat construct with a premature termination codon before a 93 CAG repeat, did not show any phenotype (McLeod et al., 2005). Based on these results, it was suggested that the toxicity in CAG triplet repeat disorders was exclusively the result of expanded polyQ protein gain of function.

From the above we can conclude that not only gain of toxicity by expanded polyQ protein, but also RNA toxicity from the expanded CAG repeat could be involved in HD pathology. However, the size of the CAG repeat is critical for RNA pathogenicity.

3.2 HTT antisense transcription

A large proportion of the genome can produce transcripts from both strands (Katayama et al., 2005). It has become clear that antisense transcripts are involved in triplet repeat disorders and bidirectional transcription has thus far been identified in DM1, spinocerebellar ataxia 8 (SCA8), and HD like 2 (HDL2) (Moseley et al., 2006; Wilburn et al., 2011).

In SCA8, which is caused by a CTG repeat expansion in a transcribed but not translated *ATXN8OS* gene, it was thought that the expanded CTG repeat caused RNA toxicity (Koob et al., 1999). Unexpectedly, bacterial artificial chromosome (BAC) transgenic SCA8 mice showed 1C2 positive inclusion bodies. The 1C2 antibody specifically recognizes expanded polyQ tracts, which are the hallmark of polyQ disorders. A novel transcript called ataxin-8, which encodes a polyQ protein, was expressed from the opposite strand, suggesting polyQ induced toxicity (Moseley et al., 2006). A BAC HDL2 mouse model with a pathogenic CTG repeat on the sense and expanded CAG repeat on the antisense strand at the *Junctophilin-3* locus showed both RNA toxicity caused by its expanded CUG repeat as well as protein toxicity by its polyQ translated expanded CAG repeat (Wilburn et al., 2011). These findings suggest that triplet repeat disorders can involve toxic gain of function of both protein and RNA by bidirectional transcription.

Recently, two natural HTT antisense (HTTAS) transcripts were identified at the HD locus (Chung et al., 2011). HTTAS was found to be 5' capped, poly A-tailed and contained 3 exons. There were two different isoforms identified of which one enclosed a functional promotor and the CTG repeat. The HTTAS containing the short CTG repeat was found to be widely expressed in multiple tissues. Remarkably, expanded CTG repeat containing HTTAS was strongly reduced in HD brains. The authors state that HTTAS acts as a negative regulator for HTT transcript expression as knock-down of HTTAS resulted in higher htt levels and overexpression of HTTAS resulted in lower HTT levels (Chung et al., 2011). This negative regulating property on HTT of HTTAS could potentially have a clinical implication by overexpressing HTTAS in HD patients, thereby alleviating pathogenicity by lowering htt levels.

4. RNA modulating therapies in HD

Although the *HTT* gene was identified in 1993, there are no treatments to cure or even slow down the progression of the disease. Most therapeutic strategies under investigation are targeting one of the many altered cellular processes caused by toxic mutant htt. Targeting a single cellular process might be inadequate to be clinically beneficial.

A more effective approach would be to reduce the expression of the causative *HTT* gene and thereby inhibiting all downstream toxic effects. Recent advances to inhibit the formation of mutant polyQ proteins using RNA modulating therapies, such as RNA interference (RNAi) and antisense oligonucleotides (AONs) look promising for HD (Sah & Aronin, 2011). RNAi is an endogenous cellular process involved in transcriptional regulation and acts as cellular defense mechanism against exogenous viral components. RNAi by introducing small interfering RNA (siRNA), short hairpin RNA (shRNA), or artificial micro RNA (miRNA), is increasingly used as a potential therapeutic tool to reduce expression of target transcripts. Specific knock-down is also achieved by introducing modified single stranded AONs that can hybridize to the target RNA, which is subsequently degraded or its translation blocked.

The most frequently used htt RNA modulating strategies for HD are: Knock-down of total htt RNA levels by targeting both wild-type and mutant htt and allele-specific reduction of mutant htt RNA only (Fig. 2).

4.1 Gene therapy to lower both htt alleles in HD

Since htt has many important wild-type functions, one of the key questions that needs to be answered for htt lowering strategies to become successful is how much htt is needed for normal function, or rather, how much can htt levels be reduced before adverse effects become apparent. Below we will first describe the studies describing lowering of both wild type and mutant htt, followed by the different approaches for allele specifically lowering mutant htt only.

Various synthetic oligonucleotides with different modifications and backbones have been used in rodents to partially lower htt expression. A partial reduction of both normal and mutant htt by 25 to 35% using shRNAs was found to be well-tolerated in wild-type rats up to 9 months without signs of toxicity or striatal degeneration (Drouet et al., 2009). Total silencing using artificial miRNAs for both wild-type and mutant htt of 75% within the striatum of a transgenic HD mouse model showed reduced toxicity, extended survival, and improved motor performance, 3 months after treatment (Boudreau et al., 2009).

Striatal injection of non allele-specific artificial miRNA in wild-type mice resulted in 70% reduction of htt levels. The high murine htt transcript reduction was sustained without adverse side effects up to the end of their study, which was set at 4 months (McBride et al., 2008). Since htt lowering strategies will be most beneficial for patients when administered over many years, the long-term safety needs to be assessed. Therefore, simultaneously lowering transcript levels from both alleles can only be applied once the role of wild-type htt in the human brain is elucidated in more detail. Moreover, to date it is not known if there is equal transcription from both the mutant and wild-type htt allele. Lowering total htt transcript levels by 70% does not necessarily mean an equal reduction of both alleles by 70%.

4.2 Allele-specific reduction of mutant htt in HD

As described in previous paragraphs, endogenous htt expression is important for normal cellular function and an ideal strategy for an autosomal dominant disorder as HD would be to specifically target the mutant allele and thereby maintaining as much wild-type htt protein as possible. Suppression of 50% to 80% using siRNA specific for human mutant htt in transgenic rodent models of HD for 4 months was found to improve motor and neuropathological abnormalities and prolonged longevity in HD mice (Harper et al., 2005; Wang et al., 2005). These studies showed that lowering mutant htt without reducing wild-type htt levels, resulted in an improved pathology. These results favored an allele-specific htt lowering approach without altering the expression of endogenous wild-type htt expression. Various studies have shown that a pronounced decrease of mutant htt levels, with only minor reductions in wild-type htt is feasible using allele-specific oligonucleotides. The different approaches, their advantages and disadvantages will be discussed in the following paragraph.

4.2.1 Targeting associated SNPs in HD

Single nucleotide polymorphisms (SNPs) are DNA sequence variations that occur when a single nucleotide is different between the two alleles of a gene. One way to distinguish between the wild-type and polyQ disease-causing allele is to target such a SNP that is unique to the mutant transcript using siRNAs (Miller et al., 2003). siRNAs are known to discriminate between transcripts that differ at a single nucleotide and various studies have shown specific reduction of mutant htt mRNA using siRNAs directed against different SNPs. The first evidence of allele-specific silencing in HD using using SNP specific RNAi was obtained in human cells overexpressing htt transgenes (Schwarz et al., 2006). The first prove of principle of endogenous mutant htt silencing using SNPs in fibroblasts derived from HD patients was acquired in 2008 (van Bilsen et al., 2008). Extensive genotyping revealed a group of 22 SNPs highly associated with mutant htt alleles in a European HD cohort (Warby et al., 2009). Since then, various groups have shown that the vast majority of the HD patient population could be treated using 5 (75% of HD patients) or 7 (85% of the HD patients) different siRNAs (Lombardi et al., 2009; Pfister et al., 2009). The most promising SNP was found to be located in exon 67 of the *HTT* gene. This SNP is strongly associated with the mutant allele and 48% of the total Western HD population was heterozygous at this site (Pfister et al., 2009).

Most of the heterozygous SNPs linked to the expanded CAG repeat in exon 1, are found remote downstream from the CAG repeat in exons 25 up to 67 (Lombardi et al., 2009; Pfister et al., 2009). To determine in HD patients whether they are heterozygous and if yes, which SNP belongs to the expanded CAG repeat, a technique called SNP linkage by circularization (SLiC) was developed (Liu et al., 2008). By circulating the DNA, the CAG repeat and SNP site were brought together, making it easy to link the SNP to the expanded CAG repeat using a single PCR.

Although the selectivity obtained from above described SNP targeting siRNAs are very promising, there are some limitations. The diversity of SNPs within patient populations would make it necessary to develop multiple siRNAs. Furthermore, for HD patients that do not exhibit any of the most frequent SNPs a different treatment needs to be developed.

4.2.2 Targeting the expanded CAG repeat in mutant HTT

Another approach to achieve allele-specific silencing is based on the common denominator of all HD patients; their expanded CAG repeat. The selective silencing is either based on the hypothesis that there are structural differences between wild-type and mutant htt mRNA, or based on the larger number of CAGs in the expanded repeat and subsequent more binding possibilities. The first prove for allele discrimination by targeting the CAG repeat was achieved in HD human fibroblasts using a siRNA with 7 consecutive CUG nucleotides (Krol et al., 2007). Further studies with CAG repeat targeting siRNAs showed a low selectivity for the mutant allele, making siRNAs incompatible for CAG repeat directed allele-specific silencing (Hu et al., 2009). Other chemical modifications and oligomers show much higher specificity for expanded CAG repeat transcripts. Single stranded peptide nucleic acids (PNA), locked nucleic acids (LNA), and AONs with a 2'O methyl addition and phosphorothioate backbone targeting CAG repeats have been used to specifically reduce expanded HD transcripts *in vitro* in patient derived skin and blood cells (Hu et al., 2009; Evers et al., 2011). However, PNA selectivity was less pronounced in CAG repeat lengths (40 to 45 CAGs) that occur most frequently in the HD patient population. The allele-specific reduction after transfection of patient cells with LNAs and AONs with 7-mer CUG repeats was more pronounced in the average HD CAG repeat length. Furthermore, other endogenous CAG repeat containing transcripts with important cellular functions were unaffected by the tested CUG oligonucleotides (Hu et al., 2009; Evers et al., 2011).

The main advantages of LNAs and AONs are that they are single stranded and do not show toxicity *in vivo*. Systemic delivery of modified AONs in Duchenne muscular dystrophy (DMD) boys carrying specific deletions in the DMD gene induced the synthesis of novel, internally deleted, but likely (semi-) functional, dystrophin proteins without clinically apparent adverse event (Goemans et al., 2011).

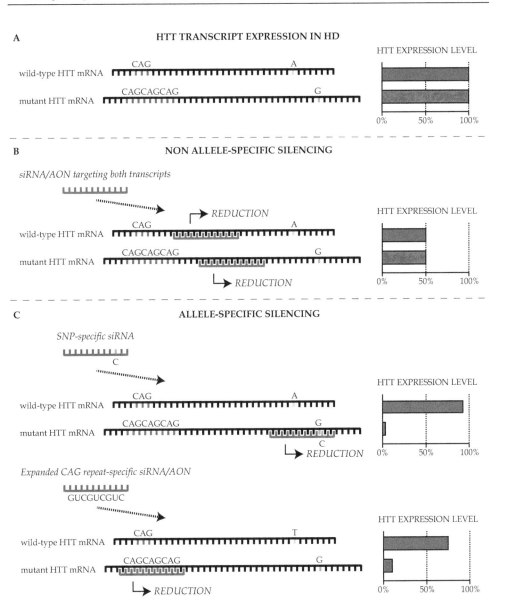

Fig. 2. RNA modulating therapeutic approaches for lowering htt. Two different HTT RNA modulating strategies used for HD are: A) Non allele-specific reduction of total HTT RNA levels by targeting a sequence that is identical in both the wild-type and mutant HTT transcript. B) Allele-specific reduction of mutant HTT RNA by targeting a unique heterozygous SNPs only present in the mutant transcript or C) Allele-specific reduction targeting the expanded CAG repeat on the mutant HTT transcripts.

Likewise, the use of only a single AON was suggested to be effective as treatment of various polyQ diseases (Hu et al., 2009; Evers et al., 2011). One expanded CAG repeat targeting AON was found to specifically reduce the expression of mutant ataxin-1 and ataxin-3 mRNA levels in SCA1 and 3, respectively, and mutant atrophin-1 in dentatorubral-pallidoluysian atrophy (DRPLA) in patient derived cells (Evers et al., 2011).

Although these results are promising, extensive research is needed to elucidate the mechanism used by those oligonucleotides to induce selective silencing and to assess specificity and safety. Likewise, the full potency of this allele-specific treatment will be revealed when the first *in vivo* results are obtained.

5. RNA modulating therapies in other neurodegenerative diseases

AONs have also been used for the treatment of neurodegenerative disorders and are found to be taken up by neurons when delivered into the cerebral lateral ventricles. Here are some examples showing therapeutic benefit in animal models and/or clinical trials.

5.1 Prevention of mutant protein translation

We will first focus on the neurodegenerative disorder amyotrophic lateral sclerosis (ALS) where RNA modulating therapeutics are used to reduce transcript levels of disease causing protein. The RNA modulating therapeutics to treat ALS are currently tested in a phase I clinical trial.

The progressive neurodegenerative muscle weakness disorder ALS is a caused by loss of motor neurons in the brain and spinal cord (Al-Chalabi & Leigh, 2000). The first mutations linked to the familial form of ALS (fALS) were found in the *superoxide dismutase 1 (SOD1)* gene. Mutated SOD1 is known to be toxic and prone to aggregation. Only approximately 1% of ALS cases is the result of mutations in the SOD1 enzyme (Bossy-Wetzel et al., 2004).

RNA modulating therapies that have been used in ALS were designed to block the translation of SOD1. In a transgenic mouse model of ALS, 2'O methoxyethyl modified AONs were used to lower mutant SOD1 levels by binding and subsequent RNase H mediated breakdown of SOD1 transcripts. Continuous ventricular infusion of the SOD1 targeting AON significantly slowed disease progression (Smith et al., 2006). The first results of a phase I study testing the safety of this SOD1 targeting AON in patients with fALS caused by mutant SOD1 are expected at the end of 2011. The outcomes of this phase I trial will be vital for future trials with RNA modulating therapies in HD.

5.2 Modulating pre-mRNA splicing

RNA modulating therapeutics are also used to modulate pre-mRNA splicing events in spinal muscular atrophy (SMA) using modified AON *in vivo*.

SMA is an autosomal recessive neuromuscular disorder caused by loss of function of the *survival motor neuron 1 (SMN1)* gene. This homozygous deletion of SMN1 results in degeneration of motor neurons in the anterior horn of the spinal cord and lower brain stem (Bowers et al., 2011). Depletion of SMN1 is not embryonic lethal because of the presence of the almost identical *SMN2* gene. However, due to a point mutation in an intron the SMN2 transcript is not correctly spliced. The majority of SMN2 transcripts are therefore lacking exon 7, which results in a truncated protein and lower expression of a functional SMN protein (Lorson et al., 2010).

Current therapeutic strategies are aimed at modulating alternative splicing of SMN2. Transfecting fibroblasts with an AON blocking intronic splicing silencers in intron 7 of SMN2 were found to result in inclusion of SMN2 exon 7 (Singh et al., 2006). Injection of differently modified AONs into the brains of SMA mouse models resulted in increased exon 7 inclusion and subsequent elevated SMN protein levels. The AON treated SMA mice displayed increased muscle size and extended survival (Williams et al., 2009; Hua et al., 2010; Passini et al., 2011).

Another modulating pre-mRNA splicing strategy involves the addition of a functional moiety to the AON to replace the missing splicing enhancer protein, thereby enhancing the inclusion of exon 7 by the splicing machinery (Cartegni & Krainer, 2003; Skordis et al., 2003). Several *in vivo* studies have shown increased SMN2 protein levels after intraventricular injection of splicing factors recruiting AONs (Dickson et al., 2008; Baughan et al., 2009).

The AONs to treat SMA show promising results *in vivo* and the progression in therapeutics will be monitored closely. Results regarding delivery of the AON to the brain in humans and how well the AON is tolerated will be very useful for the development of RNA modulating therapeutics for HD.

6. Drug delivery to the brain, how to cross the blood brain barrier?

One major challenge of AON therapies for neurodegenerative disorders is delivery of the AON to the target organ. In the following paragraph we will describe in short the blood brain barrier function and how this impairs the uptake of peripherally administered drugs. We will focus in particular on the limitations and possibilities of AON delivery to the brain and will speculate on future clinical applications.

6.1 Blood brain barrier

A unique feature of the brain is that it is separated from the blood by the blood brain barrier (BBB). This is a monolayer of endothelial cells forming tight junctions through the interaction of cell adhesion molecules (Palmer, 2010). Astrocytes with their processes surrounding the endothelial cells, pericytes located between the endothelial cells and astrocytes, macrophages, and the basement membrane, form the other structural components of the BBB. Endothelial cells of the BBB are characterized by only few fenestrae and pinocytic vesicles, limiting transport to and from the brain. In this respect, it should be noted that the BBB also separates largely the immune system from the brain. Despite this gate-controlling system, essential nutrients, such as glucose, are permitted to pass (Bernacki et al., 2008). In neurodegenerative diseases, including HD, disruption of the BBB is common (Tomkins et al., 2007; Palmer, 2010). Interestingly, in animal models, this can even lead to neurodegenerative changes itself (Tomkins et al., 2007).

The BBB has been already noticed in the work of Paul Ehrlich, Nobel Prize winning bacteriologist in the late 19th century. Injected dyes stained all organs except the brain and spinal cord. However, he did not attribute this phenomenon to the presence of a barrier but to dye characteristics. His student showed later that staining of the brain was possible when the dye was injected directly into the brain (Palmer, 2010). Subsequent studies using electron microscopy were able to directly visualize the BBB.

The BBB is a major challenge in central nervous system (CNS) drug development. When a drug is administered to the body, a fraction will be bound to proteins (e.g. serum albumin, lipoprotein etc.) and a fraction will be free. The free fraction is the pharmacologically relevant fraction, since it is available to cross the BBB (Palmer, 2010), depending on its physiochemical properties. After crossing the BBB, the drug will enter the interstitial fluid and go to the target (proteins, receptors, transporters etc.). Subsequently, the interstitial fluid drains to the cerebrospinal fluid (CSF), which is produced at a rate of 500 ml/day in humans, while the ventricle system can house only 100-150 ml. This means that there is at least 3 times CSF circulation, allowing continuous drainage of the brain's interstitial fluid.

6.2 Crossing the blood brain barrier

In the process of drug discovery, the aim is to find a substance which is potent, selective and preferably bioavailable. In addition, it needs to be able to cross the BBB, and reach the target at a sufficient concentration (Alavijeh et al., 2005). The following mechanisms are available to cross the BBB. The first one is simple diffusion. Small lipophilic substances which have a hydrogen bond are more likely to pass the BBB (Gerebtzoff & Seelig, 2006). The second mechanism is via active transport mediated by transporter molecules. The most well-known is glucose with its glucose transporter 1 (GLUT1), which is the most widely expressed among the GLUT family (13 isoforms) (Guo et al., 2005; Palmer, 2010). Other carriers are for instance lactate and amino acids. A well-known drug transported via this way is levodopa (Cotzias et al., 1967). The third mechanism to cross the BBB is via receptor-mediation. Receptor-mediated endocytosis allows macromolecules to enter the brain, such as transferrin, insulin, leptin, and insulin-like growth factor 1 (Pardridge, 2007).

Besides systemic mechanisms to cross the BBB, there are also techniques to bypass the BBB by direct infusions into the subdural space, the brain's ventricle system, or the brain parenchyma. These infusions can be single, repeated, or continuous depending on the methodology, using either simple or sophisticated pump systems. It is possible to use one probe or more probes for infusion. Using the subdural and ventricle compartments, diffuse delivery of the drug into the brain can be achieved, while using intraparenchymal delivery, a local, but well-targeted delivery can be realized

When a substance has successfully entered the brain, there are mechanisms preventing adequate functioning. One mechanism is active transport to remove the substance, also known as resistance. A superfamily of multidrug resistance proteins, belonging to the ATP-binding cassette transporters, drives substances away by an ATP-dependent process (Palmer, 2010). One of the most abundant proteins is the P-glycoprotein. This mechanism is responsible for the failure of some anticancer drugs. Another family of egress transporters is the organic anion transporting proteins.

In the field of HD, efforts are ongoing to deliver innovative drugs to the brain via the systemic route and drugs are designed to use one of the three mechanisms to cross the BBB, as explained earlier. For instance, Lee and associates described the use of a peptide nucleic acid as an antisense which was able to access endogenous transferrin transport pathways (receptor mediated endocytosis) and reach the brain in a transgenic mouse model (Lee et al., 2002). However, there are also efforts to bypass the BBB, and to deliver the drug using either the ventricle system or intraparenchymally.

7. Conclusion

To date there is no treatment to prevent or even slow down the progression of HD. Considerable research has been performed to gain more insight into HD pathology. Next to the well-known toxic gain of polyQ protein function, loss of wild-type function and a toxic gain of expanded CAG repeat RNA was also suggested recently, and needs to be examined in more detail.

Recent results using SNP specific siRNAs and CAG targeting AONs look promising both *in vitro* and *in vivo*. To develop an effective HD therapy, it is likely that a combination of different RNA modifying approaches will be optimal to lower mutant htt levels. Extensive research is required to rule out toxic off-targets effects and elucidate the exact mode of action of these RNA modulating therapeutics. Ongoing clinical trials for other neurodegenerative disorders, such as in ALS, will give us more insights in the potential of RNA modulating therapeutics.

8. Acknowledgement

MME and WvRM are supported by the Center for Biomedical Genetics (the Netherlands), AtaxiaUK (United Kingdom), Dutch ataxia charity ADCA-VN (the Netherlands), and IOP Genomics (the Netherlands). The HD related research of RV and YT received financial support from the Cure Huntington's Disease Initiative (New York, USA) and Prosensa BV (Leiden, the Netherlands).

9. References

Al-Chalabi,A. & Leigh,P.N. (2000). Recent advances in amyotrophic lateral sclerosis. *Curr. Opin. Neurol*, Vol.13, No.4, pp.397-405

Alavijeh, M.S., Chishty, M., Qaiser, M.Z. & Palmer, A.M. (2005). Drug metabolism and pharmacokinetics, the blood-brain barrier, and central nervous system drug discovery. *NeuroRx.*, Vol.2, No.4, pp.554-571

Andresen, J.M., Gayan, J., Djousse, L., Roberts, S., Brocklebank, D., Cherny, S.S., Cardon, L.R., Gusella, J.F., MacDonald, M.E., Myers, R.H., Housman, D.E. & Wexler, N.S. (2007). The relationship between CAG repeat length and age of onset differs for Huntington's disease patients with juvenile onset or adult onset. *Ann Hum. Genet*, Vol.71, No.Pt 3, pp.295-301

Arrasate, M., Mitra, S., Schweitzer, E.S., Segal, M.R. & Finkbeiner, S. (2004). Inclusion body formation reduces levels of mutant huntingtin and the risk of neuronal death. *Nature*, Vol.431, No.7010, pp.805-810

Atwal, R.S., Xia, J., Pinchev, D., Taylor, J., Epand, R.M. & Truant, R. (2007). Huntingtin has a membrane association signal that can modulate huntingtin aggregation, nuclear entry and toxicity. *Hum. Mol Genet*, Vol.16, No.21, pp.2600-2615

Baughan, T.D., Dickson, A., Osman, E.Y. & Lorson, C.L. (2009). Delivery of bifunctional RNAs that target an intronic repressor and increase SMN levels in an animal model of spinal muscular atrophy. *Hum. Mol Genet*, Vol.18, No.9, pp.1600-1611

Bernacki, J., Dobrowolska, A., Nierwinska, K. & Malecki, A. (2008). Physiology and pharmacological role of the blood-brain barrier. *Pharmacol. Rep.*, Vol.60, No.5, pp.600-622

Bossy-Wetzel, E., Schwarzenbacher, R. & Lipton, S.A. (2004). Molecular pathways to neurodegeneration. *Nat. Med.*, Vol.10 Suppl, pp.S2-S9

Boudreau, R.L., McBride, J.L., Martins, I., Shen, S., Xing, Y., Carter, B.J. & Davidson, B.L. (2009). Nonallele-specific silencing of mutant and wild-type huntingtin demonstrates therapeutic efficacy in Huntington's disease mice. *Mol Ther.*, Vol.17, No.6, pp.1053-1063

Bowers, W.J., Breakefield, X.O. & Sena-Esteves, M. (2011). Genetic therapy for the nervous system. *Hum. Mol Genet*, Vol.20, No.R1, pp.R28-R41

Browne, S.E. & Beal, M.F. (2006). Oxidative damage in Huntington's disease pathogenesis. *Antioxid. Redox. Signal.*, Vol.8, No.11-12, pp.2061-2073

Cartegni, L. & Krainer, A.R. (2003). Correction of disease-associated exon skipping by synthetic exon-specific activators. *Nat. Struct. Biol.*, Vol.10, No.2, pp.120-125

Caviston, J.P., Zajac, A.L., Tokito, M. & Holzbaur, E.L. (2011). Huntingtin coordinates the dynein-mediated dynamic positioning of endosomes and lysosomes. *Mol Biol. Cell*, Vol.22, No.4, pp.478-492

Choo, Y.S., Johnson, G.V., MacDonald, M., Detloff, P.J. & Lesort, M. (2004). Mutant huntingtin directly increases susceptibility of mitochondria to the calcium-induced permeability transition and cytochrome c release. *Hum. Mol Genet*, Vol.13, No.14, pp.1407-1420

Chung, D.W., Rudnicki, D.D., Yu, L. & Margolis, R.L. (2011). A natural antisense transcript at the Huntington's disease repeat locus regulates HTT expression. *Hum. Mol Genet*, Vol.20, No.17, pp.3467-3477

Clabough, E.B. & Zeitlin, S.O. (2006). Deletion of the triplet repeat encoding polyglutamine within the mouse Huntington's disease gene results in subtle behavioral/motor phenotypes in vivo and elevated levels of ATP with cellular senescence in vitro. *Hum. Mol Genet*, Vol.15, No.4, pp.607-623

Cooper, J.K., Schilling, G., Peters, M.F., Herring, W.J., Sharp, A.H., Kaminsky, Z., Masone, J., Khan, F.A., Delanoy, M., Borchelt, D.R., Dawson, V.L., Dawson, T.M. & Ross, C.A. (1998). Truncated N-terminal fragments of huntingtin with expanded glutamine repeats form nuclear and cytoplasmic aggregates in cell culture. *Hum. Mol Genet*, Vol.7, No.5, pp.783-790

Cornett, J., Cao, F., Wang, C.E., Ross, C.A., Bates, G.P., Li, S.H. & Li, X.J. (2005). Polyglutamine expansion of huntingtin impairs its nuclear export. *Nat. Genet*, Vol.37, No.2, pp.198-204

Cotzias, G.C., Van Woert, M.H. & Schiffer, L.M. (1967). Aromatic amino acids and modification of parkinsonism. *N Engl. J. Med.*, Vol.276, No.7, pp.374-379

Craufurd, D., Thompson, J.C. & Snowden, J.S. (2001). Behavioral changes in Huntington Disease. *Neuropsychiatry Neuropsychol. Behav. Neurol*, Vol.14, No.4, pp.219-226

Cummings, C.J. & Zoghbi, H.Y. (2000). Fourteen and counting: unraveling trinucleotide repeat diseases. *Hum. Mol Genet*, Vol.9, No.6, pp.909-916

Davies, S.W., Turmaine, M., Cozens, B.A., Difiglia, M., Sharp, A.H., Ross, C.A., Scherzinger, E., Wanker, E.E., Mangiarini, L. & Bates, G.P. (1997). Formation of neuronal intranuclear inclusions underlies the neurological dysfunction in mice transgenic for the HD mutation. *Cell*, Vol.90, No.3, pp.537-548

de Mezer M., Wojciechowska, M., Napierala, M., Sobczak, K. & Krzyzosiak, W.J. (2011). Mutant CAG repeats of Huntingtin transcript fold into hairpins, form nuclear foci and are targets for RNA interference. *Nucleic Acids Res.*, Vol.39, No.9, pp.3852-3863

de Rooij, K.E., Dorsman, J.C., Smoor, M.A., Den Dunnen, J.T. & Van Ommen, G.J. (1996). Subcellular localization of the Huntington's disease gene product in cell lines by immunofluorescence and biochemical subcellular fractionation. *Hum. Mol Genet*, Vol.5, No.8, pp.1093-1099

Dickson, A., Osman, E. & Lorson, C.L. (2008). A negatively acting bifunctional RNA increases survival motor neuron both in vitro and in vivo. *Hum. Gene Ther.*, Vol.19, No.11, pp.1307-1315

Dragatsis, I., Levine, M.S. & Zeitlin, S. (2000). Inactivation of Hdh in the brain and testis results in progressive neurodegeneration and sterility in mice. *Nat. Genet*, Vol.26, No.3, pp.300-306

Drouet, V., Perrin, V., Hassig, R., Dufour, N., Auregan, G., Alves, S., Bonvento, G., Brouillet, E., Luthi-Carter, R., Hantraye, P. & Deglon, N. (2009). Sustained effects of nonallele-specific Huntingtin silencing. *Ann Neurol*, Vol.65, No.3, pp.276-285

Evers, M.M., Pepers, B.A., van Deutekom, J.C.T., Mulders, S.A.M., Den Dunnen, J.T., Aartsma-Rus, A., Van Ommen, G.J.B. & van Roon-Mom, W.M.C. (2011). Targeting Several CAG Expansion Diseases by a Single Antisense Oligonucleotide. *PLoS. One* Vol.6, No.9,pp:e24308, Accepted

Fardaei, M., Larkin, K., Brook, J.D. & Hamshere, M.G. (2001). In vivo co-localisation of MBNL protein with DMPK expanded-repeat transcripts. *Nucleic Acids Res.*, Vol.29, No.13, pp.2766-2771

Gafni, J. & Ellerby, L.M. (2002). Calpain activation in Huntington's disease. *J. Neurosci.*, Vol.22, No.12, pp.4842-4849

Gerebtzoff, G. & Seelig, A. (2006). In silico prediction of blood-brain barrier permeation using the calculated molecular cross-sectional area as main parameter. *J. Chem. Inf. Model*, Vol.46, No.6, pp.2638-2650

Goemans, N.M., Tulinius, M., van den Akker, J.T., Burm, B.E., Ekhart, P.F., Heuvelmans, N., Holling, T., Janson, A.A., Platenburg, G.J., Sipkens, J.A., Sitsen, J.M., Aartsma-Rus, A., Van Ommen, G.J., Buyse, G., Darin, N., Verschuuren, J.J., Campion, G.V., de Kimpe, S.J. & van Deutekom, J.C. (2011). Systemic administration of PRO051 in Duchenne's muscular dystrophy. *N Engl. J. Med.*, Vol.364, No.16, pp.1513-1522

Graham, R.K., Deng, Y., Slow, E.J., Haigh, B., Bissada, N., Lu, G., Pearson, J., Shehadeh, J., Bertram, L., Murphy, Z., Warby, S.C., Doty, C.N., Roy, S., Wellington, C.L., Leavitt, B.R., Raymond, L.A., Nicholson, D.W. & Hayden, M.R. (2006). Cleavage at the caspase-6 site is required for neuronal dysfunction and degeneration due to mutant huntingtin. *Cell*, Vol.125, No.6, pp.1179-1191

Gunawardena, S., Her, L.S., Brusch, R.G., Laymon, R.A., Niesman, I.R., Gordesky-Gold, B., Sintasath, L., Bonini, N.M. & Goldstein, L.S. (2003). Disruption of axonal transport by loss of huntingtin or expression of pathogenic polyQ proteins in Drosophila. *Neuron*, Vol.40, No.1, pp.25-40

Guo, X., Geng, M. & Du, G. (2005). Glucose transporter 1, distribution in the brain and in neural disorders: its relationship with transport of neuroactive drugs through the blood-brain barrier. *Biochem. Genet*, Vol.43, No.3-4, pp.175-187

Gusella, J.F., Wexler, N.S., Conneally, P.M., Naylor, S.L., Anderson, M.A., Tanzi, R.E., Watkins, P.C., Ottina, K., Wallace, M.R., Sakaguchi, A.Y. &. (1983). A polymorphic DNA marker genetically linked to Huntington's disease. *Nature*, Vol.306, No.5940, pp.234-238

Harjes, P. & Wanker, E.E. (2003). The hunt for huntingtin function: interaction partners tell many different stories. *Trends Biochem. Sci*, Vol.28, No.8, pp.425-433

Harper, S.Q., Staber, P.D., He, X., Eliason, S.L., Martins, I.H., Mao, Q., Yang, L., Kotin, R.M., Paulson, H.L. & Davidson, B.L. (2005). RNA interference improves motor and neuropathological abnormalities in a Huntington's disease mouse model. *Proc. Natl. Acad Sci U. S. A*, Vol.102, No.16, pp.5820-5825

Hsu, R.J., Hsiao, K.M., Lin, M.J., Li, C.Y., Wang, L.C., Chen, L.K. & Pan, H. (2011). Long tract of untranslated CAG repeats is deleterious in transgenic mice. *PLoS. One.*, Vol.6, No.1, pp.e16417

Hu, J., Matsui, M., Gagnon, K.T., Schwartz, J.C., Gabillet, S., Arar, K., Wu, J., Bezprozvanny, I. & Corey, D.R. (2009). Allele-specific silencing of mutant huntingtin and ataxin-3 genes by targeting expanded CAG repeats in mRNAs. *Nat. Biotechnol.*, Vol.27, No.5, pp.478-484

Hua, Y., Sahashi, K., Hung, G., Rigo, F., Passini, M.A., Bennett, C.F. & Krainer, A.R. (2010). Antisense correction of SMN2 splicing in the CNS rescues necrosis in a type III SMA mouse model. *Genes Dev.*, Vol.24, No.15, pp.1634-1644

Huang, K., Yanai, A., Kang, R., Arstikaitis, P., Singaraja, R.R., Metzler, M., Mullard, A., Haigh, B., Gauthier-Campbell, C., Gutekunst, C.A., Hayden, M.R. & El-Husseini, A. (2004). Huntingtin-interacting protein HIP14 is a palmitoyl transferase involved in palmitoylation and trafficking of multiple neuronal proteins. *Neuron*, Vol.44, No.6, pp.977-986

Ikeda, H., Yamaguchi, M., Sugai, S., Aze, Y., Narumiya, S. & Kakizuka, A. (1996). Expanded polyglutamine in the Machado-Joseph disease protein induces cell death in vitro and in vivo. *Nat. Genet*, Vol.13, No.2, pp.196-202

Imarisio, S., Carmichael, J., Korolchuk, V., Chen, C.W., Saiki, S., Rose, C., Krishna, G., Davies, J.E., Ttofi, E., Underwood, B.R. & Rubinsztein, D.C. (2008). Huntington's disease: from pathology and genetics to potential therapies. *Biochem. J.*, Vol.412, No.2, pp.191-209

Jiang, H., Mankodi, A., Swanson, M.S., Moxley, R.T. & Thornton, C.A. (2004). Myotonic dystrophy type 1 is associated with nuclear foci of mutant RNA, sequestration of muscleblind proteins and deregulated alternative splicing in neurons. *Hum. Mol Genet*, Vol.13, No.24, pp.3079-3088

Kalchman, M.A., Graham, R.K., Xia, G., Koide, H.B., Hodgson, J.G., Graham, K.C., Goldberg, Y.P., Gietz, R.D., Pickart, C.M. & Hayden, M.R. (1996). Huntingtin is ubiquitinated and interacts with a specific ubiquitin-conjugating enzyme. *J. Biol. Chem.*, Vol.271, No.32, pp.19385-19394

Kanadia, R.N., Johnstone, K.A., Mankodi, A., Lungu, C., Thornton, C.A., Esson, D., Timmers, A.M., Hauswirth, W.W. & Swanson, M.S. (2003). A muscleblind knockout model for myotonic dystrophy. *Science*, Vol.302, No.5652, pp.1978-1980

Katayama, S., Tomaru, Y., Kasukawa, T., Waki, K., Nakanishi, M., Nakamura, M., Nishida, H., Yap, C.C., Suzuki, M., Kawai, J., Suzuki, H., Carninci, P., Hayashizaki, Y., Wells, C., Frith, M., Ravasi, T., Pang, K.C., Hallinan, J., Mattick, J., Hume, D.A., Lipovich, L., Batalov, S., Engstrom, P.G., Mizuno, Y., Faghihi, M.A., Sandelin, A., Chalk, A.M., Mottagui-Tabar, S., Liang, Z., Lenhard, B. & Wahlestedt, C. (2005). Antisense transcription in the mammalian transcriptome. *Science*, Vol.309, No.5740, pp.1564-1566

Katsuno, M., Adachi, H., Kume, A., Li, M., Nakagomi, Y., Niwa, H., Sang, C., Kobayashi, Y., Doyu, M. & Sobue, G. (2002). Testosterone reduction prevents phenotypic expression in a transgenic mouse model of spinal and bulbar muscular atrophy. *Neuron*, Vol.35, No.5, pp.843-854

Kegel, K.B., Meloni, A.R., Yi, Y., Kim, Y.J., Doyle, E., Cuiffo, B.G., Sapp, E., Wang, Y., Qin, Z.H., Chen, J.D., Nevins, J.R., Aronin, N. & Difiglia, M. (2002). Huntingtin is present in the nucleus, interacts with the transcriptional corepressor C-terminal binding protein, and represses transcription. *J. Biol. Chem.*, Vol.277, No.9, pp.7466-7476

Kegel, K.B., Sapp, E., Yoder, J., Cuiffo, B., Sobin, L., Kim, Y.J., Qin, Z.H., Hayden, M.R., Aronin, N., Scott, D.L., Isenberg, G., Goldmann, W.H. & Difiglia, M. (2005). Huntingtin associates with acidic phospholipids at the plasma membrane. *J. Biol. Chem.*, Vol.280, No.43, pp.36464-36473

Kim, Y.J., Sapp, E., Cuiffo, B.G., Sobin, L., Yoder, J., Kegel, K.B., Qin, Z.H., Detloff, P., Aronin, N. & Difiglia, M. (2006). Lysosomal proteases are involved in generation of N-terminal huntingtin fragments. *Neurobiol. Dis*, Vol.22, No.2, pp.346-356

Klement, I.A., Skinner, P.J., Kaytor, M.D., Yi, H., Hersch, S.M., Clark, H.B., Zoghbi, H.Y. & Orr, H.T. (1998). Ataxin-1 nuclear localization and aggregation: role in polyglutamine-induced disease in SCA1 transgenic mice. *Cell*, Vol.95, No.1, pp.41-53

Koob, M.D., Moseley, M.L., Schut, L.J., Benzow, K.A., Bird, T.D., Day, J.W. & Ranum, L.P. (1999). An untranslated CTG expansion causes a novel form of spinocerebellar ataxia (SCA8). *Nat. Genet*, Vol.21, No.4, pp.379-384

Kremer, B., Almqvist, E., Theilmann, J., Spence, N., Telenius, H., Goldberg, Y.P. & Hayden, M.R. (1995). Sex-dependent mechanisms for expansions and contractions of the CAG repeat on affected Huntington disease chromosomes. *Am. J. Hum. Genet*, Vol.57, No.2, pp.343-350

Kremer, B., Weber, B. & Hayden, M.R. (1992). New insights into the clinical features, pathogenesis and molecular genetics of Huntington disease. *Brain Pathol.*, Vol.2, No.4, pp.321-335

Krol, J., Fiszer, A., Mykowska, A., Sobczak, K., de, M.M. & Krzyzosiak, W.J. (2007). Ribonuclease dicer cleaves triplet repeat hairpins into shorter repeats that silence specific targets. *Mol Cell*, Vol.25, No.4, pp.575-586

Lee, H.J., Boado, R.J., Braasch, D.A., Corey, D.R. & Pardridge, W.M. (2002). Imaging gene expression in the brain in vivo in a transgenic mouse model of Huntington's disease with an antisense radiopharmaceutical and drug-targeting technology. *J. Nucl. Med.*, Vol.43, No.7, pp.948-956

Legleiter, J., Mitchell, E., Lotz, G.P., Sapp, E., Ng, C., Difiglia, M., Thompson, L.M. & Muchowski, P.J. (2010). Mutant huntingtin fragments form oligomers in a polyglutamine length-dependent manner in vitro and in vivo. *J. Biol. Chem.*, Vol.285, No.19, pp.14777-14790

Levesque, M., Bedard, A., Cossette, M. & Parent, A. (2003). Novel aspects of the chemical anatomy of the striatum and its efferents projections. *J. Chem. Neuroanat.*, Vol.26, No.4, pp.271-281

Li, L.B., Yu, Z., Teng, X. & Bonini, N.M. (2008). RNA toxicity is a component of ataxin-3 degeneration in Drosophila. *Nature*, Vol.453, No.7198, pp.1107-1111

Li, W., Serpell, L.C., Carter, W.J., Rubinsztein, D.C. & Huntington, J.A. (2006). Expression and characterization of full-length human huntingtin, an elongated HEAT repeat protein. *J. Biol. Chem.*, Vol.281, No.23, pp.15916-15922

Liu, W., Kennington, L.A., Rosas, H.D., Hersch, S., Cha, J.H., Zamore, P.D. & Aronin, N. (2008). Linking SNPs to CAG repeat length in Huntington's disease patients. *Nat. Methods*, Vol.5, No.11, pp.951-953

Lombardi, M.S., Jaspers, L., Spronkmans, C., Gellera, C., Taroni, F., Di, M.E., Donato, S.D. & Kaemmerer, W.F. (2009). A majority of Huntington's disease patients may be treatable by individualized allele-specific RNA interference. *Exp. Neurol*, Vol.217, No.2, pp.312-319

Lorson, C.L., Rindt, H. & Shababi, M. (2010). Spinal muscular atrophy: mechanisms and therapeutic strategies. *Hum. Mol Genet*, Vol.19, No.R1, pp.R111-R118

McBride, J.L., Boudreau, R.L., Harper, S.Q., Staber, P.D., Monteys, A.M., Martins, I., Gilmore, B.L., Burstein, H., Peluso, R.W., Polisky, B., Carter, B.J. & Davidson, B.L. (2008). Artificial miRNAs mitigate shRNA-mediated toxicity in the brain: implications for the therapeutic development of RNAi. *Proc. Natl. Acad Sci U. S. A*, Vol.105, No.15, pp.5868-5873

McLeod, C.J., O'Keefe, L.V. & Richards, R.I. (2005). The pathogenic agent in Drosophila models of 'polyglutamine' diseases. *Hum. Mol Genet*, Vol.14, No.8, pp.1041-1048

McNeil, S.M., Novelletto, A., Srinidhi, J., Barnes, G., Kornbluth, I., Altherr, M.R., Wasmuth, J.J., Gusella, J.F., MacDonald, M.E. & Myers, R.H. (1997). Reduced penetrance of the Huntington's disease mutation. *Hum. Mol Genet*, Vol.6, No.5, pp.775-779

Mende-Mueller, L.M., Toneff, T., Hwang, S.R., Chesselet, M.F. & Hook, V.Y. (2001). Tissue-specific proteolysis of Huntingtin (htt) in human brain: evidence of enhanced levels of N- and C-terminal htt fragments in Huntington's disease striatum. *J. Neurosci.*, Vol.21, No.6, pp.1830-1837

Miller, V.M., Xia, H., Marrs, G.L., Gouvion, C.M., Lee, G., Davidson, B.L. & Paulson, H.L. (2003). Allele-specific silencing of dominant disease genes. *Proc. Natl. Acad Sci U. S. A*, Vol.100, No.12, pp.7195-7200

Modregger, J., DiProspero, N.A., Charles, V., Tagle, D.A. & Plomann, M. (2002). PACSIN 1 interacts with huntingtin and is absent from synaptic varicosities in presymptomatic Huntington's disease brains. *Hum. Mol Genet*, Vol.11, No.21, pp.2547-2558

Morfini, G., Pigino, G., Brady, S.T. (2005). Polyglutamine expansion diseases: failing to deliver. *Trends Mol Med* 11, pp.64–70.

Moseley, M.L., Zu, T., Ikeda, Y., Gao, W., Mosemiller, A.K., Daughters, R.S., Chen, G., Weatherspoon, M.R., Clark, H.B., Ebner, T.J., Day, J.W. & Ranum, L.P. (2006). Bidirectional expression of CUG and CAG expansion transcripts and intranuclear polyglutamine inclusions in spinocerebellar ataxia type 8. *Nat. Genet*, Vol.38, No.7, pp.758-769

Mykowska, A., Sobczak, K., Wojciechowska, M., Kozlowski, P. & Krzyzosiak, W.J. (2011). CAG repeats mimic CUG repeats in the misregulation of alternative splicing. *Nucleic Acids Res.*

Nucifora, F.C., Jr., Sasaki, M., Peters, M.F., Huang, H., Cooper, J.K., Yamada, M., Takahashi, H., Tsuji, S., Troncoso, J., Dawson, V.L., Dawson, T.M. & Ross, C.A. (2001). Interference by huntingtin and atrophin-1 with cbp-mediated transcription leading to cellular toxicity. *Science*, Vol.291, No.5512, pp.2423-2428

Orr, A.L., Li, S., Wang, C.E., Li, H., Wang, J., Rong, J., Xu, X., Mastroberardino, P.G., Greenamyre, J.T. & Li, X.J. (2008). N-terminal mutant huntingtin associates with mitochondria and impairs mitochondrial trafficking. *J. Neurosci.*, Vol.28, No.11, pp.2783-2792

Orr, H.T. & Zoghbi, H.Y. (2007). Trinucleotide repeat disorders. *Annu. Rev. Neurosci.*, Vol.30, pp.575-621

Palmer, A.M. (2010). The blood-brain barrier. *Neurobiol. Dis*, Vol.37, No.1, pp.1-2

Panov, A.V., Gutekunst, C.A., Leavitt, B.R., Hayden, M.R., Burke, J.R., Strittmatter, W.J. & Greenamyre, J.T. (2002). Early mitochondrial calcium defects in Huntington's disease are a direct effect of polyglutamines. *Nat. Neurosci.*, Vol.5, No.8, pp.731-736

Pardridge, W.M. (2007). Blood-brain barrier delivery. *Drug Discov. Today*, Vol.12, No.1-2, pp.54-61

Passini, M.A., Bu, J., Richards, A.M., Kinnecom, C., Sardi, S.P., Stanek, L.M., Hua, Y., Rigo, F., Matson, J., Hung, G., Kaye, E.M., Shihabuddin, L.S., Krainer, A.R., Bennett, C.F. & Cheng, S.H. (2011). Antisense oligonucleotides delivered to the mouse CNS ameliorate symptoms of severe spinal muscular atrophy. *Sci Transl. Med.*, Vol.3, No.72, pp.72ra18

Paulsen, J.S., Ready, R.E., Hamilton, J.M., Mega, M.S. & Cummings, J.L. (2001). Neuropsychiatric aspects of Huntington's disease. *J. Neurol Neurosurg. Psychiatry*, Vol.71, No.3, pp.310-314

Perutz, M.F., Johnson, T., Suzuki, M. & Finch, J.T. (1994). Glutamine repeats as polar zippers: their possible role in inherited neurodegenerative diseases. *Proc. Natl. Acad Sci U. S. A*, Vol.91, No.12, pp.5355-5358

Pfister, E.L., Kennington, L., Straubhaar, J., Wagh, S., Liu, W., Difiglia, M., Landwehrmeyer, B., Vonsattel, J.P., Zamore, P.D. & Aronin, N. (2009). Five siRNAs targeting three SNPs may provide therapy for three-quarters of Huntington's disease patients. *Curr. Biol.*, Vol.19, No.9, pp.774-778

Rawlins, M. (2010). Huntington's disease out of the closet? *Lancet*, Vol.376, No.9750, pp.1372-1373

Rigamonti, D., Bauer, J.H., De-Fraja, C., Conti, L., Sipione, S., Sciorati, C., Clementi, E., Hackam, A., Hayden, M.R., Li, Y., Cooper, J.K., Ross, C.A., Govoni, S., Vincenz, C. & Cattaneo, E. (2000). Wild-type huntingtin protects from apoptosis upstream of caspase-3. *J. Neurosci.*, Vol.20, No.10, pp.3705-3713

Rockabrand, E., Slepko, N., Pantalone, A., Nukala, V.N., Kazantsev, A., Marsh, J.L., Sullivan, P.G., Steffan, J.S., Sensi, S.L. & Thompson, L.M. (2007). The first 17 amino acids of Huntingtin modulate its sub-cellular localization, aggregation and effects on calcium homeostasis. *Hum. Mol Genet*, Vol.16, No.1, pp.61-77

Roos, R.A. (2010). Huntington's disease: a clinical review. *Orphanet. J. Rare. Dis*, Vol.5, No.1, pp.40

Rosas, H.D., Koroshetz, W.J., Chen, Y.I., Skeuse, C., Vangel, M., Cudkowicz, M.E., Caplan, K., Marek, K., Seidman, L.J., Makris, N., Jenkins, B.G. & Goldstein, J.M. (2003). Evidence for more widespread cerebral pathology in early HD: an MRI-based morphometric analysis. *Neurology*, Vol.60, No.10, pp.1615-1620

Rosas, H.D., Salat, D.H., Lee, S.Y., Zaleta, A.K., Pappu, V., Fischl, B., Greve, D., Hevelone, N. & Hersch, S.M. (2008). Cerebral cortex and the clinical expression of Huntington's disease: complexity and heterogeneity. *Brain*, Vol.131, No.Pt 4, pp.1057-1068

Ryan, A. & Scrable, H. (2008). Mutant alleles of HD improve the life span of p53(-/-) mice. *Mech Ageing Dev.*, Vol.129, No.4, pp.238-241

Ryan, A.B., Zeitlin, S.O. & Scrable, H. (2006). Genetic interaction between expanded murine Hdh alleles and p53 reveal deleterious effects of p53 on Huntington's disease pathogenesis. *Neurobiol. Dis*, Vol.24, No.2, pp.419-427

Sah, D.W. & Aronin, N. (2011). Oligonucleotide therapeutic approaches for Huntington disease. *J. Clin. Invest*, Vol.121, No.2, pp.500-507

Saudou, F., Finkbeiner, S., Devys, D. & Greenberg, M.E. (1998). Huntingtin acts in the nucleus to induce apoptosis but death does not correlate with the formation of intranuclear inclusions. *Cell*, Vol.95, No.1, pp.55-66

Schwarz, D.S., Ding, H., Kennington, L., Moore, J.T., Schelter, J., Burchard, J., Linsley, P.S., Aronin, N., Xu, Z. & Zamore, P.D. (2006). Designing siRNA that distinguish between genes that differ by a single nucleotide. *PLoS. Genet*, Vol.2, No.9, pp.e140

Shoulson, I. & Young, A.B. (2011). Milestones in huntington disease. *Mov Disord.*, Vol.26, No.6, pp.1127-1133

Simpson, S.A. (2007). Late stage care in Huntington's disease. *Brain Res. Bull.*, Vol.72, No.2-3, pp.179-181

Singh, N.K., Singh, N.N., Androphy, E.J. & Singh, R.N. (2006). Splicing of a critical exon of human Survival Motor Neuron is regulated by a unique silencer element located in the last intron. *Mol Cell Biol.*, Vol.26, No.4, pp.1333-1346

Skordis, L.A., Dunckley, M.G., Yue, B., Eperon, I.C. & Muntoni, F. (2003). Bifunctional antisense oligonucleotides provide a trans-acting splicing enhancer that stimulates SMN2 gene expression in patient fibroblasts. *Proc. Natl. Acad Sci U. S. A*, Vol.100, No.7, pp.4114-4119

Smith, R., Klein, P., Koc-Schmitz, Y., Waldvogel, H.J., Faull, R.L., Brundin, P., Plomann, M. & Li, J.Y. (2007). Loss of SNAP-25 and rabphilin 3a in sensory-motor cortex in Huntington's disease. *J. Neurochem.*, Vol.103, No.1, pp.115-123

Smith, R.A., Miller, T.M., Yamanaka, K., Monia, B.P., Condon, T.P., Hung, G., Lobsiger, C.S., Ward, C.M., McAlonis-Downes, M., Wei, H., Wancewicz, E.V., Bennett, C.F. & Cleveland, D.W. (2006). Antisense oligonucleotide therapy for neurodegenerative disease. *J. Clin. Invest*, Vol.116, No.8, pp.2290-2296

Snowden, J.S., Craufurd, D., Thompson, J. & Neary, D. (2002). Psychomotor, executive, and memory function in preclinical Huntington's disease. *J. Clin. Exp. Neuropsychol.*, Vol.24, No.2, pp.133-145

Steffan, J.S., Agrawal, N., Pallos, J., Rockabrand, E., Trotman, L.C., Slepko, N., Illes, K., Lukacsovich, T., Zhu, Y.Z., Cattaneo, E., Pandolfi, P.P., Thompson, L.M. & Marsh, J.L. (2004). SUMO modification of Huntingtin and Huntington's disease pathology. *Science*, Vol.304, No.5667, pp.100-104

Steffan, J.S., Kazantsev, A., Spasic-Boskovic, O., Greenwald, M., Zhu, Y.Z., Gohler, H., Wanker, E.E., Bates, G.P., Housman, D.E. & Thompson, L.M. (2000). The Huntington's disease protein interacts with p53 and CREB-binding protein and represses transcription. *Proc. Natl. Acad Sci U. S. A*, Vol.97, No.12, pp.6763-6768

Strehlow, A.N., Li, J.Z. & Myers, R.M. (2007). Wild-type huntingtin participates in protein trafficking between the Golgi and the extracellular space. *Hum. Mol Genet*, Vol.16, No.4, pp.391-409

Strong, T.V., Tagle, D.A., Valdes, J.M., Elmer, L.W., Boehm, K., Swaroop, M., Kaatz, K.W., Collins, F.S. & Albin, R.L. (1993). Widespread expression of the human and rat Huntington's disease gene in brain and nonneural tissues. *Nat. Genet*, Vol.5, No.3, pp.259-265

Tabrizi, S.J., Langbehn, D.R., Leavitt, B.R., Roos, R.A., Durr, A., Craufurd, D., Kennard, C., Hicks, S.L., Fox, N.C., Scahill, R.I., Borowsky, B., Tobin, A.J., Rosas, H.D., Johnson, H., Reilmann, R., Landwehrmeyer, B. & Stout, J.C. (2009). Biological and clinical manifestations of Huntington's disease in the longitudinal TRACK-HD study: cross-sectional analysis of baseline data. *Lancet Neurol*, Vol.8, No.9, pp.791-801

Takano, H. & Gusella, J.F. (2002). The predominantly HEAT-like motif structure of huntingtin and its association and coincident nuclear entry with dorsal, an NF-kB/Rel/dorsal family transcription factor. *BMC. Neurosci.*, Vol.3, pp.15

The Huntington's Disease Collaborative Research Group (1993). A novel gene containing a trinucleotide repeat that is expanded and unstable on Huntington's disease chromosomes. *Cell*, Vol.72, No.6, pp.971-983

Tomkins, O., Friedman, O., Ivens, S., Reiffurth, C., Major, S., Dreier, J.P., Heinemann, U. & Friedman, A. (2007). Blood-brain barrier disruption results in delayed functional and structural alterations in the rat neocortex. *Neurobiol. Dis*, Vol.25, No.2, pp.367-377

van Bilsen, P.H., Jaspers, L., Lombardi, M.S., Odekerken, J.C., Burright, E.N. & Kaemmerer, W.F. (2008). Identification and allele-specific silencing of the mutant huntingtin allele in Huntington's disease patient-derived fibroblasts. *Hum. Gene Ther.*, Vol.19, No.7, pp.710-719

van Roon-Mom, W.M., Hogg, V.M., Tippett, L.J. & Faull, R.L. (2006). Aggregate distribution in frontal and motor cortex in Huntington's disease brain. *Neuroreport*, Vol.17, No.6, pp.667-670

van Roon-Mom, W.M., Reid, S.J., Jones, A.L., MacDonald, M.E., Faull, R.L. & Snell, R.G. (2002). Insoluble TATA-binding protein accumulation in Huntington's disease cortex. *Brain Res. Mol Brain Res.*, Vol.109, No.1-2, pp.1-10

Vonsattel, J.P., Myers, R.H., Stevens, T.J., Ferrante, R.J., Bird, E.D. & Richardson, E.P., Jr. (1985). Neuropathological classification of Huntington's disease. *J. Neuropathol. Exp. Neurol*, Vol.44, No.6, pp.559-577

Walker, F.O. (2007). Huntington's disease. *Lancet*, Vol.369, No.9557, pp.218-228

Wang, L.C., Chen, K.Y., Pan, H., Wu, C.C., Chen, P.H., Liao, Y.T., Li, C., Huang, M.L. & Hsiao, K.M. (2011). Muscleblind participates in RNA toxicity of expanded CAG and CUG repeats in Caenorhabditis elegans. *Cell Mol Life Sci*, Vol.68, No.7, pp.1255-1267

Wang, Y.L., Liu, W., Wada, E., Murata, M., Wada, K. & Kanazawa, I. (2005). Clinico-pathological rescue of a model mouse of Huntington's disease by siRNA. *Neurosci. Res.*, Vol.53, No.3, pp.241-249

Wanker, E.E. (2000). Protein aggregation and pathogenesis of Huntington's disease: mechanisms and correlations. *Biol. Chem.*, Vol.381, No.9-10, pp.937-942

Warby, S.C., Montpetit, A., Hayden, A.R., Carroll, J.B., Butland, S.L., Visscher, H., Collins, J.A., Semaka, A., Hudson, T.J. & Hayden, M.R. (2009). CAG expansion in the Huntington disease gene is associated with a specific and targetable predisposing haplogroup. *Am. J. Hum. Genet*, Vol.84, No.3, pp.351-366

Weiss, A., Klein, C., Woodman, B., Sathasivam, K., Bibel, M., Regulier, E., Bates, G.P. & Paganetti, P. (2008). Sensitive biochemical aggregate detection reveals aggregation onset before symptom development in cellular and murine models of Huntington's disease. *J. Neurochem.*, Vol.104, No.3, pp.846-858

Wellington, C.L., Ellerby, L.M., Gutekunst, C.A., Rogers, D., Warby, S., Graham, R.K., Loubser, O., van, R.J., Singaraja, R., Yang, Y.Z., Gafni, J., Bredesen, D., Hersch, S.M., Leavitt, B.R., Roy, S., Nicholson, D.W. & Hayden, M.R. (2002). Caspase cleavage of mutant huntingtin precedes neurodegeneration in Huntington's disease. *J. Neurosci.*, Vol.22, No.18, pp.7862-7872

Wilburn, B., Rudnicki, D.D., Zhao, J., Weitz, T.M., Cheng, Y., Gu, X., Greiner, E., Park, C.S., Wang, N., Sopher, B.L., La Spada, A.R., Osmand, A., Margolis, R.L., Sun, Y.E. & Yang, X.W. (2011). An antisense CAG repeat transcript at JPH3 locus mediates expanded polyglutamine protein toxicity in Huntington's disease-like 2 mice. *Neuron*, Vol.70, No.3, pp.427-440

Williams, J.H., Schray, R.C., Patterson, C.A., Ayitey, S.O., Tallent, M.K. & Lutz, G.J. (2009). Oligonucleotide-mediated survival of motor neuron protein expression in CNS improves phenotype in a mouse model of spinal muscular atrophy. *J. Neurosci.*, Vol.29, No.24, pp.7633-7638

Zeitlin, S., Liu, J.P., Chapman, D.L., Papaioannou, V.E. & Efstratiadis, A. (1995). Increased apoptosis and early embryonic lethality in mice nullizygous for the Huntington's disease gene homologue. *Nat. Genet*, Vol.11, No.2, pp.155-163

Zhang, S., Feany, M.B., Saraswati, S., Littleton, J.T. & Perrimon, N. (2009). Inactivation of Drosophila Huntingtin affects long-term adult functioning and the pathogenesis of a Huntington's disease model. *Dis Model Mech*, Vol.2, No.5-6, pp.247-266

Zhang, Y., Li, M., Drozda, M., Chen, M., Ren, S., Mejia Sanchez, R.O., Leavitt, B.R., Cattaneo, E., Ferrante, R.J., Hayden, M.R. & Friedlander, R.M. (2003). Depletion of wild-type huntingtin in mouse models of neurologic diseases. *J. Neurochem.*, Vol.87, No.1, pp.101-106

Zuccato, C., Ciammola, A., Rigamonti, D., Leavitt, B.R., Goffredo, D., Conti, L., MacDonald, M.E., Friedlander, R.M., Silani, V., Hayden, M.R., Timmusk, T., Sipione, S. & Cattaneo, E. (2001). Loss of huntingtin-mediated BDNF gene transcription in Huntington's disease. *Science*, Vol.293, No.5529, pp.493-498

7

BDNF in Huntington's Disease: Role in Pathogenesis and Treatment

Maryna Baydyuk and Baoji Xu
Georgetown University
USA

1. Introduction

Huntington's Disease (HD) is a neurodegenerative disorder characterized by motor, cognitive, and psychiatric abnormalities, and is inherited in an autosomal dominant fashion (Borrell-Pages et al., 2006). HD is caused by the CAG trinucleotide repeat expansion in the first exon of the gene encoding huntingtin (htt) (The Huntington's Disease Collaborative Research Group, 1993). This mutation is translated into a polyglutamine (poly Q) stretch near the amino terminus of htt, which results in a toxic gain of function (Gusella & MacDonald, 2000). Although htt is widely expressed in the human body and its mutation is not tissue-specific, the striatum is preferentially affected. The pathological changes in the striatum develop first in the caudate nucleus and then in the putamen, causing a 50-60% neuronal loss in these areas (Mann et al., 1993; Vonsattel & DiFiglia, 1998). Striatal atrophy is due to selective degeneration of medium-sized spiny neurons (MSNs), which comprise 90% of striatal neurons. Interestingly, the MSNs of the indirect pathway, responsible for inhibition of involuntary movement, are preferentially affected, causing motor symptoms of HD such as uncontrollable sequence of movements called "chorea". In the course of the disease, atrophy spreads to other brain regions, including the cerebral cortex, the globus pallidus (GP), and the thalamus (Mann et al., 1993).

The mechanism behind selective degeneration of striatal neurons remains to be elucidated, but it has been suggested that reduced trophic support renders striatal neurons more vulnerable to the toxic actions of mutant htt. Numerous *in vitro* and *in vivo* studies have shown that striatal neurons require brain-derived neurotrophic factor (BDNF) for their survival and function. A deficiency in BDNF-mediated signaling alone is sufficient to cause dendritic abnormalities and neuronal loss in the cerebral cortex and striatum (Baquet et al., 2004; Gorski et al., 2003). Moreover, reduced levels of striatal BDNF were detected in both HD animal models (Apostol et al., 2008; Gharami et al., 2008; Spires et al., 2004) and HD patients (Ferrer et al., 2000). These observations raise the possibility that reduced levels of striatal BDNF may significantly contribute to HD pathogenesis. In support of this view, the progression of HD is accelerated in *Bdnf* heterozygous mice (Canals et al., 2004). Furthermore, alterations of gene expression profile in the striatum have been shown to be similar in HD patients and mice in which the *Bdnf* gene is deleted in the cerebral cortex (Strand et al., 2007). Importantly, the receptor for BDNF, tropomyosin related kinase B (TrkB), is preferentially expressed in striatal MSNs of the indirect pathway, which may explain why this population of neurons is degenerated first in HD patients (Baydyuk et al., 2011).

BDNF found in the striatum is synthesized and anterogradely transported from the cell bodies located in the cerebral cortex, substantia nigra pars compacta, amygdala, and thalamus (Altar et al., 1997; Baquet et al., 2004). Since striatum does not produce BDNF but depends on it for proper function, abnormalities in anterograde transport and reduced gene expression in brain regions supplying BDNF to the striatum might contribute to neuronal dysfunction and death seen in HD (Gauthier et al., 2004; Zuccato et al., 2001). In light of these findings, efforts have been made to test whether increasing BDNF expression represents a valuable strategy for treatment of Huntington's Disease. Indeed, increasing striatal BDNF levels by a transgene, viral delivery, or stimulations that induce *Bdnf* gene expression have been shown to improve disease phenotypes in several HD mouse models (Cho et al., 2007; Gharami et al., 2008; Xie et al., 2010).

This book chapter will review these recent discoveries regarding the role of BDNF deficiency in the pathogenesis of HD and BDNF as a potential therapeutic agent for HD.

2. Wild-type but not mutant htt promotes *Bdnf* gene expression

The pathogenic mechanisms induced by mutant htt are not fully understood but are thought to involve the gain of toxic function and/or the loss of normal activities. Htt is a ubiquitously expressed protein, highly enriched in the brain (DiFiglia et al., 1995). While its exact functions are unknown, htt has been shown to be essential during embryogenesis and possess anti-apoptotic properties during adulthood (Dragatsis et al., 2000; O'Kusky et al., 1999; Rigamonti et al., 2000). Several mechanisms have been proposed for the neurodegenerative effect of the expanded polyQ tract in htt (Rubinsztein, 2002). Discovery of neuronal intranuclear inclusions in HD patients and HD mouse models led to the hypothesis that these protein aggregates might cause neuronal death. However, studies in mice and cultured neurons indicate that the formation of nuclear inclusions does not correlate with neuronal death (Hodgson et al., 1999; Kim et al., 1999; Laforet et al., 2001; Rubinsztein, 2002; Saudou et al., 1998). At present, the molecular basis for the toxic gain of function associated with mutant htt remains unclear.

The loss of a beneficial activity of normal htt has been proposed to contribute to the pathogenesis of HD. Wild type htt is known to regulate transcription of multiple genes, among which the gene encoding BDNF has received special attention (Zuccato et al., 2001). BDNF is a member of the neurotrophin family, which also includes nerve growth factor (NGF), neurotrophin-3 (NT-3) and neurotrophin-4/5 (NT-4/5) (Reichardt, 2006). BDNF has been shown to promote neuronal growth, survival, and differentiation by activating its TrkB receptor tyrosine kinase (Patapoutian & Reichardt, 2001). Upon binding to BDNF, activated full-length TrkB triggers multiple intracellular signaling cascades through protein-protein interactions (Chao, 2003). TrkB-initiated signaling pathways have been shown to promote cell survival by up-regulating the activity of survival genes and inhibiting the function of the proteins that lead to programmed cell death (Bhave et al., 1999; Encinas et al., 1999; Yamada et al., 2001). TrkB signaling pathways can also mediate various synaptic reorganization processes, including formation and maintenance of dendrites and dendritic spines (McAllister et al., 1999). In support of these in *vitro* observations, deletion of either the *TrkB* or *Bdnf* gene leads to cell atrophy, dendritic degeneration, and neuronal loss, as shown in the excitatory neurons of the dorsal forebrain (Gorski et al., 2003; Xu et al., 2000).

In rodents and humans, the *Bdnf* gene is transcribed from at least 8 discrete promoters, producing many different *Bdnf* mRNA species that encode the same protein (Aid et al., 2007). The different transcripts are generated in different tissues in a stimulus- and development-specific manner and may have differential subcellular localizations and targets (Metsis et al., 1993; Pattabiraman et al., 2005; Timmusk et al., 1993). Zuccato et al. have shown that wild-type htt enhances *Bdnf* transcription from promoter II, whereas mutant htt suppresses *Bdnf* transcription from promoter II as well as two other *Bdnf* promoters in cultured cells and the cerebral cortex of YAC72 transgenic mice expressing mutant htt with an expanded tract of 72 glutamines (Zuccato et al., 2001). The same group further investigated the mechanism underlying *Bdnf* gene regulation by wild-type and mutant htt, and found that wild-type htt promotes transcription of promoter II by sequestering the repressor element-1 transcription factor/neuron restrictive silencer factor (REST/NRSF) in the cytoplasm, thereby freeing the nucleus of the inhibitory complex and allowing transcription to occur (Zuccato et al., 2003). In contrast, mutant htt is unable to retain REST/NRSF complex in the cytoplasm, leading to aberrant accumulation of REST/NRSF in the nucleus and inhibition of *Bdnf* gene transcription. Interestingly, the effect of htt on *Bdnf* gene expression in cortical neurons is specific since the protein does not affect expression of two other neurotrophins, NGF and NT-3, in cortical neurons (Zuccato et al., 2003). In agreement with these findings, levels of *Bdnf* mRNA are reduced in the cerebral cortices of HD patients (Zuccato et al., 2008). It also has been shown that lower levels of BDNF are associated with higher numbers of CAG repeats in mutant *htt* alleles and correlate with the severity of the disease (Ciammola et al., 2007). It is important to note, however, that this autopsy data should be interpreted with caution. As mutant htt alters electrophysiological properties of cortical neurons (Cummings et al., 2009) and neuronal activity regulates *Bdnf* gene expression (Aid et al., 2007), we should not exclude the possibility that the observed reduction in cortical *Bdnf* mRNA levels may be secondary to neurodegeneration.

Although the contribution of suppressed *Bdnf* transcription to reduced BDNF levels in HD striatum is a widely accepted hypothesis, there are studies that contradict this idea. A reduction in *Bdnf* transcription would predict reduced levels of BDNF protein in cerebral cortices of both HD patients and mouse models. This prediction has been confirmed in one study (Zuccato et al., 2008) but not in another study (Gauthier et al., 2004) using post-mortem tissues from multiple control subjects and HD patients. Furthermore, *in situ hybridization* revealed normal levels of cortical *Bdnf* mRNA in aging YAC128 mice that express the whole human *htt* gene with 128 CAG repeats (Xie et al., 2010). Consistent with this observation, levels of cortical BDNF in YAC128 mice and R6/1 mice, another HD model, were found to be similar to those in WT mice (Gharami et al., 2008; Xie et al., 2010). Further analysis of *Bdnf* gene expression in other HD mouse models at various ages is necessary to clear the discrepancy. Despite the discrepancy in determining cortical *Bdnf* mRNA levels, a significant reduction in striatal BDNF has been consistently shown in both HD patients and animal models.

3. Htt promotes axonal BDNF transport

Studies by Gauthier et al. indicate that in addition to controlling *Bdnf* mRNA production in the cortex, wild-type htt may also regulate BDNF transport along the corticostriatal axes (Gauthier et al., 2004). The idea that htt is involved in intracellular trafficking arose from the subcellular localization of htt and its association with various proteins of molecular motors. Although present in the nucleus, htt is predominantly found in the cytoplasm, where it interacts with the huntingtin-associated protein-1 (HAP1), a protein involved in axonal transport via association with p150^{glued} subunit of dynactin, which is an essential part of the microtubule-based motor complex (Block-Galarza et al., 1997; Engelender et al., 1997; Li et al., 1998). While htt and other pathogenic polyQ-containing proteins have been shown to affect fast axonal transport (Gunawardena et al., 2003; Szebenyi et al., 2003), the link between deficient trafficking and selective neuronal degeneration has not been established. Gauthier and colleagues show that in normal condition wild-type htt promotes neuronal survival by facilitating the transport of BDNF-containing vesicles along microtubules. Consistent with a loss of function hypothesis, reduction in wild-type htt levels leads to attenuated BDNF trafficking. On the other hand, mutation in htt increases association of polyQ-htt and p150^{glued} via HAP1 and prevents efficient movement of BDNF-containing vesicles along microtubules. They also demonstrate that disruption of BDNF transport leads to decreased neurotrophic support and neurotoxicity, which can be rescued by wild-type htt (Gauthier et al., 2004).

BDNF synthesized in the cortex and transported to the striatum via corticostriatal projections provides the main support for survival of striatal neurons in the adult brain (Altar et al., 1997; Baquet et al., 2004). Importantly, it has been shown that BDNF levels are reduced in the striatum but not in the cortex of HD patients (Gauthier et al., 2004). These observations are in agreement with the notion that both mechanisms, suppressed *Bdnf* gene expression and deficient BDNF transport, might concomitantly contribute to reduced levels of BDNF in the striata of HD patients and mouse models, thus providing strong evidence for BDNF as a crucial factor in the pathogenesis of HD.

4. Possible effects of mutant htt on BDNF maturation

One additional cause for reduced neurotrophic support of striatal neurons in HD may be due to deficits in processing of proBDNF. The proBDNF is a 32-kDa precursor protein that is cleaved to generate the mature BDNF protein of 14 kDa. Whereas the mature form binds to its TrkB receptor and promotes neuronal survival, the uncleaved proBDNF preferentially activates the low-affinity neurotrophin receptor p75NTR (Hempstead 2006), which is a member of the tumor necrosis factor receptor subfamily and is known to induce neuronal death via apoptosis (Frade & Barde, 1998; Teng et al., 2005).

As discussed earlier, immunoblotting analysis has consistently found a reduction in striatal levels of mature BDNF in HD mouse models (Apostol et al., 2008; Gharami et al., 2008; Spires et al., 2004; Xie et al., 2010) and HD patients (Ferrer et al., 2000; Gauthier et al., 2004). However, studies using ELISA assays reported normal striatal levels of BDNF in R6/1 HD mice (Canals et al., 2004; Pang et al., 2006) and increased striatal levels of BDNF in YAC72 mice (Seo et al., 2008). As ELISA assays detect both mature BDNF and proBDNF, this discrepancy suggests that maturation of proBDNF may be impaired in the striatum, leading to accumulation of proBDNF in the striatum. Impaired proBDNF maturation could be detrimental to striatal neurons, because they lose the protective effect of mature BDNF via TrkB receptor signaling and are subject to the apoptotic effect of proBDNF via the p75NTR receptor (Teng et al., 2005). As current BDNF antibodies are still problematic in detecting proBDNF on immunoblots, utilization of tagged *Bdnf* knockin mice (Matsumoto et al., 2008; Yang et al., 2009) will help uncover the effect of mutant htt on BDNF maturation.

A recent study has suggested that proteins involved in proBDNF axonal transport might also play a role in BDNF maturation (Yang et al., 2011). As discussed earlier, htt facilitates axonal transport via its interaction with HAP1 and the mutation in htt alters the formation of proper motor complex and inhibits BDNF transport (Gauthier et al., 2004). Yang et al. found that proBDNF interacts with both HAP1 and sortilin, a binding partner of p75NTR, to form a complex that prevents proBDNF degradation and modulates proBDNF targeting to dendrites and axonal organelles. Furthermore, their data suggest that the complex of proBDNF-HAP1-sortilin might facilitate cleavage and release of mature BDNF (Yang et al., 2011). Thus, it is possible that mutant htt can affect both BDNF maturation and trafficking via its interaction with HAP1.

5. BDNF and selectivity of striatal degeneration

Striatal neurons are not uniformly affected in HD. Immunohistochemical studies using tissues from HD patients have shown a greater decrease in the number of neurons co-expressing the dopamine receptor D2 (Drd2) and enkephalin (Enk) (Reiner et al., 1988). These neurons comprise the indirect pathway, projecting to the external segment of globus pallidus. The indirect pathway acts to terminate basal ganglia associated movements or suppress unwanted sequences of movements (Bolam et al., 2000). Hence, the loss of the indirect pathway neurons leads to disinhibition of the thalamus and increased facilitation of the motor cortex, producing hyperkinesias in HD patients (Calabresi et al., 1996). On the other hand, the direct pathway neurons co-expressing the dopamine receptor D1 (Drd1) and substance P (SP) are less affected in HD. In contrast, striatal interneurons containing acetylcholine, somatostatin/neuropeptide Y, or parvalbumin are spared in patients with HD; a striking phenomenon considering the fact that these cell populations comprise only 5% of striatal neurons (Ferrante et al., 1987a; Ferrante et al., 1987b). These findings suggest that the Drd2/Enk neurons of the striatum may be more vulnerable to the deleterious effects of mutated htt. However, the precise mechanism of this selective neuronal loss is unknown.

Genetic studies using HD mouse models with altered levels of BDNF indicate that BDNF plays an important role in this specificity of degeneration. Depletion of BDNF using heterozygous or forebrain-specific knockout mice results in alterations of striatal gene expression profiling that more closely recapitulates human HD than any other HD models (Strand et al., 2007). Deletion of one copy of the Bdnf gene in R6/1 HD mice resulted in early onset of the disease, more severe motor dysfunction, and led to a significant and selective loss of Drd2/Enk striatal neurons (Canals et al., 2004). Data originated in our laboratory show that the loss of striatal neurons was associated with reduced levels of mRNAs for both Enk and Drd2 in YAC128 HD mice (Xie et al., 2010), indicating selective degeneration of striatal neurons in the indirect pathway. Our recent data suggest that selective vulnerability of striatal neurons in the indirect pathway is due to differential expression of the TrkB receptor among striatal neurons. We found that the majority of the TrkB receptor was localized in striatal neurons of the indirect pathway in the adult mouse brain and deletion of TrkB receptor in the developing striatum caused selective loss of this neuronal population (Baydyuk et al., 2011). Together, all these findings indicate that a decrease in striatal BDNF can lead to dysfunction and death of MSNs in the indirect pathway, producing severe motor phenotype as seen in HD. Hence, restoring BDNF levels in the striatum may delay or even stop disease progression.

6. Increasing BDNF expression rescues disease phenotypes in HD mouse models

The evidence discussed above clearly indicates that the reduction in striatal BDNF levels plays a pivotal role in the pathogenesis of HD. Therefore, it is not surprising that efforts have been made to examine whether increasing BDNF expression represents a valuable strategy for treatment of Huntington's Disease. Indeed, increasing striatal BDNF levels via stimulation that induces *Bdnf* gene expression (Duan et al., 2003; Peng et al., 2008; Simmons et al., 2009; Spires et al., 2004) or by viral delivery (Cho et al., 2007) has been shown to improve disease phenotypes in several HD mouse models.

Early symptoms of HD are manifested by cognitive and memory deficits that start before characteristic motor dysfunction (Ho et al., 2003; Lawrence et al., 1998). In HD mouse models, impaired learning and memory, measured as hippocampal long-term potentiation (LTP), occur prior to motor deficits and neuronal loss (Mazarakis et al., 2005; Murphy et al., 2000; Van Raamsdonk et al., 2005). LTP, a form of synaptic plasticity, is potentiated by release of BDNF. Thus, reduced levels of BDNF in HD patients and mice can disrupt synaptic changes important for learning and memory formation. Applying low concentrations of BDNF to hippocampal slices prepared from HD mice fully restores LTP (Lynch et al., 2007). Furthermore, up-regulation of endogenous BDNF levels with an ampakine, a positive modulator of AMPA-type glutamate receptors, rescues synaptic plasticity and reduces learning deficits in HD mice (Simmons et al., 2009).

Altered neurogenesis has been reported in HD mouse models and in human postmortem brains (Curtis et al., 2003; Gil et al., 2005; Phillips et al., 2005). It has been shown that in addition to promoting survival and inducing synaptic plasticity, BDNF also regulates adult neurogenesis (Bath et al., 2011; Henry et al., 2007; Scharfman et al., 2005). The adenoviral delivery of BDNF and Noggin (a known suppressor of gliogenesis) to the striatum of R6/2 HD mice resulted in induction of striatal neurogenesis (Cho et al., 2007). The majority of the newly born neurons differentiated to MSNs and became functional, leading to delayed motor impairment and prolonged survival in R6/2 mice. Similar improvements have been seen in the same HD mouse model after administration of the antidepressant sertraline (Peng et al., 2008). By increasing BDNF levels and stimulating neurogenesis, sertraline treatment resulted in improved motor performance, reduced striatal atrophy, and prolonged survival.

To more directly evaluate the effect of increasing cortical BDNF supply to the striatum on the progression of HD, we overexpressed BDNF in the mouse forebrain by employing a *Bdnf* transgene under the control of the promoter for Ca^{2+}/calmodulin-dependent protein kinase II alpha (Gharami et al., 2008; Xie et al., 2010). This transgene starts to express BDNF in the cerebral cortex in the first postnatal week and reaches plateau in the third postnatal week, as does the endogenous *Bdnf* gene (Huang et al., 1999). It also expresses at low levels in the striatum where the endogenous *Bdnf* gene is mostly inactive (Gharami et al., 2008; Xie et al., 2010). We found that the *Bdnf* transgene was able to greatly increase BDNF levels in the striata of R6/1 and YAC128 mice, indicating that overexpressed BDNF in the cortex is efficiently transported to the striatum despite expression of mutant htt. Importantly, BDNF overexpression reversed brain atrophy, normalized the expression of several important genes in the striatum, and ameliorated deficits in motor coordination in these two HD mouse models (Gharami et al., 2008; Xie et al., 2010). In addition, overexpression of BDNF in YAC128 mice prevented loss of striatal neurons, normalized spine abnormalities of medium-sized spiny neurons, and significantly improved procedural learning (Xie et al., 2010). In summary, these studies suggest that increasing striatal BDNF supply may have therapeutic potential for HD.

7. Conclusion

Many pathways have been proposed to contribute to the pathogenesis of HD. Recent studies have identified complex molecular mechanisms that mediate neuronal dysfunction and death; these include transcriptional dysregulation, excitotoxicity, impaired axonal transport, and altered synaptic transmission. The findings presented in this chapter support the hypothesis that reduced striatal BDNF plays a crucial role in HD pathogenesis. Currently, drugs used to treat HD act on the symptoms and do not slow or stop the disease progression. Attempting to restore striatal BDNF levels or activate downstream signaling pathways may have therapeutic potential in treating HD patients.

8. Acknowledgment

This work was supported by a grant from the National Institutes of Health (R01 NS050596) to BX.

9. References

Aid T, Kazantseva A, Piirsoo M, Palm K, Timmusk T. (2007). Mouse and rat BDNF gene structure and expression revisited. *Journal of Neuroscience Research*, Vol.85, No.3, (Feb 15), pp.525-535, ISSN 0360-4012

Altar CA, Cai N, Bliven T, Juhasz M, Conner JM, et al. (1997). Anterograde transport of brain-derived neurotrophic factor and its role in the brain. *Nature*, Vol.389, No.6653, (Oct 23), pp.856-860, ISSN 0028-0836

Apostol BL, Simmons DA, Zuccato C, Illes K, Pallos J, et al. (2008). CEP-1347 reduces mutant huntingtin-associated neurotoxicity and restores BDNF levels in R6/2 mice. *Molecular and Cellular Neuroscience*, Vol.39, No.1, (Sep), pp.8-20, ISSN 1095-9327

Baquet ZC, Gorski JA, Jones KR. (2004). Early striatal dendrite deficits followed by neuron loss with advanced age in the absence of anterograde cortical brain-derived neurotrophic factor. *Journal of Neuroscience*, Vol.24, No.17, (Apr 28), pp.4250-4258, ISSN 1529-2401

Bath KG, Akins MR, Lee FS. (2011). BDNF control of adult SVZ neurogenesis. *Developmental Psychobiology*, (Mar 22), ISSN 1098-2302

Baydyuk M, Russell T, Liao GY, Zang K, An JJ, et al. (2011). TrkB receptor controls striatal formation by regulating the number of newborn striatal neurons. *Proceedings of National Academy of Sciences U S A*, Vol.108, No.4, (Jan 25), pp.1669-1674, ISSN 1091-6490

Bhave SV, Ghoda L, Hoffman PL. (1999). Brain-derived neurotrophic factor mediates the anti-apoptotic effect of NMDA in cerebellar granule neurons: signal transduction cascades and site of ethanol action. *Journal of Neuroscience*, Vol.19, No.9, (May 1), pp.3277-3286, ISSN 0270-6474

Block-Galarza J, Chase KO, Sapp E, Vaughn KT, Vallee RB, et al. (1997). Fast transport and retrograde movement of huntingtin and HAP 1 in axons. *Neuroreport*, Vol.8, No.9-10, (Jul 7), pp.2247-2251, ISSN 0959-4965

Bolam JP, Hanley JJ, Booth PA, Bevan MD. (2000). Synaptic organisation of the basal ganglia. *Journal of Anatomy*, Vol.196 (Pt 4), (May), pp.527-542, ISSN 0021-8782

Borrell-Pages M, Zala D, Humbert S, Saudou F. (2006). Huntington's disease: from huntingtin function and dysfunction to therapeutic strategies. *Cellular and Molecular Life Science*, Vol.63, No.22, (Nov), pp.2642-2660, ISSN 1420-682X

Calabresi P, Pisani A, Mercuri NB, Bernardi G. (1996). The corticostriatal projection: from synaptic plasticity to dysfunctions of the basal ganglia. *Trends in Neuroscience*, Vol.19, No.1, (Jan), pp.19-24, ISSN 0166-2236

Canals JM, Pineda JR, Torres-Peraza JF, Bosch M, Martin-Ibanez R, et al. (2004). Brain-derived neurotrophic factor regulates the onset and severity of motor dysfunction associated with enkephalinergic neuronal degeneration in Huntington's disease. *Journal of Neuroscience*, Vol.24, No.35, (Sep 1), pp.7727-7739, ISSN 1529-2401

Chao MV. (2003). Neurotrophins and their receptors: a convergence point for many signalling pathways. *Nature Reviews Neuroscience*, Vol.4, No.4, (Apr), pp.299-309, ISSN 1471-003X

Cho SR, Benraiss A, Chmielnicki E, Samdani A, Economides A, Goldman SA. (2007). Induction of neostriatal neurogenesis slows disease progression in a transgenic murine model of Huntington disease. *Journal of Clinical Investigations*, Vol.117, No.10, (Oct), pp.2889-2902, ISSN 0021-9738

Ciammola A, Sassone J, Cannella M, Calza S, Poletti B, et al. (2007). Low brain-derived neurotrophic factor (BDNF) levels in serum of Huntington's disease patients. *Am J Med Genet B Neuropsychiatr Genet*, Vol.144B, No.4, (Jun 5), pp.574-577, ISSN 1552-4841

Cummings DM, Andre VM, Uzgil BO, Gee SM, Fisher YE, et al. (2009). Alterations in cortical excitation and inhibition in genetic mouse models of Huntington's disease. *Journal of Neuroscience*, Vol.29, No.33, (Aug 19), pp.10371-10386, ISSN 1529-2401

Curtis MA, Penney EB, Pearson AG, van Roon-Mom WM, Butterworth NJ, et al. (2003). Increased cell proliferation and neurogenesis in the adult human Huntington's disease brain. *Proceedings of National Academy of Science U S A*, Vol.100, No.15, (Jul 22), pp.9023-9027, ISSN 0027-8424

DiFiglia M, Sapp E, Chase K, Schwarz C, Meloni A, et al. (1995). Huntingtin is a cytoplasmic protein associated with vesicles in human and rat brain neurons. *Neuron*, Vol.14, No.5, (May), pp.1075-1081, ISSN 0896-6273

Dragatsis I, Levine MS, Zeitlin S. (2000). Inactivation of Hdh in the brain and testis results in progressive neurodegeneration and sterility in mice. *Nature Genetics*, Vol.26, No.3, (Nov), pp.300-306, ISSN 1061-4036

Duan W, Guo Z, Jiang H, Ware M, Li XJ, Mattson MP. (2003). Dietary restriction normalizes glucose metabolism and BDNF levels, slows disease progression, and increases survival in huntingtin mutant mice. *Proceedings of National Academy of Science U S A*, Vol.100, No.5, (Mar 4), pp.2911-2916, ISSN 0027-8424

Encinas M, Iglesias M, Llecha N, Comella JX. (1999). Extracellular-regulated kinases and phosphatidylinositol 3-kinase are involved in brain-derived neurotrophic factor-mediated survival and neuritogenesis of the neuroblastoma cell line SH-SY5Y. *Journal of Neurochemistry*, Vol.73, No.4, (Oct), pp.1409-1421, ISSN 0022-3042

Engelender S, Sharp AH, Colomer V, Tokito MK, Lanahan A, et al. (1997). Huntingtin-associated protein 1 (HAP1) interacts with the p150Glued subunit of dynactin. *Human Molecular Genetics*, Vol.6, No.13, (Dec), pp.2205-2212, ISSN 0964-6906

Ferrante RJ, Beal MF, Kowall NW, Richardson EP, Jr., Martin JB. (1987a). Sparing of acetylcholinesterase-containing striatal neurons in Huntington's disease. *Brain Research*, Vol.411, No.1, (May 12), pp.162-166, ISSN 0006-8993

Ferrante RJ, Kowall NW, Beal MF, Martin JB, Bird ED, Richardson EP, Jr. (1987b). Morphologic and histochemical characteristics of a spared subset of striatal neurons in Huntington's disease. *Journal of Neuropathology and Experimental Neurology*, Vol.46, No.1, (Jan), pp.12-27, ISSN 0022-3069

Ferrer I, Goutan E, Marin C, Rey MJ, Ribalta T. (2000). Brain-derived neurotrophic factor in Huntington disease. *Brain Research*, Vol.866, No.1-2, (Jun 2), pp.257-261, ISSN 0006-8993

Frade JM, Barde YA. (1998). Nerve growth factor: two receptors, multiple functions. *Bioessays*, Vol.20, No.2, (Feb), pp.137-145, ISSN 0265-9247

Gauthier LR, Charrin BC, Borrell-Pages M, Dompierre JP, Rangone H, et al. (2004). Huntingtin controls neurotrophic support and survival of neurons by enhancing BDNF vesicular transport along microtubules. *Cell*, Vol.118, No.1, (Jul 9), pp.127-138, ISSN 0092-8674

Gharami K, Xie Y, An JJ, Tonegawa S, Xu B. (2008). Brain-derived neurotrophic factor over-expression in the forebrain ameliorates Huntington's disease phenotypes in mice. *Journal of Neurochemistry*, Vol.105, No.2, (Apr), pp.369-379, ISSN 1471-4159

Gil JM, Mohapel P, Araujo IM, Popovic N, Li JY, et al. (2005). Reduced hippocampal neurogenesis in R6/2 transgenic Huntington's disease mice. *Neurobiology of Disease*, Vol.20, No.3, (Dec), pp.744-751, ISSN 0969-9961

Gorski JA, Zeiler SR, Tamowski S, Jones KR. (2003). Brain-derived neurotrophic factor is required for the maintenance of cortical dendrites. *Journal of Neuroscience*, Vol.23, No.17, (Jul 30), pp.6856-6865, ISSN 1529-2401

Gunawardena S, Her LS, Brusch RG, Laymon RA, Niesman IR, et al. (2003). Disruption of axonal transport by loss of huntingtin or expression of pathogenic polyQ proteins in Drosophila. *Neuron*, Vol.40, No.1, (Sep 25), pp.25-40, ISSN 0896-6273

Gusella JF, MacDonald ME. (2000). Molecular genetics: unmasking polyglutamine triggers in neurodegenerative disease. *Nature Reviews Neuroscience*, Vol.1, No.2, (Nov), pp.109-115, ISSN 1471-003X

Hempstead BL. (2006). Dissecting the diverse actions of pro- and mature neurotrophins. *Current Alzheimer Research*, Vol.3, No.1, (Feb), pp.19-24, ISSN 1567-2050

Henry RA, Hughes SM, Connor B. (2007). AAV-mediated delivery of BDNF augments neurogenesis in the normal and quinolinic acid-lesioned adult rat brain. *European Journal of Neuroscience*, Vol.25, No.12, (Jun), pp.3513-3525, ISSN 0953-816X

Ho AK, Sahakian BJ, Brown RG, Barker RA, Hodges JR, et al. (2003). Profile of cognitive progression in early Huntington's disease. *Neurology*, Vol.61, No.12, (Dec 23), pp.1702-1706, ISSN 1526-632X

Hodgson JG, Agopyan N, Gutekunst CA, Leavitt BR, LePiane F, et al. (1999). A YAC mouse model for Huntington's disease with full-length mutant huntingtin, cytoplasmic toxicity, and selective striatal neurodegeneration. *Neuron*, Vol.23, No.1, (May), pp.181-192, ISSN 0896-6273

Huang ZJ, Kirkwood A, Pizzorusso T, Porciatti V, Morales B, et al. (1999). BDNF regulates the maturation of inhibition and the critical period of plasticity in mouse visual cortex. *Cell*, Vol.98, No.6, (Sep 17), pp.739-755, ISSN 0092-8674

Kim M, Lee HS, LaForet G, McIntyre C, Martin EJ, et al. (1999). Mutant huntingtin expression in clonal striatal cells: dissociation of inclusion formation and neuronal survival by caspase inhibition. *Journal of Neuroscience*, Vol.19, No.3, (Feb 1), pp.964-973, ISSN 0270-6474

Laforet GA, Sapp E, Chase K, McIntyre C, Boyce FM, et al. (2001). Changes in cortical and striatal neurons predict behavioral and electrophysiological abnormalities in a transgenic murine model of Huntington's disease. *Journal of Neuroscience*, Vol.21, No.23, (Dec 1), pp.9112-9123, ISSN 1529-2401

Lawrence AD, Hodges JR, Rosser AE, Kershaw A, ffrench-Constant C, et al. (1998). Evidence for specific cognitive deficits in preclinical Huntington's disease. *Brain*, Vol.121 (Pt 7), (Jul), pp.1329-1341, ISSN 0006-8950

Li SH, Gutekunst CA, Hersch SM, Li XJ. (1998). Interaction of huntingtin-associated protein with dynactin P150Glued. *Journal of Neuroscience*, Vol.18, No.4, (Feb 15), pp.1261-1269, ISSN 0270-6474

Lynch G, Kramar EA, Rex CS, Jia Y, Chappas D, et al. (2007). Brain-derived neurotrophic factor restores synaptic plasticity in a knock-in mouse model of Huntington's disease. *Journal of Neuroscience*, Vol.27, No.16, (Apr 18), pp.4424-4434, ISSN 1529-2401

Mann DM, Oliver R, Snowden JS. (1993). The topographic distribution of brain atrophy in Huntington's disease and progressive supranuclear palsy. *Acta Neuropathologica*, Vol.85, No.5, pp.553-559, ISSN 0001-6322

Matsumoto T, Rauskolb S, Polack M, Klose J, Kolbeck R, et al. (2008). Biosynthesis and processing of endogenous BDNF: CNS neurons store and secrete BDNF, not pro-BDNF. *Nature Neuroscience*, Vol.11, No.2, (Feb), pp.131-133, ISSN 1097-6256

Mazarakis NK, Cybulska-Klosowicz A, Grote H, Pang T, Van Dellen A, et al. (2005). Deficits in experience-dependent cortical plasticity and sensory-discrimination learning in presymptomatic Huntington's disease mice. *Journal of Neuroscience*, Vol.25, No.12, (Mar 23), pp.3059-3066, ISSN 1529-2401

McAllister AK, Katz LC, Lo DC. (1999). Neurotrophins and synaptic plasticity. *Annual Reviews Neuroscience*, Vol.22, pp.295-318, ISSN 0147-006X

Metsis M, Timmusk T, Arenas E, Persson H. (1993). Differential usage of multiple brain-derived neurotrophic factor promoters in the rat brain following neuronal activation. *Proceedings of National Academy of Science U S A*, Vol.90, No.19, (Oct 1), pp.8802-8806, ISSN 0027-8424

Murphy KP, Carter RJ, Lione LA, Mangiarini L, Mahal A, et al. (2000). Abnormal synaptic plasticity and impaired spatial cognition in mice transgenic for exon 1 of the human Huntington's disease mutation. *Journal of Neuroscience*, Vol.20, No.13, (Jul 1), pp.5115-5123, ISSN 1529-2401

O'Kusky JR, Nasir J, Cicchetti F, Parent A, Hayden MR. (1999). Neuronal degeneration in the basal ganglia and loss of pallido-subthalamic synapses in mice with targeted disruption of the Huntington's disease gene. *Brain Research*, Vol.818, No.2, (Feb 13), pp.468-479, ISSN 0006-8993

Pang TY, Stam NC, Nithianantharajah J, Howard ML, Hannan AJ. (2006). Differential effects of voluntary physical exercise on behavioral and brain-derived neurotrophic factor expression deficits in Huntington's disease transgenic mice. *Neuroscience*, Vol.141, No.2, (Aug 25), pp.569-584, ISSN 0306-4522

Patapoutian A, Reichardt LF. (2001). Trk receptors: mediators of neurotrophin action. *Current Opinions in Neurobiology*, Vol.11, No.3, (Jun), pp.272-280, ISSN 0959-4388

Pattabiraman PP, Tropea D, Chiaruttini C, Tongiorgi E, Cattaneo A, Domenici L. (2005). Neuronal activity regulates the developmental expression and subcellular localization of cortical BDNF mRNA isoforms in vivo. *Molecular and Cellular Neuroscience*, Vol.28, No.3, (Mar), pp.556-570, ISSN 1044-7431

Peng Q, Masuda N, Jiang M, Li Q, Zhao M, et al. (2008). The antidepressant sertraline improves the phenotype, promotes neurogenesis and increases BDNF levels in the R6/2 Huntington's disease mouse model. *Experimental Neurology*, Vol.210, No.1, (Mar), pp.154-163, ISSN 0014-4886

Phillips W, Morton AJ, Barker RA. (2005). Abnormalities of neurogenesis in the R6/2 mouse model of Huntington's disease are attributable to the in vivo microenvironment. *Journal of Neuroscience*, Vol.25, No.50, (Dec 14), pp.11564-11576, ISSN 1529-2401

Reichardt LF. (2006). Neurotrophin-regulated signalling pathways. *Philos Trans R Soc Lond B Biol Sci*, Vol.361, No.1473, (Sep 29), pp.1545-1564, ISSN 0962-8436

Reiner A, Albin RL, Anderson KD, D'Amato CJ, Penney JB, Young AB. (1988). Differential loss of striatal projection neurons in Huntington disease. *Proceedings of National Academy of Science U S A*, Vol.85, No.15, (Aug), pp.5733-5737, ISSN 0027-8424

Rigamonti D, Bauer JH, De-Fraja C, Conti L, Sipione S, et al. (2000). Wild-type huntingtin protects from apoptosis upstream of caspase-3. *Journal of Neuroscience*, Vol.20, No.10, (May 15), pp.3705-3713, ISSN 1529-2401

Rubinsztein DC. (2002). Lessons from animal models of Huntington's disease. *Trends in Genetics*, Vol.18, No.4, (Apr), pp.202-209, ISSN 0168-9525

Saudou F, Finkbeiner S, Devys D, Greenberg ME. (1998). Huntingtin acts in the nucleus to induce apoptosis but death does not correlate with the formation of intranuclear inclusions. *Cell*, Vol.95, No.1, pp.55-66, ISSN 0092-8674

Scharfman H, Goodman J, Macleod A, Phani S, Antonelli C, Croll S. (2005). Increased neurogenesis and the ectopic granule cells after intrahippocampal BDNF infusion in adult rats. *Experimental Neurology*, Vol.192, No.2, (Apr), pp.348-356, ISSN 0014-4886

Seo H, Kim W, Isacson O. (2008). Compensatory changes in the ubiquitin-proteasome system, brain-derived neurotrophic factor and mitochondrial complex II/III in YAC72 and R6/2 transgenic mice partially model Huntington's disease patients. *Human Molecular Genetics*, Vol.17, No.20, (Oct 15), pp.3144-3153, ISSN 1460-2083

Simmons DA, Rex CS, Palmer L, Pandyarajan V, Fedulov V, et al. (2009). Up-regulating BDNF with an ampakine rescues synaptic plasticity and memory in Huntington's disease knockin mice. *Proceedings of National Academy of Science U S A*, Vol.106, No.12, (Mar 24), pp.4906-4911, ISSN 1091-6490

Spires TL, Grote HE, Varshney NK, Cordery PM, van Dellen A, et al. (2004). Environmental enrichment rescues protein deficits in a mouse model of Huntington's disease, indicating a possible disease mechanism. *Journal of Neuroscience*, Vol.24, No.9, (Mar 3), pp.2270-2276, ISSN 1529-2401

Strand AD, Baquet ZC, Aragaki AK, Holmans P, Yang L, et al. (2007). Expression profiling of Huntington's disease models suggests that brain-derived neurotrophic factor depletion plays a major role in striatal degeneration. *Journal of Neuroscience*, Vol.27, No.43, (Oct 24), pp.11758-11768, ISSN 1529-2401

Szebenyi G, Morfini GA, Babcock A, Gould M, Selkoe K, et al. (2003). Neuropathogenic forms of huntingtin and androgen receptor inhibit fast axonal transport. *Neuron*, Vol.40, No.1, (Sep 25), pp.41-52, ISSN 0896-6273

Teng HK, Teng KK, Lee R, Wright S, Tevar S, et al. (2005). ProBDNF induces neuronal apoptosis via activation of a receptor complex of p75NTR and sortilin. *Journal of Neuroscience*, Vol.25, No.22, (Jun 1), pp.5455-5463, ISSN 1529-2401

The Huntington's Disease Collaborative Research Group. (1993). A novel gene containing a trinucleotide repeat that is expanded and unstable on Huntington's disease chromosomes. *Cell*, Vol.72, No.6, (Mar 26), pp.971-983, ISSN 8458085

Timmusk T, Palm K, Metsis M, Reintam T, Paalme V, et al. (1993). Multiple promoters direct tissue-specific expression of the rat BDNF gene. *Neuron*, Vol.10, No.3, (Mar), pp.475-489, ISSN 0896-6273

Van Raamsdonk JM, Pearson J, Slow EJ, Hossain SM, Leavitt BR, Hayden MR. (2005). Cognitive dysfunction precedes neuropathology and motor abnormalities in the YAC128 mouse model of Huntington's disease. *Journal of Neuroscience*, Vol.25, No.16, (Apr 20), pp.4169-4180, ISSN 1529-2401

Vonsattel JP, DiFiglia M. (1998). Huntington disease. *Journal of Neuropathology and Experimental Neurology*, Vol.57, No.5, (May), pp.369-384, ISSN 0022-3069

Xie Y, Hayden MR, Xu B. (2010). BDNF overexpression in the forebrain rescues Huntington's disease phenotypes in YAC128 mice. *Journal of Neuroscience*, Vol.30, No.44, (Nov 3), pp.14708-14718, ISSN 1529-2401

Xu B, Zang K, Ruff NL, Zhang YA, McConnell SK, et al. (2000). Cortical degeneration in the absence of neurotrophin signaling: dendritic retraction and neuronal loss after removal of the receptor TrkB. *Neuron*, Vol.26, No.1, (Apr), pp.233-245, ISSN 0896-6273

Yamada M, Tanabe K, Wada K, Shimoke K, Ishikawa Y, et al. (2001). Differences in survival-promoting effects and intracellular signaling properties of BDNF and IGF-1 in cultured cerebral cortical neurons. *Journal of Neurochemistry*, Vol.78, No.5, (Sep), pp.940-951, ISSN 0022-3042

Yang J, Siao CJ, Nagappan G, Marinic T, Jing D, et al. (2009). Neuronal release of proBDNF. *Nature Neuroscience*, Vol.12, No.2, (Feb), pp.113-115, ISSN 1546-1726

Yang M, Lim Y, Li X, Zhong JH, Zhou XF. (2011). Precursor of brain-derived neurotrophic factor (proBDNF) forms a complex with Huntingtin-associated protein-1 (HAP1) and sortilin that modulates proBDNF trafficking, degradation, and processing. *Journal of Biological Chemistry*, Vol.286, No.18, (May 6), pp.16272-16284, ISSN 1083-351X

Zuccato C, Ciammola A, Rigamonti D, Leavitt BR, Goffredo D, et al. (2001). Loss of huntingtin-mediated BDNF gene transcription in Huntington's disease. *Science*, Vol.293, No.5529, (Jul 20), pp.493-498, ISSN 0036-8075

Zuccato C, Marullo M, Conforti P, MacDonald ME, Tartari M, Cattaneo E. (2008). Systematic assessment of BDNF and its receptor levels in human cortices affected by Huntington's disease. *Brain Pathology*, Vol.18, No.2, (Apr), pp.225-238, ISSN 1015-6305

Zuccato C, Tartari M, Crotti A, Goffredo D, Valenza M, et al. (2003). Huntingtin interacts with REST/NRSF to modulate the transcription of NRSE-controlled neuronal genes. *Nature Genetics*, Vol.35, No.1, (Sep), pp.76-83, ISSN 1061-4036

8

Don't Take Away My P: Phosphatases as Therapeutic Targets in Huntington's Disease

Ana Saavedra[1,2,3], Jordi Alberch[1,2,3] and Esther Pérez-Navarro[1,2,3]
[1]Departament de Biologia Cellular, Immunologia i Neurociències,
Facultat de Medicina, Universitat de Barcelona, Barcelona,
[2]Institut d'Investigacions Biomèdiques August Pi i Sunyer (IDIBAPS), Barcelona,
[3]Centro de Investigación Biomédica en Red sobre,
Enfermedades Neurodegenerativas (CIBERNED),
Spain

1. Introduction

The molecular bases that account for the preferential neurodegeneration of striatal medium-sized spiny neurons (MSNs) in Huntington's Disease (HD) are still unknown, and different mechanisms have been proposed to contribute to the neurodegenerative process. These include mitochondrial dysfunction and metabolic impairment, transcriptional dysregulation, altered expression of trophic factors, dopamine toxicity, oxidative stress, and changes in autophagy, and huntingtin (htt) phosphorylation. In addition, excitotoxicity through the overactivation of N-methyl-D-aspartate (NMDA) receptors (NMDARs) has also been proposed to contribute to the preferential loss of these neurons (for review see Ehrnhoefer et al., 2011; Jin & Johnson, 2010; Perez-Navarro et al., 2006; Renna et al., 2010; Rosenstock et al., 2010; Weir et al., 2011).

Some of these mechanisms are controlled by the attachment/removal of phosphate groups through the action of protein kinases and protein phosphatases, respectively. Therefore, alterations in their levels/activity in the presence of mutant htt (mhtt) can impact on cell survival.

Htt is expressed in almost all tissues, has a widespread distribution in the brain, its expression levels are similar in control individuals and in HD patients, with no evidence of increased htt expression in the brain regions most affected in HD (reviewed by Han et al., 2010). These evidences indicate that differences in mhtt expression do not contribute to the increased vulnerability of MSNs in HD. Conversely, several cell-type specific features including morphological, biochemical, and functional characteristics might play a role in rendering MSNs more vulnerable to the toxic effects of mhtt (Han et al., 2010). In this line, it is relevant in context of the present review to mention that the phosphatases calcineurin (also known as protein phosphatase 2B – PP2B) (Goto et al., 1987) and striatal-enriched protein tyrosine phosphatase (STEP) (Lombroso et al., 1991) are enriched in MSNs, suggesting that variations in their expression levels/activity can impact seriously in the function and viability of these neurons.

Here, we will revisit the excitotoxic hypothesis in HD through the phosphatase point of view, and we will also pay attention to the importance of phosphorylation in reducing the toxicity of mhtt. We will discuss the results obtained in both exon-1 and full-length HD models, and we will integrate the potential contribution of an imbalance between the activity of phosphatases and kinases to HD pathophysiology.

1.1 Excitotoxicity

Glutamate, the major excitatory neurotransmitter in the central nervous system (CNS), is important for neural development, synaptic plasticity, and learning and memory under physiological conditions. Dysregulation of glutamate levels and/or glutamate receptor activity can result in an overstimulation of glutamate receptors leading to cell death via excitotoxicity (Olney, 1969). In HD, excitotoxicity induced by overactivation of NMDARs has been proposed to explain the preferential neurodegeneration of MSNs (reviewed by Fan & Raymond, 2007; Milnerwood & Raymond, 2010; Perez-Navarro et al., 2006). Functional NMDARs are tetrameric structures (Laube et al., 1998) composed of two NR1 and at least two NR2 subunits (Ozawa et al., 1998), and the striatum is enriched in NR2B compared with other NR2 subunits (Landwehrmeyer et al., 1995). The presence of mhtt in striatal neurons leads to a number of alterations that can explain changes in the susceptibility to excitotoxicity. These include: (1) Selective increase of the current flowing through NMDARs comprising NR1/NR2B subunits (Zeron et al., 2001, 2002); (2) Changes in NMDAR scaffolding proteins (Jarabek et al., 2004; Sun et al., 2001; Torres-Peraza et al., 2008); (3) Altered phosphorylation of NMDAR subunits (Jarabek et al., 2004; Song et al., 2003) and (4) Imbalance between synaptic and extra-synaptic NMDARs (Milnerwood et al., 2010; Okamoto, 2009). In addition to alterations at the level of NMDARs, mhtt also alters intracellular mechanisms regulated by NMDAR stimulation, such as the activity of kinases and phosphatases. Calcineurin, PP1, PP2A, and STEP are phosphatases regulated by NMDARs stimulation (Figure 1) whose levels/activity have been shown to be altered in neurons expressing exon-1 or full-length mhtt (Table 1).

1.2 Phosphorylation of htt

Htt has several known sites of phosphorylation, all of them less phosphorylated in the mutant than in the wild-type protein (reviewed by Ernhoefer et al., 2011). Among the htt phosphorylation sites identified, serine 421 (Ser421) is the most studied and thus, the best characterized. This site can be phosphorylated by Akt (Humbert et al., 2002) and serum and glucocorticoid-induced kinase (SGK) (Rangone et al., 2004), whereas calcineurin (Pardo et al., 2006; Pineda et al., 2009), PP1 and PP2A (Metzler et al., 2010) dephosphorylate it. Until now, phosphatases known to regulate htt phosphorylation at Ser421 have been shown to be altered in HD models (Table 1). Phosphorylation of Ser421 regulates htt's toxicity (Humbert et al., 2002; Pardo et al., 2006), htt's role in vesicle transport (Colin et al., 2008; Pineda et al., 2009; Zala et al., 2008), and htt cleavage by caspases (Metzler et al., 2010; Warby et al., 2009). In addition, phosphorylation of htt and mhtt at Ser421 is significantly reduced in neurons after excitotoxic stimulation of NMDARs (Metzler et al., 2010) (Figure 1). Moreover, there are other Ser and threonine (Thr) residues of htt that can be phosphorylated, and all of them regulate its toxicity. Most of the kinases that phosphorylate these sites have been identified, and include IKK (Thompson et al., 2009), cyclin-dependent kinase 5 (Cdk5) (Anne et al.,

2007; Luo et al., 2005), ERK1 (Schilling et al., 2006), and CK2 (Atwal et al., 2011). In contrast, the phosphatases acting on these residues are still unknown (reviewed by Ernhoefer et al., 2011).

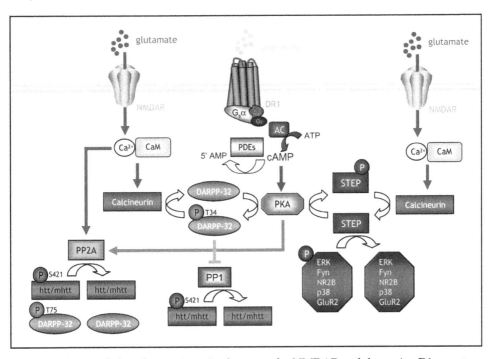

Fig. 1. Regulation of phosphatases in striatal neurons by NMDAR and dopamine D1 receptor (DR1) stimulation. Stimulation of NMDARs activates PP2A and calcineurin, which in turn will activate STEP and PP1. DR1 stimulation activates PP2A, and indirectly blocks PP1 activity. Several pathways and targets have been omitted for simplification. PDEs: Phosphodiesterases; AC: Adenylyl cyclase; PKA: cAMP-dependent protein kinase; CaM: calmodulin; DARPP-32: dopamine- and cAMP-regulated phosphoprotein of 32 kDa

2. Ser/Thr phosphatases

Ser/Thr phosphatases catalyze dephosphorylation reactions on phospho-Ser and phospho-Thr residues. They are classified into three families: protein phosphatase Mg^{2+}-activated (PPM), phosphoprotein phosphatases (PPPs) and the aspartate-based phosphatases represented by FCP/SCP (TFIIF-associating component of RNA polymerase II CTD phosphatase/small CTD phosphatase). The PPM family includes PP2C, pyruvate dehydrogenase phosphatase, and PP2C-"like" phosphatases, and the major phosphatases in the PPP family are PP1, PP2A and calcineurin (reviewed by McConnell & Wadzinski, 2009). PP1, PP2A and calcineurin are composed of catalytic and regulatory subunits, whereas PP2C exists as a monomer devoid of regulatory subunits. In the brain, the activity of these phosphatases is regulated by the regulatory subunit, interacting partners, scaffolding proteins and/or specific endogenous activators/inhibitors (reviewed by Gee & Mansuy,

2005). These phosphatases are implicated in the regulation of excitotoxicity, synaptic plasticity and cell survival, and are altered in neurodegenerative disorders such as Alzheimer's Disease (Ducruet et al., 2005; Iqbal & Grundke-Iqbal, 2007; F. Liu et al., 2006; Tian & Wang, 2002), Parkinson's Disease (Lou et al., 2010; Wera & Neyts, 1994) and HD (Metzler et al., 2010; Pineda et al., 2009; Saavedra et al., 2010; Xifro et al., 2008; 2009).

Type of phosphatase	Phosphatase	Change	HD model	Reference
Ser/Thr Phosphatase	Calcineurin	Increased	STHdh $^{Q7/Q111}$ cells and Hdh$^{Q111/Q111}$ mice	Xifro et al., 2008 Pineda et al., 2009
		Reduced	R6/1; YAC128	Xifro et al., 2009 Metzler et al., 2010
	PHLPP1	Reduced	R6/1; R6/1:BDNF; R6/2; Tet/HD94; Hdh$^{Q111/Q111}$ and STHdh $^{Q111/Q111}$ cells	Saavedra et al., 2010
	PHLPP2	Unchanged/Reduced	R6/1	Rue et al., unpublished
	PP1	Unchanged Reduced	YAC128 YAC128	Metzler et al., 2010 Ehrnhoefer et al., 2011
	PP2A	Unchanged	YAC128; R6/1	Metzler et al., 2010 Saavedra et al., 2010
		Reduced	YAC128	Ehrnhoefer et al., 2011
Tyr Phosphatase	STEP	Decreased	R6/1; R6/2; Tet/HD94; Hdh$^{Q111/Q111}$, primary striatal neurons overexpressing htt171-82Q	Saavedra et al., 2011 Runne et al., 2008
	MKP1 and MKP3	Increased	PC12 cells overexpressing exon-1 mhtt 118Q	Z. L. Wu et al., 2002
	MKP-2	Intracellular redistribution	HEK 293 cells overexpressing mhtt 138Q and NR1/NR2B	Fan et al., 2008

Calcineurin (Xifro et al., 2009) and PHLPP1 (Saavedra et al., 2010) protein levels, and STEP mRNA levels (Hodges et al., 2006) are also decreased in the caudate/putamen of HD patients. HEK: human embryonic kidney; Q: glutamine; Tet/HD94: conditional mouse model of HD

Table 1. Phosphatases altered in HD models.

2.1 Calcineurin

Calcineurin is a Ser/Thr phosphatase activated by calcium/calmodulin, highly expressed in the brain, and abundant in the cytosol, and in pre-synaptic and post-synaptic terminals (Mansuy, 2003; Shibasaki et al., 2002). It is a heterodimer composed by a calmodulin-binding catalytic subunit, calcineurin A, and an intrinsic calcium-binding regulatory subunit, calcineurin B. The dependence on calcium distinguishes calcineurin from spontaneously active PP2A and from Mg^{2+}-dependent PP2C. The binding of the calcium/calmodulin complex to calcineurin A with high affinity leads to the release of the auto-inhibitory domain from the active site and calcineurin activation. In addition to activation by calcium, calcineurin can also be activated by caspase- or calpain-mediated proteolysis, which originate a constitutively active form, insensitive to calcium/calmodulin (reviewed by A. Mukherjee & Soto, 2011).

Calcineurin is the only calcium-dependent phosphatase present in neurons, which confers it an important role in the maintenance of cellular homeostasis, and in neuronal activity (Mansuy, 2003; Shibasaki et al., 2002). Calcineurin also modulates gene expression by the regulation of transcription factors such as the cAMP responsive element binding protein (CREB) and the nuclear factor of activated T-cell (NFAT) (reviewed by A. Mukherjee & Soto, 2011).

Calcineurin is highly expressed in the striatum, and in particular in MSNs (Goto et al., 1987). The participation of calcineurin in neuronal death induced by insults that elevate intracellular calcium levels (Ankarcrona et al., 1996; Butcher et al., 1997; Dawson et al., 1993; Shamloo et al., 2005; Shibasaki & McKeon 1995; Wood & Bristow 1998; H. Y. Wu et al., 2004) suggests that this phosphatase might be a good candidate to participate in the excitotoxic events associated with HD.

The pro-apoptotic function of calcineurin has been linked to the dephosphorylation of selected substrates related to apoptosis, such as Bad (a pro-apoptotic Bcl-2 family member) (Springer et al., 2000; H. G. Wang et al., 1999), death-associated protein kinase (Shamloo et al., 2005; Xifro et al., 2008), cdk5 (Nishi et al., 2002) or transcription factors, such as NFAT (Beals et al., 1997). Importantly, calcineurin also dephosphorylates mhtt at Ser421 (Pardo et al., 2006). Consistent with the neuroprotective role of htt phosphorylation at Ser421 (Humbert et al., 2002; Rangone et al., 2004; Warby et al., 2005), inhibition of calcineurin activity in HD neuronal cells restores htt phosphorylation levels at Ser421, and prevents polyglutamine (polyQ)-mediated cell death of striatal neurons (Pardo et al., 2006). Moreover, inhibition of calcineurin by FK506 leads to sustained phosphorylation of mhtt at Ser421 and reestablishes BDNF transport in rat primary neuronal cultures expressing mhtt, and in mouse cortical neurons from $Hdh^{Q111/Q111}$ mice (Pineda et al., 2009). Recently, calcineurin has been shown to dephosphorylate the pro-fission dynamin related protein 1 (Cereghetti et al., 2008), which increases its mitochondrial translocation and activation, leading to mitochondrial fragmentation and contributing to the hypersensitivity of HD mitochondria to apoptosis (Costa et al., 2010). In fact, mitochondrial fragmentation can be prevented by genetic or pharmacological inhibition of calcineurin (Costa et al., 2010).

Studies using primary striatal cultures from YAC transgenic mice show that NMDAR stimulation produces a polyQ length-dependent increase in cell death (Shehadeh et al., 2006; Zeron et al., 2002). These observations were extended by our studies showing that

STHdh$^{Q111/Q111}$ cells are more susceptible to NMDA-mediated cell death than STHdh$^{Q7/Q7}$ cells, a phenomenon related to higher calcineurin A protein levels and calcineurin activity in mhtt knock-in striatal cells than in wild-type cells (Xifro et al., 2008). Interestingly, although calcineurin protein levels are similar in mouse brains containing wild-type and mhtt, Hdh$^{Q111/Q111}$ and Hdh$^{Q111/Q7}$ mice have significantly higher levels of calcineurin activity in the cortex than Hdh$^{Q7/Q7}$ mice (Pineda et al., 2009). In agreement with these reports showing increased calcineurin activity, the levels of the negative regulator of calcineurin RCAN1-1L are significantly down-regulated in HD brain samples (Ermak et al., 2009). Additionally, a dysregulation in the levels of cytosolic calcium, the calcineurin activator, was also reported in primary cultures from YAC128 mice (Tang et al., 2005). Calcineurin can play a toxic role in striatal cells expressing full-length mhtt at two different levels. High levels of calcineurin increase the susceptibility to excitotoxicity (Xifro et al., 2008) and, on the other hand, calcineurin can increase mhtt toxicity directly by dephosphorylation of its Ser421 (Ermak et al., 2009; Pardo et al., 2006; Pineda et al., 2009), or indirectly by regulating proteins that modulate mhtt toxicity, such as cdk5 (Luo et al., 2005) or calpain (Gafni et al., 2004).

Conversely, calcineurin A mRNA levels are decreased in human HD samples (Hodges et al., 2006). Similarly, in the striatum of R6 mouse models of HD, which express the exon-1 mhtt fragment, calcineurin levels are lower than in the wild-type mice striatum (Hernandez-Espinosa & Morton, 2006; Lievens et al., 2002; Luthi-Carter et al., 2000; Xifro et al., 2009). Interestingly, these mice are resistant to excitotoxicity (Hansson et al., 1999, 2001; Torres-Peraza et al., 2008). These findings suggest a dual regulation of calcineurin A expression during the progression of the disease, with high levels at early stages resulting in high susceptibility to excitotoxicity (Xifro et al., 2008), and low levels at end stages participating in the resistance to excitotoxic-induced cell death (Xifro et al., 2009) (Figure 2). Thus, it would be relevant to study whether this dual calcineurin regulation also occurs in full-length mouse models of HD as YAC128 mice, which were reported to be more sensitive to excitotoxicity than controls at presymptomatic stages, but resistant to intrastriatal quinolinic acid (an NMDAR agonist) injection when signs of HD are obvious (Graham et al., 2009). Consistent with resistance to excitotoxicity (Graham et al., 2009), reduced calcineurin activity has been shown in the striatum of YAC128 mice at 12 months of age (Metzler et al., 2010).

Studies performed in *in vivo* models of HD confirm the important role played by calcineurin in the excitotoxic-mediated cell death of striatal neurons. Calcineurin inhibition in wild-type mice drastically reduces quinolinic acid-induced striatal cell death (Xifro et al., 2009). Moreover, calcineurin activation induced by intrastriatal quinolinic acid injection in R6/1 mice is lower than in wild-type mice (Xifro et al., 2009), which is consistent with R6/1 animals being resistant to excitotoxicity (Hansson et al., 1999, 2001).

However, the role of calcineurin in HD remains controversial as calcineurin inhibition has been reported to have protective (Costa et al., 2010; Ermak et al., 2009; Pardo et al., 2006; Pineda et al., 2009; Xifro et al., 2008) or worsening (Hernandez-Espinosa & Morton, 2006) effects in HD models. The participation of reduced calcineurin activity caused by alteration of calcineurin A expression in the pathophysiology of HD, and in the excitotoxic resistance observed in exon-1 mouse models (Xifro et al., 2009), together with the finding that treatment with calcineurin inhibitors accelerates the progression of the disease in R6/2 mice (Hernandez-Espinosa & Morton, 2006) suggest that decreased levels of calcineurin could result in striatal neuronal dysfunction affecting the onset of motor alterations. However, since both FK506 and cyclosporine A, that does not cross the blood–brain barrier, have the same negative effect (Hernandez-Espinosa & Morton, 2006) the harmful effect of calcineurin inhibition reported in this study might be unrelated to the effect of these inhibitors in the CNS.

Taken together, these findings suggest calcineurin as an important therapeutic target for HD, by its participation in excitotoxic events, as well as by its action on phosphorylated mhtt (Ser421) to increase toxicity.

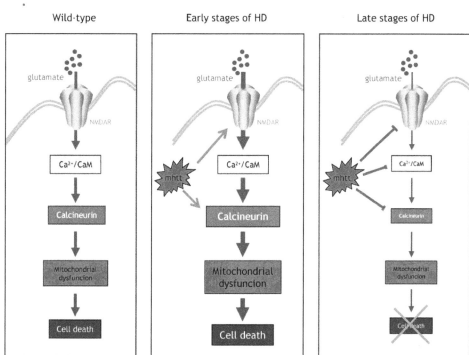

Fig. 2. Changes in striatal calcineurin levels during HD progression, and involvement in excitotoxicity. Results from Xifro et al. (2008) suggest that at early stages of HD calcineurin levels are increased and striatal neurons are more susceptible to NMDA-induced excitotoxicity. In contrast, at late stages, calcineurin levels are decreased and participate in the resistance of striatal neurons to NMDA-induced excitotoxicity (Xifro et al., 2009). CaM: calmodulin.

2.2 Pleckstrin homology (PH) domain leucine-rich repeat protein phosphatase (PHLPP)

PHLPPs constitute a subfamily within the PP2C phosphatase family. PHLPPs require Mg^{2+} and Mn^{2+} for their catalytic activity, and are not inhibited by traditional phosphatase inhibitors such as okadaic acid (Brognard et al., 2007; Gao et al., 2005). This family comprises three members: PHLPP1α, PHLPP1β and PHLPP2. PHLPP1α and PHLPP1β are splice variants from the same gene but have different sizes, whereas PHLPP2 is a different gene product and has the same domain composition of PHLPP1 (Brognard et al., 2007). PHLPP1 and PHLPP2 have an identical domain structure with a PH domain (sharing 63% amino identity) followed by a region of leucine-rich repeats, a PP2C phosphatase domain (sharing 58% amino identity) and a C terminal PDZ ligand. In addition, PHLPP1β and PHLPP2 contain a Ras-association domain preceding the PH domain (Brognard & Newton, 2008).

PHLPPs are expressed in the majority of human tissues and are localized in different cellular compartments such as cytosol, nucleus and membrane (Brognard et al., 2007; Brognard & Newton, 2008). In the CNS, PHLPP1β was the first identified as an mRNA that oscillated in a circadian rhythm-dependent manner in the suprachiasmatic nucleus (SCN) and was named SCOP (SCN circadian oscillatory protein) (Shimizu et al., 1999). PHLPP1β/SCOP is expressed in various brain regions with a relative enrichment in hippocampus and cerebellum (Shimizu et al., 1999). Its expression is highly concentrated in neurons, and is present in nuclear, mitochondrial and cytosolic fractions (Shimizu et al., 1999), as well as in membrane rafts (Shimizu et al., 2003). Recently, PHLPP1α and PHLPP2 have been shown to be also expressed in hippocampal neurons (Jackson et al., 2009; 2010) with PHLPP1α as the most abundantly expressed in the adult (Jackson et al., 2010). Although PHLPP1 and 2 can be found in the cytosolic fraction, only PHLPP1α can be localized in the nucleus of hippocampal neurons (Jackson et al., 2010). In addition, we have detected PHLPP1α in the cortex and striatum of adult mice (Saavedra et al., 2010).

So far, the known substrates for PHLPPs are the kinases Akt (also known as protein kinase B), and protein kinase C (PKC). Akt, the first identified substrate of PHLPP (Gao et al., 2005), is a key regulator of a wide range of cellular processes including growth, proliferation, metabolism, cell cycle progression, and survival. Thus, altered Akt activity has been associated with cancer and other disease conditions such as diabetes and neurodegenerative diseases (Liao & Hung, 2010). For its full catalytic activity, Akt requires phosphorylation at Thr308 in the activation loop and at Ser473 in the hydrophobic motif (Brazil & Hemmings, 2001). Its activation depends on the PI3-kinase, which produces the lipid second messenger PtdIns-3, 4, 5-P3 (PIP3) that interacts with the PH domain of Akt and recruits the kinase to the plasma membrane (Sancak et al., 2008). Subsequently, the Thr308 residue is phosphorylated by membrane-localized 3-phosphoinositide-dependent protein kinase 1 (PDK1) (Alessi et al., 1997; Calleja et al., 2007) and the Ser473 residue is phosphorylated by mTORC2 (Sarbassov et al., 2005) (Figure 3). PHLPPs specifically dephosphorylate the hydrophobic motif of Akt, resulting in a decrease of its activity (Gao et al., 2005), whereas the Thr308 site is dephosphorylated by PP2A (Bayascas & Alessi, 2005). PKC, the other PHLPPs substrate, consists in a Ser/Thr family of phosphorylating enzymes ubiquitously expressed and implicated in multiple cellular functions. There are 12 isoforms of PKC termed (1) calcium-dependent or classical PKCs, cPKCs (2) calcium-independent or novel PKCs, nPKCs, and (3) atypical PKCs, aPKCs (Amadio et al., 2006; Pearce et al., 2010). PKC isoforms, like Akt, are also activated by the phosphorylation of the activation segment and hydrophobic motif (Newton, 2003). PDK1 phosphorylates the activation segment (Dutil et al., 1998; Le Good et al., 1998), and there is increasing evidence that mTORC2 phosphorylates the hydrophobic motif of at least some isoforms (Sarbassov et al., 2004; Guertin et al., 2006). The phosphorylation of the hydrophobic motif regulates the amplitude of PKC signaling by controlling the stability of the kinase. Both PHLPP1 and PHLPP2 dephosphorylate the hydrophobic motif of conventional and novel PKC isoforms, but not atypical PKC isoforms (Gao et al., 2008). This dephosphorylation induces the degradation of PKC. Thus, depletion of PHLPP1 or PHLPP2 leads to a robust increase in PKC levels (Gao et al., 2008).

Members of the AGC kinase family like p70S6K, SGK or p90RSK, which have hydrophobic phosphorylation motifs, are other potential substrates of PHLPPs (Brognard & Newton, 2008). In addition to the dephosphorylation of Akt and PKC, PHLPP1β/SCOP negatively regulates the Ras–Raf–MEK–ERK pathway by interacting directly with Ras (Shimizu et al., 2003).

In the CNS, PHLPPs participate in the regulation of the circadian clock (Shimizu et al., 1999), learning and memory (Shimizu et al., 2007), and survival (Jackson et al., 2009; 2010; Saavedra et al., 2010). In HD, we have shown that PHLPP1α is reduced in cellular as well as in HD mouse models, and in the putamen of HD patients (Saavedra et al., 2010). STHdh$^{Q111/Q111}$ cells display decreased levels of PHLPP1α compared with STHdh$^{Q7/Q7}$ cells. Similarly, we detected reduced levels of PHLPP1α in the striatum of Hdh$^{Q111/Q111}$ mice (at 5 months of age), and also in the striatum of the exon-1 mouse models R6/1 (from 12 to 30 weeks of age), R6/1:BDNF +/- (from 12 to 30 weeks of age), R6/2 (at 12 weeks of age) and Tet/HD94 (at 22 months of age). In addition, PHLPP1α levels are also decreased in the cortex and hippocampus of R6/1 mice at 12 and 30 weeks of age. PHLPP1 expression was regulated by mhtt at the transcriptional level since we also detected decreased PHLPP1 mRNA levels in the striatum of R6/1 mice (Saavedra et al., 2010). We speculated that the down-regulation of PHLPP1 mRNA levels could be related with decreased activity of the transcription factor NF-Y, since this transcription factor is sequestered in mhtt aggregates (Yamanaka et al., 2008). It has recently been shown that the expression of PHLPP is controlled by mammalian target of rapamycin (mTOR)-dependent protein translation in colon and breast cancer cells (J. Liu et al., 2011). Interestingly, mTOR activity is reduced in HD (Ravikumar et al., 2004). Thus, it is tempting to speculate that this mechanism could also be involved in the down-regulation of PHLPP1α levels. In good correlation with decreased levels of PHLPP1α in the striatum, we observed increased phosphorylation levels of Akt (Ser473) and of its targets GSK3β (Ser9) and FoxO (Ser256). Although PHLPP1α levels were down-regulated in the cortex and hippocampus of R6/1 mice we did not observe changes in pAkt (Ser473) levels indicating that a reduction of PHLPP1α levels may not be enough to increase pAkt (Ser473) levels *in vivo* (Saavedra et al., 2010). In addition, in the striatum of Tet/HD94 mice, we observed that after shutting-down the expression of mhtt, PHLPP1α protein levels returned to wild-type levels but pAkt (Ser473) up-regulation was only partially reduced (Saavedra et al., 2010). Taken together, these results suggest that increased levels of pAkt is a specific mechanism taking place in striatal neurons expressing mhtt, which could be the sum of increased activation of kinases that phosphorylate Akt and decreased levels of PHLPP1α. Since Akt activation is one of the main mechanisms to prevent neuronal death during injury (Chong et al., 2005), and many transgenic HD mouse models show little, if any, striatal cell death (Canals et al., 2004; Diaz-Hernandez et al., 2005; Garcia-Martinez et al., 2007; Mangiarini et al., 1996; Martin-Aparicio et al., 2001), our results suggest that increased Akt activation could counteract mhtt toxicity.

In addition, we showed that decreased levels of PHLPP1α could help to maintain high levels of pAkt (Ser473) in R6/1 striatum after excitotoxicity, contributing to prevent cell death induced by NMDARs overstimulation (Saavedra et al., 2010).

Conversely, we found unchanged levels of PHLPP2 in the striatum in R6/1 mice at different stages of the disease (8, 12, 20 and 30 weeks of age), while cortical levels are decreased at 12 and 30 weeks of age.

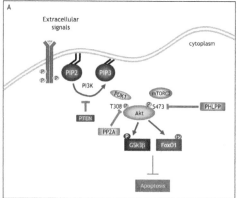
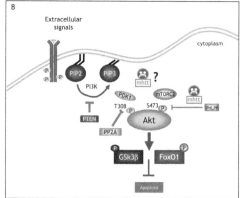

Fig. 3. PHLPP1α is down-regulated in HD striatum. (A) Scheme showing pathways that control Akt phosphorylation in wild-type cells. Akt is phosphorylated at Thr308 (T308) by PDK1 and dephosphorylated by PP2A, whereas the Ser473 residue (S473) is phosphorylated by mTORC2 and dephosphorylated by PHLPP. Once activated, Akt prevents apoptosis through the phosphorylation of several targets such as GSK3β and FoxO1. (B) Control of Akt phosphorylation in striatal cells expressing mhtt. In the presence of mhtt PHLPP1α levels are decreased and contribute to maintain high levels of Akt phosphorylated at S473 that through increased levels of phosphorylated GSK3β and FoxO1 may delay striatal cell death. Results obtained by analyzing different brain regions suggest that mhtt could also affect the activation of kinases that phosphorylate Akt in the striatum, but not in other brain regions (Saavedra et al., 2010).

2.3 PP1 and PP2A

PP1 and PP2A account for the majority of Ser/Thr phosphatase activity in mammalian cells, and are involved in diverse cellular processes such as cell growth and proliferation, development, DNA replication and repair, metabolism, neural signaling, and apoptosis. The activity of these two phosphatases can be blocked by okadaic acid and caliculin at different IC50 values (Sheppeck et al., 1997). The specific oligomeric composition of PP1 and PP2A holoenzyme is important to control their phosphatase activity. Functional PP1 enzyme consists of a catalytic subunit (PP1c) and a regulatory subunit (R subunit). The PP1c associates with more than 50 proteins that regulate substrate specificity and subcellular localization (Ceulemans & Bollen, 2004; P.T. Cohen, 2002). The interaction of PP1c with its regulatory subunit can also influence substrate specificity. In addition, its activity is regulated by endogenous inhibitory proteins like inhibitor-1 (P. Cohen & Nimmo, 1978), inhibitor-2 (Foulkes & P. Cohen, 1980), CPI-17 (Eto et al., 1997), and DARPP-32 (Walaas & Greengard, 1991), which is highly expressed in MSNs. PP2A exists in two forms: a core dimer and a heterotrimeric holoenzyme. The PP2A core dimer is composed by the scaffolding A subunit and the catalytic C subunit and associates with a regulatory B subunit to generate the heterotrimeric holoenzyme, which is the predominant form of PP2A in the cell. PP2A regulatory B subunits are divided into four different families and play a crucial role in the subcellular localization of PP2A. They can also alter the overall shape of the catalytic subunit as well as enzyme kinetics (reviewed by McConnell & Wadzinski, 2009; Shi, 2009).

In the CNS, PP1 and PP2A dephosphorylate neurotransmitter receptors and proteins localized at the post-synaptic site, thus participating in the regulation of excitatory and inhibitory transmission. PP1 dephosphorylates CaMKII when bound to post-synaptic density, whereas soluble or synaptosomal CaMKII is deposphorylated by PP2A (Shields et al., 1985; Strack et al., 1997). In addition, both phosphatases regulate NMDARs-mediated synaptic currents in an activity-dependent manner (L. Y. Wang et al., 1994; Westphal et al., 1999). PP1 dephosphorylates GABA receptor subunits (X. Wang et al., 2002) and down-regulates AMPA receptor activity and trafficking by dephosphorylation of the GluR1 subunit (reviewed by Mansuy & Shenolikar, 2006). In addition, PP1 and PP2A activity can promote apoptosis (reviewed by Garcia et al., 2003; Klumpp & Krieglstein, 2002). PP1 dephosphorylates the pro-apoptotic protein Bad with its consequent activation, and PP2A dephosphorylates the anti-apoptotic proteins Akt and Bcl-2 inactivating them. PP2A can also regulate the activity of a large number of kinases, such as ERK, PKA and p38 (reviewed by Millward et al., 1999), all of them important to neuronal survival and function.

Recently, the number of targets of PP1 and PP2A has been extended since both proteins dephosphorylate htt *in situ* and after excitotoxic stimulation of NMDARs (Metzler et al., 2010; see Figure 1). Metzler and colleagues (2010) showed that NMDARs overstimulation induces a decrease of phtt (Ser421) in primary neurons from wild-type and YAC128 transgenic mice. In addition, dephosphorylation of htt (Ser421) was also observed in YAC128 transgenic mice after quinolinic acid injection in the striatum. Dephosphorylation of htt after excitotoxicity seems to participate in the induction of cell death since blockade of PP1 and PP2A activity protects YAC128 striatal neurons from NMDA-induced cell death *in vitro*. Moreover, they showed that dopamine modulates htt phosphorylation in the striatum through the regulation of the PP1 inhibitor DARPP-32. These authors also observed a decrease in the PP1 substrate pCREB, which together with decreased levels of DARPP-32 in YAC128 striatum suggested an altered regulation of phosphatase activity in HD. However, they could not detect changes in the activity of PP1 and PP2A in YAC128 mice striatum. Although these results point to a role of htt dephosphorylation in excitotoxic-induced cell death in the striatum, it remains to be shown whether inhibition of PP1 and PP2A is also neuroprotective *in vivo*. In addition, it would be interesting to investigate whether dephosphorylation of mhtt takes place in the striatum of YAC128 mice when they are resistant to excitotoxicity. PP2A protein levels have also been analyzed in the striatum of R6/1 mice. Similarly to that observed in YAC128 mice striatum (Metzler et al., 2010), no changes in PP2A protein levels have been detected in R6/1 mouse striatum at 4, 8, 12, 16 and 30 weeks of age compared with their littermate controls (Saavedra et al., 2010).

3. Tyrosine phosphatases

Tyrosine (Tyr) phosphatases, encoded by about 107 genes in the human genome (Alonso et al., 2004; Andersen et al., 2004), have the ability to hydrolyze p-nitrophenyl phosphate, are inhibited by vanadate and are insensitive to okadaic acid. They are classified into three groups: (1) Cytoplasmic, (2) Receptor-like, and (3) Dual specificity phosphatases, which dephosphorylate Ser, Thr and Tyr residues that are in close proximity. The specificity of Tyr phosphatases is regulated by several molecular strategies such as preferential recognition of phosphopeptides, cell-type and organelle-specific expression, and assembly with other proteins (for review see S. Paul & Lombroso, 2003; Z. Y. Zhang, 2002). These phosphatases play important roles in the development and function of the CNS (Ensslen-Craig & Brady-Kalnay, 2004; S. Paul & Lombroso, 2003), and have been suggested to function as neuroprotectants. STEP, the SH2-containing Tyr phosphatases SHP1 and SHP2, and protein Tyr phosphatase alpha are among the protective candidates. However, protein Tyr phosphatase alpha and phosphatase and tensin homolog deleted from chromosome 10 (PTEN) may also induce neurotoxicity (Gee & Mansuy, 2005). Increased Tyr phosphorylation has been suggested to induce neuronal cell death in cerebral ischemia (Ohtsuki et al., 1996; R. Paul et al., 2001) and after epileptiform activity (Chun et al., 2004; Sanna et al., 2000). In addition, alterations in protein Tyr phosphatases are considered to be involved in the etiology of neural disorders such as Alzheimer's Disease (Kerr et al., 2006; Lee et al., 2004), Parkinson's Disease (Herradon & Ezquerra, 2009) and HD (Saavedra et al., 2011; Z. L. Wu et al., 2002).

3.1 STEP

STEP, encoded by the *Ptpn5* gene, is a brain-specific Tyr phosphatase involved in neuronal signal transduction. STEP plays an important role in synaptic plasticity through the opposition to synaptic strengthening (Braithwaite et al., 2006a). Additionally, STEP has been implicated in susceptibility to cell death through the modulation of ERK1/2 signaling (Choi et al., 2007; Saavedra et al., 2011), while other studies suggest that STEP can play a role in neuroprotection through the regulation of the p38 pathway (Poddar et al., 2010; Xu et al., 2009). The mechanism underlying the ability of STEP to regulate both pro-survival and pro-cell death pathways has been recently elucidated (Xu et al., 2009; see details below).

STEP is enriched in MSNs (Lombroso et al., 1991), and expressed at lower levels in the cortex, hippocampus and amygdala (Boulanger et al., 1995). STEP mRNA is alternatively spliced into several STEP isoforms (Bult et al., 1997; Sharma et al., 1995) that are differentially targeted to the post-synaptic density (Oyama et al., 1995), extra-synaptic and cytosolic compartments (Goebel-Goody et al., 2009; Xu et al., 2009). The major isoforms are $STEP_{46}$, the cytosolic isoform, and $STEP_{61}$, which is membrane-associated through the additional 172 amino acids in the N-terminus (Bult et al., 1997). Both isoforms are expressed in the striatum, whereas other brain regions only express $STEP_{61}$ (Boulanger et al., 1995).

STEP activity is regulated through phosphorylation/dephosphorylation of a Ser residue within its kinase interacting motif (KIM) domain. Stimulation of D1Rs activates PKA (Stoof & Kebabian, 1981), which phosphorylates STEP thereby inactivating it (S. Paul et al., 2000) (Figure 1). In contrast, stimulation of NMDARs results in the dephosphorylation and activation of STEP through a calcineurin/PP1 pathway (S. Paul et al., 2003; Valjent et al., 2005) (Figure 1). Additionally, STEP activity is also regulated by proteolytic cleavage (Xu et al., 2009), ubiquitin-proteasome degradation (Kurup et al., 2010; S. Mukherjee et al., 2011; Xu et al., 2009), local translation (Y. Zhang et al., 2008), and oligomerization (Deb et al., 2011).

Once activated, STEP dephosphorylates the glutamate receptor subunits NR2B (Braithwaite et al., 2006b; Pelkey et al., 2002; Snyder et al., 2005) and GluR2 (Y. Zhang et al., 2008), leading to their endocytosis, and the kinases ERK1/2, p38 and Fyn, thereby controlling the duration of their signal (Munoz et al., 2003; Nguyen et al., 2002; S. Paul et al., 2003; Pulido et al., 1998) (Figure 1).

The enrichment of STEP in MSNs, its role in the regulation of key substrates implicated in neuronal function, together with the fact that both dopaminergic and glutamatergic systems regulate STEP activity and are affected in HD patients and mouse models (Andre et al., 2010; Fan & Raymond, 2007; Jakel & Maragos, 2000) prompted us to study the possible role of STEP in the pathophysiology of HD (Saavedra et al., 2011). In fact, previous studies showed decreased mRNA levels of STEP in the caudate nucleus and cortex of HD patients (Hodges et al., 2006), in the striatum of R6 mice (Desplats et al., 2006; Luthi-Carter et al., 2000), and in primary striatal neurons overexpressing htt171-82Q (Runne et al., 2008). Our results show that R6/1 mice display reduced STEP protein levels in the striatum and cortex, and increased phosphorylation levels in the striatum, cortex and hippocampus. R6/2, Tet/HD94 and Hdh$^{Q7/Q111}$ mice striatum also displays decreased STEP protein and increased STEP phosphorylation levels (Saavedra et al., 2011). The early increase in striatal STEP phosphorylation levels correlates with a dysregulation of the PKA pathway that together with decreased calcineurin activity at later stages further contributes to an enhancement of STEP inactivation. Accordingly, the levels of phosphorylated ERK2 and p38, two targets of STEP, are increased in R6/1 mice striatum at advanced stages of the disease (Saavedra et al., 2011).

HD mouse models develop resistance to excitotoxicity (Graham et al., 2009; Hansson et al., 1999, 2001; Jarabek et al., 2004; Torres-Peraza et al., 2008), and reduced levels of calcineurin expression and activity can contribute to this phenomenon (Xifro et al., 2009). Stimulation of NMDARs activates STEP in a calcineurin-dependent manner (S. Paul et al., 2003), and disruption of STEP activity has been shown to lead to the activation of ERK1/2 signaling and to the attenuation of excitotoxic-induced cell death in the hippocampus (Choi et al., 2007). Therefore, we wondered whether STEP acts as a calcineurin target after an excitotoxic stimulus to the striatum thereby contributing to the resistance to excitotoxicity observed in HD mouse models. After intrastriatal quinolinic acid injection, we observed higher and unaltered pSTEP levels, and more sustained ERK signaling in R6/1 than in wild-type mice suggesting that STEP inactivation could mediate neuroprotection in R6/1 striatum (Saavedra et al., 2011). These findings are consistent with lower calcineurin activation which, importantly, correlates with reduced cell death in R6/1 mice striatum after quinolinic acid injection (Xifro et al., 2009). In agreement with a protective role for STEP inactivation, blockade of STEP activity with FK-506 (an inhibitor of calcineurin) allows ERK activation and confers protection to hilar interneurons of the hippocampus against excitotoxicity (Choi et al., 2007), and intrastriatal infusion of TAT-STEP, a cell-permeable form, increases quinolic acid-induced cell death in the striatum (Saavedra et al., 2011). Conversely, low striatal STEP levels and activity (increased pSTEP levels) in R6/1 mice can contribute to their reduced vulnerability to excitotoxicity (Saavedra et al., 2011).

Activation of extra-synaptic NMDARs in primary cortical neurons leads to calpain-mediated cleavage of STEP$_{61}$. This prevents STEP from binding to its substrates and contributes to the selective activation of extra-synaptically concentrated p38 (Xu et al., 2009). In contrast, synaptic NMDAR stimulation leads to the ubiquitination and degradation of STEP$_{61}$ and ERK1/2 activation (Xu et al., 2009). We did not observe STEP$_{61}$ cleavage or p38 activation which, together with ERK2 activation, suggests a preferential stimulation of synaptic NMDARs in our model (Saavedra et al., 2011). This is relevant because an imbalance between synaptic and extra-synaptic NMDARs has been shown to occur in YAC128 mice (Milnerwood et al., 2010; Okamoto et al., 2009). However, these mice develop resistance to excitotoxicity with age (Graham et al., 2009), and those studies were performed in vulnerable mice. Thus, it is likely that increased extra-synaptic NMDARs during excitotoxicity-sensitive stages might increase $STEP_{61}$ cleavage to $STEP_{33}$ enabling higher activation of p38 than in wild-type mice. In contrast, in resistant mice other mechanisms should regulate striatal cell survival in response to excitotoxicity and, according with our findings, STEP regulation of ERK activity seems to play an important role (Saavedra et al., 2011).

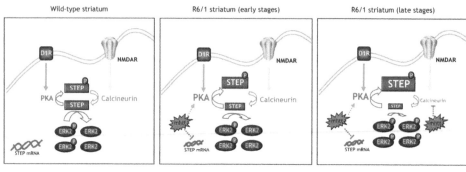

Fig. 4. Regulation of STEP levels and activity in the R6/1 mouse striatum during the progression of the disease. The presence of mhtt in the striatum alters this system at different levels: (1) At early stages mhtt induces a down-regulation of STEP mRNA and protein levels, and a dysregulation of the PKA pathway that correlates with increased STEP phosphorylation. (2) At late stages, calcineurin activity is also reduced further inactivating STEP with a consequent increase of pERK2 levels (p-p38 levels and possibly other non-analyzed STEP targets). Decreased STEP activity, through the regulation of its targets, could be involved in the development of resistance to excitotoxicity in R6/1 mice striatum. (scheme from Saavedra et al., 2011).

STEP has recently been implicated in the etiology of Alzheimer's Disease (Kurup et al., 2010; Snyder et al., 2005; Y. Zhang et al., 2010) but the alterations in the STEP pathway found in HD mouse models are specific because STEP protein levels and activity, in contrast to that observed in Alzheimer's Disease, are reduced in HD (Saavedra et al., 2011). Since the genetic reduction of STEP levels reverses cognitive and cellular deficits in Alzheimer's Disease mice (Y. Zhang et al., 2010), the modulation of STEP levels might be a good therapeutic strategy in HD. Nevertheless, the possibility of restoring STEP expression in HD is presently hampered by the lack of data about the regulation of *STEP* gene expression.

3.2 MAP kinase phosphatases (MKPs)

MKPs are intracellular dual Tyr phosphatases with an expression restricted to different subcellular compartments (S. Paul & Lombroso, 2003). Some of these MKPs, such as MKP-1, -2, -3 and -X, have been shown to be expressed in the brain with a specific distribution and different substrate preferences. MKP-1 is expressed in the cortex, thalamus, striatum and cerebellum with the following substrate specificity: p38>JNK/SAPK>>ERK (Boschert et al., 1998; Franklin & Kraft, 1997; Misra-Press et al., 1995; Takaki et al., 2001). MKP-2 is localized in the prefrontal cortex, hippocampus and cerebellum and inactivates ERK and JNK/SAPK with the same specificity, but it can also act on p38 (Chu et al., 1996; Dwivedi et al., 2001; Groom et al., 1996; Misra-Press et al., 1995). MKP-3 is detected in the cerebral cortex, striatum and hippocampus acting preferentially on ERK, but it can also inactivate JNK/SAPK and p38 with the same specificity (Boschert et al., 1998; Muda et al., 1996a,b; Takaki et al., 2001). Finally, MKP-X is expressed throughout the brain and acts preferentially on ERK, although it can also dephosphorylate p38 (Boschert et al., 1998; Dowd et al., 1998; Muda et al., 1996b; Shin et al., 1997).

Although they are expressed in the brain, their role in neuronal function is not well established. MKP-1 increases in rat brain after limbic epilepsy (Gass et al., 1996) and, together with MKP-3, upon cerebral hypoxia in neuronal nuclei of newborn piglets (Mishra & Delivoria-Papadopoulos, 2004). Moreover, both MKP-1 and -3 play important roles in neural plastic modifications after drug exposure (Takaki et al., 2001), whereas MKP-2 is increased in postmortem brains of suicide subjects with major depression (Dwivedi et al., 2001). Recently, it has been shown that MKP-1 controls axon branching of cortical neurons in response to the trophic factor BDNF (Jeanneteau et al., 2010). In addition, in PC12 cells, oxidative stress and hypoxia increase MPK-1 expression, while trophic factor treatment up-regulates both MKP-1 and -3 (Camps et al., 1998; Keyse & Emslie, 1992; Seta et al., 2001). Thus, regulation of MPKs seems to be important not only after brain injury, but also during development.

In a stable PC12 cell line expressing truncated mhtt with 118Q, Z. L. Wu and colleagues (2002) showed that MKP-1 and -3 mRNA levels, and MKP-1 protein levels, were increased at different time points after mhtt expression. In good correlation with changes in MKPs levels, they observed a substantial reduction of ERK1/2 phosphorylation. Interestingly, treatment with sodium orthovanadate and bp V (pic), two general Tyr phosphatase inhibitors, rescues cells from polyQ-induced cell death suggesting that these phosphatases are involved in mhtt-induced toxicity (Z. L. Wu et al., 2002). In HEK 293 cells transfected with NR1/NR2B and htt containing 138Q, MKP-2 has been shown to be reduced in the soluble fraction and increased in the particulate-derived fraction when compared with cells expressing htt with 15Q (Fan et al., 2008). However, the mechanism underlying this redistribution and the physiological significance of this event are presently unknown.

4. Conclusion

Understanding the pathways by which mhtt causes neuronal dysfunction and death is essential to develop efficient treatments for HD. Great progress has been made over the last years in highlighting the molecular mechanisms affected by mhtt. Here, we have reviewed the existing data about changes in the expression and regulation of phosphatases in HD models and human HD brain. From these results, it is becoming increasingly clear that alterations in phosphatases are involved in the pathogenesis of HD. So far, the phosphatases analyzed participate in the regulation of excitotoxicity and neuronal survival (through the regulation of the PI3K/Akt pathway, ERK2 and/or htt phosphorylation). In mouse models, most of them are decreased, which seems to be a compensatory mechanism induced in response to mhtt expression in order to prevent neuronal cell death. However, how this might translate to humans is still unknown as we cannot follow the disease from the beginning, and analysis of phosphatase levels and activity can be performed only at late stages of the disease. We believe that the regulation of phosphatases is a new and promising approach to treat HD. Therefore, our future challenge is to develop novel tools to treat HD based on these findings. In addition, phosphatases are also involved in the pathogenesis of other neurodegenerative disorders, and ongoing investigations of disease mechanisms in HD can also provide new therapeutic approaches to Parkinson's or Alzheimer's Diseases.

5. Acknowledgements

Research in our group is supported by Fondo de Investigaciones Sanitarias (Instituto de Salud Carlos III, PI10/01072 to E.P.-N.), Ministerio de Educación y Ciencia (Grant SAF2008-04360 to J.A.), and Generalitat de Catalunya (group of excellence; Grant 2009SGR-00326). A.S. is supported by Ministerio de Ciencia e Innovación, Juan de la Cierva subprograme, Spain (JCI-2010-08207).

6. References

Alessi D. R., James S. R., Downes C. P., Holmes A. B., Gaffney P. R., Reese C. B. & Cohen P. (1997) Characterization of a 3-phosphoinositide-dependent protein kinase which phosphorylates and activates protein kinase Balpha. *Current Biology*, Vol. 7, No. 4, pp. 261-269, ISSN 0960-9822

Alonso A., Sasin J., Bottini N., Friedberg I., Osterman A., Godzik A., Hunter T., Dixon J. & Mustelin T. (2004) Protein tyrosine phosphatases in the human genome. *Cell*, Vol. 117, No. 6, pp. 699-711, ISSN 0092-8674

Amadio M., Battaini F. & Pascale A. (2006) The different facets of protein kinases C: old and new players in neuronal signal transduction pathways. *Pharmacological Research*, Vol. 54, No. 5, pp. 317-325, ISSN 1043-6618

Andersen J. N., Jansen P. G., Echwald S. M., Mortensen O. H., Fukada T., Del Vecchio R., Tonks N. K. & Moller N. P. (2004) A genomic perspective on protein tyrosine phosphatases: gene structure, pseudogenes, and genetic disease linkage. *FASEB Journal*, Vol. 18, No. 1, pp. 8-30, ISSN 0892-6638

Andre V. M., Cepeda C. & Levine M. S. (2010) Dopamine and glutamate in Huntington's disease: A balancing act. *CNS Neuroscience & Therapeutics*, Vol. 16, No. 3, pp. 163-178, ISSN 1755-5930

Ankarcrona M., Dypbukt J. M., Orrenius S. & Nicotera P. (1996) Calcineurin and mitochondrial function in glutamate-induced neuronal cell death. *FEBS Letters*, Vol. 394, No. 3, pp. 321-324, ISSN 0014-5793

Anne S. L., Saudou F. & Humbert S. (2007) Phosphorylation of huntingtin by cyclin-dependent kinase 5 is induced by DNA damage and regulates wild-type and mutant huntingtin toxicity in neurons. *Journal of Neuroscience*, Vol. 27, No. 27, pp. 7318-7328, ISSN 0270-6474

Atwal R. S., Desmond C. R., Caron N., Maiuri T., Xia J., Sipione S. & Truant R. (2011) Kinase inhibitors modulate huntingtin cell localization and toxicity. *Nature Chemical Biology*, Vol. 7, No. 7, pp. 453-460, ISSN 1552-4450

Bayascas J. R. & Alessi D. R. (2005) Regulation of Akt/PKB Ser473 phosphorylation. *Molecular Cell*, Vol. 18, No. 2, pp. 143-145, ISSN 1097-2765

Beals C. R., Clipstone N. A., Ho S. N. & Crabtree G. R. (1997) Nuclear localization of NF-ATc by a calcineurin-dependent, cyclosporin-sensitive intramolecular interaction. *Genes & Development*, Vol. 11, No. 7, pp. 824-834, ISSN 0890-9369

Boschert U., Dickinson R., Muda M., Camps M. & Arkinstall S. (1998) Regulated expression of dual specificity protein phosphatases in rat brain. *Neuroreport*, Vol. 9, No. 18, pp. 4081-4086, ISSN 0959- 4965

Boulanger L. M., Lombroso P. J., Raghunathan A., During M. J., Wahle P. & Naegele J. R. (1995) Cellular and molecular characterization of a brain-enriched protein tyrosine phosphatase. *Journal of Neuroscience*, Vol. 15, No. 2, pp. 1532-1544, ISSN 0270-6474

Braithwaite S. P., Paul S., Nairn A. C. & Lombroso P. J. (2006a) Synaptic plasticity: one STEP at a time. *Trends in Neuroscience*, Vol. 29, No. 8, pp. 452-458, ISSN 0166-2236

Braithwaite S. P., Adkisson M., Leung J., Nava A., Masterson B., Urfer R., Oksenberg D. & Nikolich K. (2006b) Regulation of NMDA receptor trafficking and function by striatal-enriched tyrosine phosphatase (STEP). *European Journal of Neuroscience*, Vol. 23, No. 11, pp. 2847-2856, ISSN 0953-816X

Brazil D. P. & Hemmings B. A. (2001) Ten years of protein kinase B signalling: a hard Akt to follow. *Trends in Biochemical Sciences*, Vol. 26, No. 11, pp. 657-664, ISSN 0968-0004

Brognard J. & Newton A. C. (2008) PHLiPPing the switch on Akt and protein kinase C signaling. *Trends in Endocrinology and Metabolism*, Vol. 19, No. 6, pp. 223-230, ISSN 1043-2760

Brognard J., Sierecki E., Gao T. & Newton A. C. (2007) PHLPP and a second isoform, PHLPP2, differentially attenuate the amplitude of Akt signaling by regulating distinct Akt isoforms. *Molecular Cell*, Vol. 25, No. 6, pp. 917-931, ISSN 1097-2765

Bult A., Zhao F., Dirkx R., Jr., Raghunathan A., Solimena M. & Lombroso P. J. (1997) STEP: a family of brain-enriched PTPs. Alternative splicing produces transmembrane, cytosolic and truncated isoforms. *European Journal of Cell Biology*, Vol. 72, No. 4, pp. 337-344, ISSN 0171-9335

Butcher S. P., Henshall D. C., Teramura Y., Iwasaki K. & Sharkey J. (1997) Neuroprotective actions of FK506 in experimental stroke: in vivo evidence against an antiexcitotoxic mechanism. *Journal of Neuroscience*, Vol. 17, No. 18, pp. 6939-6946, ISSN 0270-6474

Calleja V., Alcor D., Laguerre M., Park J., Vojnovic B., Hemmings B. A., Downward J., Parker P. J. & Larijani B. (2007) Intramolecular and intermolecular interactions of protein kinase B define its activation in vivo. *PLoS Biology*, Vol. 5, No. 4, pp. e95, ISSN 1544-9173

Camps M., Chabert C., Muda M., Boschert U., Gillieron C. & Arkinstall S. (1998) Induction of the mitogen-activated protein kinase phosphatase MKP3 by nerve growth factor in differentiating PC12. *FEBS Letters*, Vol. 425, No. 2, pp. 271-276, ISSN 0014-5793

Canals J. M., Pineda J. R., Torres-Peraza J. F., Bosch M., Martin-Ibanez R., Munoz M. T., Mengod G., Ernfors P. & Alberch J. (2004) Brain-derived neurotrophic factor regulates the onset and severity of motor dysfunction associated with enkephalinergic neuronal degeneration in Huntington's disease. *Journal of Neuroscience*, Vol. 24, No. 35, pp. 7727-7739, ISSN 0270-6474

Cereghetti G. M., Stangherlin A., Martins d. B., Chang C. R., Blackstone C., Bernardi P. & Scorrano L. (2008) Dephosphorylation by calcineurin regulates translocation of Drp1 to mitochondria. *Proceedings of the National Academy of Sciences USA* , Vol. 105, No. 41, pp. 15803-15808, ISSN 0027-8424

Ceulemans H. & Bollen M. (2004) Functional diversity of protein phosphatase-1, a cellular economizer and reset button. *Physiological Reviews*, Vol. 84, No. 1, pp. 1-39, ISSN 0031-9333

Choi Y. S., Lin S. L., Lee B., Kurup P., Cho H. Y., Naegele J. R., Lombroso P. J. & Obrietan K. (2007) Status epilepticus-induced somatostatinergic hilar interneuron degeneration is regulated by striatal enriched protein tyrosine phosphatase. *Journal of Neuroscience*, Vol. 27, No. 11, pp. 2999-3009, ISSN 0270-6474

Chong Z. Z., Li F. & Maiese K. (2005) Activating Akt and the brain's resources to drive cellular survival and prevent inflammatory injury. *Histology and Histopathology*, Vol. 20, No. 1, pp. 299-315, ISSN 0213- 3911

Chu Y., Solski P. A., Khosravi-Far R., Der C. J. & Kelly K. (1996) The mitogen-activated protein kinase phosphatases PAC1, MKP-1, and MKP-2 have unique substrate specificities and reduced activity in vivo toward the ERK2 sevenmaker mutation. *Journal of Biological Chemistry*, Vol. 271, No. 11, pp. 6497-6501, ISSN 0021-9258

Chun J. T., Crispino M. & Tocco G. (2004) The dual response of protein kinase Fyn to neural trauma: early induction in neurons and delayed induction in reactive astrocytes. *Experimental Neurology*, Vol. 185, No. 1, pp. 109–119, ISSN 0014-4886

Cohen P. & Nimmo G. A. (1978) The purification and characterization of protein phosphatase inhibitor-1 from rabbit skeletal muscle. *Biochemical Society Transactions*, Vol. 6, No. 1, pp. 17-20, ISSN 0300-5127

Cohen P. T. (2002) Protein phosphatase 1 - targeted in many directions. *Journal of Cell Science*, Vol. 115, Pt 2, pp. 241-256, ISSN 0021-9533

Colin E., Zala D., Liot G., Rangone H., Borrell-Pages M., Li X. J., Saudou F. & Humbert S. (2008) Huntingtin phosphorylation acts as a molecular switch for anterograde/retrograde transport in neurons. *EMBO Journal*, Vol. 27, No. 15, pp. 2124-2134, ISSN 0261-4189

Costa V., Giacomello M., Hudec R., Lopreiato R., Ermak G., Lim D., Malorni W., Davies K. J., Carafoli E. & Scorrano L. (2010) Mitochondrial fission and cristae disruption increase the response of cell models of Huntington's disease to apoptotic stimuli. *EMBO Molecular Medicine*, Vol. 2, No. 12, pp. 490-503, ISSN 1757-4676

Dawson T. M., Steiner J. P., Dawson V. L., Dinerman J. L., Uhl G. R. & Snyder S. H. (1993) Immunosuppressant FK506 enhances phosphorylation of nitric oxide synthase and protects against glutamate neurotoxicity. *Proceedings of the National Academy of Sciences USA* , Vol. 90, No. 21, pp. 9808-9812, ISSN 0027-8424

Deb I., Poddar R. & Paul S. (2011) Oxidative stress-induced oligomerization inhibits the activity of the non-receptor tyrosine phosphatase STEP61. *Journal of Neurochemistry*, Vol. 116, No. 6, pp. 1097-1111, ISSN 0022-3042

Desplats P. A., Kass K. E., Gilmartin T., Stanwood G. D., Woodward E. L., Head S. R., Sutcliffe J. G. & Thomas E. A. (2006) Selective deficits in the expression of striatal-enriched mRNAs in Huntington's disease. *Journal of Neurochemistry*, Vol. 96, No. 3, pp. 743-757, ISSN 0022-3042

Diaz-Hernandez M., Torres-Peraza J., Salvatori-Abarca A., Moran M. A., Gomez-Ramos P., Alberch J. & Lucas J. J. (2005) Full motor recovery despite striatal neuron loss and formation of irreversible amyloid-like inclusions in a conditional mouse model of Huntington's disease. *Journal of Neuroscience*, Vol. 25, No. 42, pp. 9773-9781, ISSN 0270-6474

Dowd S., Sneddon A. A. & Keyse S. M. (1998) Isolation of the human genes encoding the pyst1 and Pyst2 phosphatases: characterisation of Pyst2 as a cytosolic dual-specificity MAP kinase phosphatase and its catalytic activation by both MAP and SAP kinases. *Journal of Cell Science*, Vol. 111 (Pt 22), No. pp. 3389-3399, ISSN 0021-9533

Ducruet A. P., Vogt A., Wipf P. & Lazo J. S. (2005) Dual specificity protein phosphatases: therapeutic targets for cancer and Alzheimer's disease. *Annual Review of Pharmacology and Toxicology*, Vol. 45, No. pp. 725-750, ISSN 0362-1642

Dutil E. M., Toker A. & Newton A. C. (1998) Regulation of conventional protein kinase C isozymes by phosphoinositide-dependent kinase 1 (PDK-1). *Current Biology*, Vol. 8, No. 25, pp. 1366-1375, ISSN 0960-9822

Dwivedi Y., Rizavi H. S., Roberts R. C., Conley R. C., Tamminga C. A. & Pandey G. N. (2001) Reduced activation and expression of ERK1/2 MAP kinase in the post-mortem brain of depressed suicide subjects. *Journal of Neurochemistry*, Vol. 77, No. 3, pp. 916-928, ISSN 0022-3042

Ehrnhoefer D. E., Sutton L. & Hayden M. R. (2011) Small Changes, Big Impact: Posttranslational Modifications and Function of Huntingtin in Huntington Disease. *Neuroscientist*, Vol. No. pp. ISSN 1073-8584

Ensslen-Craig S. E. & Brady-Kalnay S. M. (2004) Receptor protein tyrosine phosphatases regulate neural development and axon guidance. *Developmental Biology*, Vol. 275, No. 1, pp. 12-22, ISSN 0012-1606

Ermak G., Hench K. J., Chang K. T., Sachdev S. & Davies K. J. (2009) Regulator of calcineurin (RCAN1-1L) is deficient in Huntington disease and protective against mutant huntingtin toxicity in vitro. *Journal of Biological Chemistry*, Vol. 284, No. 18, pp. 11845-11853, ISSN 0021-9258

Eto M., Senba S., Morita F. & Yazawa M (1997) Molecular cloning of a novel phosphorylation-dependent inhibitory protein of protein phosphatase-1 (CPI17) in smooth muscle: its specific localization in smooth muscle. *FEBS Letters*, Vol. 410, No. 2-3, pp. 356-360, ISSN 0014-5793

Fan M. M. & Raymond L. A. (2007) N-methyl-D-aspartate (NMDA) receptor function and excitotoxicity in Huntington's disease. *Progress in Neurobiology*, Vol. 81, No. 5-6, pp. 272-293, ISSN 0301-0082

Fan M. M., Zhang H., Hayden M. R., Pelech S. L. & Raymond L. A. (2008) Protective up-regulation of CK2 by mutant huntingtin in cells co-expressing NMDA receptors. *Journal of Neurochemistry*, Vol. 104, No. 3, pp. 790-805, ISSN 0022-3042

Foulkes J. G. & Cohen P. (1980) The regulation of glycogen metabolism. Purification and properties of protein phosphatase inhibitor-2 from rabbit skeletal muscle. *European Journal of Biochemistry*, Vol. 105, No. 1, pp. 195-203, ISSN 0014-2956

Franklin C. C. & Kraft A.S. (1997) Conditional expression of the mitogen-activated protein kinase (MAPK) phosphatase MKP-1 preferentially inhibits p38 MAPK and stress-activated protein kinase in U937 cells. *Journal of Biological Chemistry*, Vol. 272, No. 27, pp. 16917-16923, ISSN 0021-9258

Gafni J., Hermel E., Young J. E., Wellington C. L., Hayden M. R. & Ellerby L. M. (2004) Inhibition of calpain cleavage of huntingtin reduces toxicity: accumulation of calpain/caspase fragments in the nucleus. *Journal of Biological Chemistry*, Vol. 279, No. 19, pp. 20211-20220, ISSN 0021-9258

Gao T., Furnari F. & Newton A. C. (2005) PHLPP: a phosphatase that directly dephosphorylates Akt, promotes apoptosis, and suppresses tumor growth. *Molecular Cell*, Vol. 18, No. 1, pp. 13-24, ISSN 1097-2765

Gao T., Brognard J. & Newton A. C. (2008) The phosphatase PHLPP controls the cellular levels of protein kinase C. *Journal of Biological Chemistry*, Vol. 283, No. 10, pp. 6300-6311, ISSN 0021-9258

Garcia-Martinez J. M., Perez-Navarro E., Xifro X., Canals J. M., Diaz-Hernandez M., Trioulier Y., Brouillet E., Lucas J. J. & Alberch J. (2007) BH3-only proteins Bid and Bim(EL) are differentially involved in neuronal dysfunction in mouse models of Huntington's disease. *Journal of Neuroscience Research*, Vol. 85, No. 12, pp. 2756-2769, ISSN 0360-4012

Garcia A., Cayla X., Guergnon J., Dessauge F., Hospital V., Rebollo M. P., Fleischer A. & Rebollo A. (2003) Serine/threonine protein phosphatases PP1 and PP2A are key players in apoptosis. *Biochimie*, Vol. 85, No. 8, pp. 721-726, ISSN 0300-9084

Gass P., Eckhardt A., Schroder H., Bravo R. & Herdegen T. (1996) Transient expression of the mitogen-activated protein kinase phosphatase MKP-1 (3CH134/ERP1) in the rat brain after limbic epilepsy. *Brain Research Molecular Brain Research*, Vol. 41, No. 1-2, pp. 74-80, ISSN 0169-328X

Gee C. E. & Mansuy I. M. (2005) Protein phosphatases and their potential implications in neuroprotective processes. *Cellular and Molecular Life Sciences*, Vol. 62, No. 10, pp. 1120-1130, ISSN 1420-682X

Goebel-Goody S. M., Davies K. D., Alvestad Linger R. M., Freund R. K. & Browning M. D. (2009) Phospho-regulation of synaptic and extrasynaptic N-methyl-d-aspartate receptors in adult hippocampal slices. *Neuroscience*, Vol. 158, No. 4, pp. 1446-1459, ISSN 0306-4522

Goto S., Matsukado Y., Miyamoto E. & Yamada M. (1987) Morphological characterization of the rat striatal neurons expressing calcineurin immunoreactivity. *Neuroscience*, Vol. 22, No. 1, pp. 189-201, ISSN 0306-4522

Graham R. K., Pouladi M. A., Joshi P., Lu G., Deng Y., Wu N. P., Figueroa B. E., Metzler M., Andre V. M., Slow E. J., Raymond L., Friedlander R., Levine M. S., Leavitt B. R. & Hayden M. R. (2009) Differential susceptibility to excitotoxic stress in YAC128 mouse models of Huntington disease between initiation and progression of disease. *Journal of Neuroscience*, Vol. 29, No. 7, pp. 2193-2204, ISSN 0270-6474

Groom L. A., Sneddon A. A., Alessi D. R., Dowd S. & Keyse S. M. (1996) Differential regulation of the MAP, SAP and RK/p38 kinases by Pyst1, a novel cytosolic dual-specificity phosphatase. *EMBO Journal* Vol. 15, No. 14, pp. 3621-3632, ISSN 0261-4189

Guertin D. A., Stevens D. M., Thoreen C. C., Burds A. A., Kalaany N. Y., Moffat J., Brown M., Fitzgerald K. J. & Sabatini D. M. (2006) Ablation in mice of the mTORC components raptor, rictor, or mLST8 reveals that mTORC2 is required for signaling to Akt-FOXO and PKCalpha, but not S6K1. *Developmental Cell*, Vol. 11, No. 6, pp. 859-871, ISSN 1534-5807

Han I., You Y., Kordower J. H., Brady S. T. & Morfini G. A. (2010) Differential vulnerability of neurons in Huntington's disease: the role of cell type-specific features. *Journal of Neurochemistry*, Vol. 113, No. 5, pp. 1073-1091, ISSN 0022-3042

Hansson O., Petersen A., Leist M., Nicotera P., Castilho R. F. & Brundin P. (1999) Transgenic mice expressing a Huntington's disease mutation are resistant to quinolinic acid-induced striatal excitotoxicity. *Proceedings of the National Academy of Sciences USA,* Vol. 96, No. 15, pp. 8727-8732, ISSN 0027-8424

Hansson O., Guatteo E., Mercuri N. B., Bernardi G., Li X. J., Castilho R. F. & Brundin P. (2001) Resistance to NMDA toxicity correlates with appearance of nuclear inclusions, behavioural deficits and changes in calcium homeostasis in mice transgenic for exon 1 of the huntington gene. *European Journal of Neuroscience,* Vol. 14, No. 9, pp. 1492-1504, ISSN 0953-816X

Hernandez-Espinosa D. & Morton A. J. (2006) Calcineurin inhibitors cause an acceleration of the neurological phenotype in a mouse transgenic for the human Huntington's disease mutation. *Brain Research Bulletin* Vol. 69, No. 6, pp. 669-679, ISSN 0361-9230

Herradon G. & Ezquerra L. (2009) Blocking receptor protein tyrosine phosphatase beta/zeta: a potential therapeutic strategy for Parkinson's disease. *Current Medicinal Chemistry,* Vol. 16, No. 25, pp. 3322-3329, ISSN 0929-8673

Hodges A., Strand A. D., Aragaki A. K., Kuhn A., Sengstag T., Hughes G., Elliston L. A., Hartog C., Goldstein D. R., Thu D., Hollingsworth Z. R., Collin F., Synek B., Holmans P. A., Young A. B., Wexler N. S., Delorenzi M., Kooperberg C., Augood S. J., Faull R. L., Olson J. M., Jones L. & Luthi-Carter R. (2006) Regional and cellular gene expression changes in human Huntington's disease brain. *Human Molecular Genetics,* Vol. 15, No. 6, pp. 965-977, ISSN 0964-6906

Humbert S., Bryson E. A., Cordelieres F. P., Connors N. C., Datta S. R., Finkbeiner S., Greenberg M. E., Saudou F. (2002) The IGF-1/Akt pathway is neuroprotective in Huntington's disease and involves Huntingtin phosphorylation by Akt. *Developmental Cell,* Vol. 2, No. 6, pp 831-837, ISSN 1534-5807

Iqbal K. & Grundke-Iqbal I. (2007) Developing pharmacological therapies for Alzheimer disease. *Cellular and Molecular Life Sciences,* Vol. 64, No. 17, pp. 2234-2244, ISSN 1420-682X

Jackson T. C., Rani A., Kumar A. & Foster T. C. (2009) Regional hippocampal differences in AKT survival signaling across the lifespan: implications for CA1 vulnerability with aging. *Cell Death & Differentiation,* Vol. 16, No. 3, pp. 439-448, ISSN 1350-9047

Jackson T. C., Verrier J. D., Semple-Rowland S., Kumar A. & Foster T. C. (2010) PHLPP1 splice variants differentially regulate AKT and PKCalpha signaling in hippocampal neurons: characterization of PHLPP proteins in the adult hippocampus. *Journal of Neurochemistry,* Vol. 115, No. 4, pp. 941-955, ISSN 0022-3042

Jakel R. J. & Maragos W. F. (2000) Neuronal cell death in Huntington's disease: a potential role for dopamine. *Trends in Neurosciences,* Vol. 23, No. 6, pp. 239-245, ISSN 0166-2236

Jarabek B. R., Yasuda R. P. & Wolfe B. B. (2004) Regulation of proteins affecting NMDA receptor-induced excitotoxicity in a Huntington's mouse model. *Brain,* Vol. 127, Pt 3, pp. 505-516, ISSN 0006-8950

Jeanneteau F., Deinhardt K., Miyoshi G., Bennett A. M. & Chao M. V. (2010) The MAP kinase phosphatase MKP-1 regulates BDNF-induced axon branching. *Nature Neuroscience,* Vol. 13, No. 11, pp. 1373-1379, ISSN 1097-6256

Jin Y. N. & Johnson G. V. (2010) The interrelationship between mitochondrial dysfunction and transcriptional dysregulation in Huntington disease. *Journal of Bioenergetics and Biomembranes*, Vol. 42, No. 3, pp. 199-205, ISSN 0145-479X

Kerr F., Rickle A., Nayeem N., Brandner S., Cowburn R. F. & Lovestone S. (2006) PTEN, a negative regulator of PI3 kinase signalling, alters tau phosphorylation in cells by mechanisms independent of GSK-3. *FEBS Letters*, Vol. 580, No. 13, pp. 3121-3128, ISSN 0014-5793

Keyse S. M. & Emslie E. A. (1992) Oxidative stress and heat shock induce a human gene encoding a protein-tyrosine phosphatase. *Nature*, Vol. 359, No. 6396, pp. 644-647, ISSN 0028-0836

Klumpp S. & Krieglstein J. (2002) Serine/threonine protein phosphatases in apoptosis. *Current Opinion in Pharmacology*, Vol. 2, No. 4, pp. 458-462, ISSN 1471-4892

Kurup P., Zhang Y., Xu J., Venkitaramani D. V., Haroutunian V., Greengard P., Nairn A. C. & Lombroso P. J. (2010) Abeta-mediated NMDA receptor endocytosis in Alzheimer's disease involves ubiquitination of the tyrosine phosphatase STEP61. *Journal of Neuroscience*, Vol. 30, No. 17, pp. 5948-5957, ISSN 0270-6474

Landwehrmeyer G. B., Standaert D. G., Testa C. M., Penney J. B. Jr. & Young A. B. (1995) NMDA receptor subunit mRNA expression by projection neurons and interneurons in rat striatum. *Journal of Neuroscience*, Vol. 15, No. 7, pp. 5297-5307, ISSN 0270-6474

Laube B., Kuhse J. & Betz H. (1998) Evidence for a tetrameric structure of recombinant NMDA receptors. *Journal of Neuroscience*, Vol. 18, No. 8, pp. 2954-2961, ISSN 0270-6474

Le Good J. A., Ziegler W. H., Parekh D. B., Alessi D. R., Cohen P. & Parker P. J. (1998) Protein kinase C isotypes controlled by phosphoinositide 3-kinase through the protein kinase PDK1. *Science*, Vol. 281, No. 3585, pp. 2042-2045, ISSN 0036-8075

Lee G., Thangavel R., Sharma V. M., Litersky J. M., Bhaskar K., Fang S. M., Do L. H., Andreadis A., Van Hoesen G. & Ksiezak-Reding H. (2004) Phosphorylation of tau by fyn: implications for Alzheimer's disease. *Journal of Neuroscience*, Vol. 24, No. 9, pp. 2304-2312, ISSN 0270-6474

Liao Y. & Hung M. C. (2010) Physiological regulation of Akt activity and stability. *American Journal of Translational Research*, Vol. 2, No. 1, pp. 19-42, ISSN 1943-8141

Lievens J. C., Woodman B., Mahal A. & Bates G. P. (2002) Abnormal phosphorylation of synapsin I predicts a neuronal transmission impairment in the R6/2 Huntington's disease transgenic mice. *Molecular and Cellular Neuroscience*, Vol. 20, No. 4, pp. 638-648, ISSN 1044-7431

Liu F., Liang Z. & Gong C. X. (2006) Hyperphosphorylation of tau and protein phosphatases in Alzheimer disease. *Panminerva Medica*, Vol. 48, No. 2, pp. 97-108, ISSN 0031-0808

Liu J., Stevens P. D. & Gao T. (2011) mTOR-dependent regulation of PHLPP expression controls the rapamycin sensitivity in cancer cells. *Journal of Biological Chemistry*, Vol. 286, No. 8, pp. 6510-6520, ISSN 0021-9258

Lombroso P. J., Murdoch G. & Lerner M. (1991) Molecular characterization of a protein-tyrosine-phosphatase enriched in striatum. *Proceedings of the National Academy of Sciences USA* , Vol. 88, No. 16, pp. 7242-7246, ISSN 0027-8424

Lou H., Montoya S. E., Alerte T. N., Wang J., Wu J., Peng X., Hong C. S., Friedrich E. E., Mader S. A., Pedersen C. J., Marcus B. S., McCormack A. L., Di Monte D. A., Daubner S. C. & Perez R. G. (2010) Serine 129 phosphorylation reduces the ability of alpha-synuclein to regulate tyrosine hydroxylase and protein phosphatase 2A in vitro and in vivo. *Journal of Biological Chemistry*, Vol. 285, No. 23, pp. 17648-17661, ISSN 0021-9258

Luo S., Vacher C., Davies J. E. & Rubinsztein D. C. (2005) Cdk5 phosphorylation of huntingtin reduces its cleavage by caspases: implications for mutant huntingtin toxicity. *Journal of Cell Biology*, Vol. 169, No. 4, pp. 647-656, ISSN 0021-9525

Luthi-Carter R., Strand A., Peters N. L., Solano S. M., Hollingsworth Z. R., Menon A. S., Frey A. S., Spektor B. S., Penney E. B., Schilling G., Ross C. A., Borchelt D. R., Tapscott S. J., Young A. B., Cha J. H. & Olson J. M. (2000) Decreased expression of striatal signaling genes in a mouse model of Huntington's disease. *Human Molecular Genetics*, Vol. 9, No. 9, pp. 1259-1271, ISSN 0964-6906

Mangiarini L., Sathasivam K., Seller M., Cozens B., Harper A., Hetherington C., Lawton M., Trottier Y., Lehrach H., Davies S. W. & Bates G. P. (1996) Exon 1 of the HD gene with an expanded CAG repeat is sufficient to cause a progressive neurological phenotype in transgenic mice. *Cell*, Vol. 87, No. 3, pp. 493-506, ISSN 0092-8674

Mansuy I. M. (2003) Calcineurin in memory and bidirectional plasticity. *Biochemical and Biophysical Research Communications*, Vol. 311, No. 4, pp. 1195-1208, ISSN: 0006-291X

Mansuy I. M. & Shenolikar S. (2006) Protein serine/threonine phosphatases in neuronal plasticity and disorders of learning and memory. *Trends in Neuroscience*, Vol. 29, No. 12, pp. 679-686, ISSN 0166-2236

Martin-Aparicio E., Yamamoto A., Hernandez F., Hen R., Avila J. & Lucas J. J. (2001) Proteasomal-dependent aggregate reversal and absence of cell death in a conditional mouse model of Huntington's disease. *Journal of Neuroscience*, Vol. 21, No. 22, pp. 8772-8781, ISSN 0270-6474

McConnell J. L. & Wadzinski B. E. (2009) Targeting protein serine/threonine phosphatases for drug development. *Molecular Pharmacology*, Vol. 75, No. 6, pp. 1249-1261, ISSN 0026-895X

Metzler M., Gan L., Mazarei G., Graham R. K., Liu L., Bissada N., Lu G., Leavitt B. R. & Hayden M. R. (2010) Phosphorylation of huntingtin at Ser421 in YAC128 neurons is associated with protection of YAC128 neurons from NMDA-mediated excitotoxicity and is modulated by PP1 and PP2A. *Journal of Neuroscience*, Vol. 30, No. 43, pp. 14318-14329, ISSN 0270-6474

Millward T. A., Zolnierowicz S. & Hemmings B. A. (1999) Regulation of protein kinase cascades by protein phosphatase 2A. *Trends in Biochemical Sciences*, Vol. 24, No. 5, pp. 186-191, ISSN 0968-0004

Milnerwood A. J. & Raymond L. A. (2010) Early synaptic pathophysiology in neurodegeneration: insights from Huntington's disease. *Trends in Neurosciences*, Vol. 33, No. 11, pp. 513-523, ISSN 0166-2236

Milnerwood A. J., Gladding C. M., Pouladi M. A., Kaufman A. M., Hines R. M., Boyd J. D., Ko R. W., Vasuta O. C., Graham R. K., Hayden M. R., Murphy T. H. & Raymond L. A. (2010) Early increase in extrasynaptic NMDA receptor signaling and expression contributes to phenotype onset in Huntington's disease mice. *Neuron*, Vol. 65, No. 2, pp. 178-190, ISSN 0896-6273

Mishra O. P. & Delivoria-Papadopoulos M. (2004) Effect of hypoxia on protein tyrosine kinase activity in cortical membranes of newborn piglets--the role of nitric oxide. *Neuroscience Letters*, Vol. 372, No. 1-2, pp. 114-118, ISSN 0304-3940

Misra-Press A., Rim C. S., Yao H., Roberson M. S. & Stork P. J. (1995) A novel mitogen-activated protein kinase phosphatase. Structure, expression, and regulation. *Journal of Biological Chemistry*, Vol. 270, No. 24, pp. 14587-14596, ISSN 0021-9258

Muda M., Boschert U., Dickinson R., Martinou J. C., Martinou I., Camps M., Schlegel W. & Arkinstall S. (1996a) MKP-3, a novel cytosolic protein-tyrosine phosphatase that exemplifies a new class of mitogen-activated protein kinase phosphatase. *Journal of Biological Chemistry*, Vol. 271, No. 8, pp. 4319-4326, ISSN 0021-9258

Muda M., Theodosiou A., Rodrigues N., Boschert U., Camps M., Gillieron C., Davies K., Ashworth A. & Arkinstall S. (1996b) The dual specificity phosphatases M3/6 and MKP-3 are highly selective for inactivation of distinct mitogen-activated protein kinases. *Journal of Biological Chemistry*, Vol. 271, No. 44, pp. 27205-27208, ISSN 0021-9258

Mukherjee A. & Soto C. (2011) Role of calcineurin in neurodegeneration produced by misfolded proteins and endoplasmic reticulum stress. *Current Opinion in Cell Biology*, Vol. 23, No. 2, pp. 223-230, ISSN 0955-0674

Mukherjee S., Poddar R., Deb I. & Paul S. (2011) Dephosphorylation of specific sites in the KIS domain leads to ubiquitin-mediated degradation of the tyrosine phosphatase STEP. *Biochemical Journal*, doi:10.1042/BJ20110240, ISSN 0264-6021

Munoz J. J., Tarrega C., Blanco-Aparicio C. & Pulido R. (2003) Differential interaction of the tyrosine phosphatases PTP-SL, STEP and HePTP with the mitogen-activated protein kinases ERK1/2 and p38alpha is determined by a kinase specificity sequence and influenced by reducing agents. *Biochemical Journal*, Vol. 372, Pt 1, pp. 193-201, ISSN 0264-6021

Newton A. C. (2003) Regulation of the ABC kinases by phosphorylation: protein kinase C as a paradigm. *Biochemical Journal*, Vol. 370, Pt 2, pp. 361-371, ISSN 0264-6021

Nguyen T. H., Liu J. & Lombroso P. J. (2002) Striatal enriched phosphatase 61 dephosphorylates Fyn at phosphotyrosine 420. *Journal of Biological Chemistry*, Vol. 277, No. 27, pp. 24274-24279, ISSN 0021-9258

Nishi A., Bibb J. A., Matsuyama S., Hamada M., Higashi H., Nairn A. C. & Greengard P. (2002) Regulation of DARPP-32 dephosphorylation at PKA- and Cdk5-sites by NMDA and AMPA receptors: distinct roles of calcineurin and protein phosphatase-2A. *Journal of Neurochemistry*, Vol. 81, No. 4, pp. 832-841, ISSN 0022-3042

Ohtsuki T., Matsumoto M., Kitagawa K., Mabuchi T., Mandai K., Matsushita K., Kuwabara K., Tagaya M., Ogawa S., Ueda H., Kamada T. & Yanagihara T. (1996) Delayed neuronal death in ischemic hippocampus involves stimulation of protein tyrosine phosphorylation. *American Journal of Physiology*, Vol. 271, No. 4 Pt 1, pp. C1085-C1097, ISSN 0363-6143

Okamoto S., Pouladi M. A., Talantova M., Yao D., Xia P., Ehrnhoefer D. E., Zaidi R., Clemente A., Kaul M., Graham R. K., Zhang D., Vincent Chen H. S., Tong G., Hayden M. R. & Lipton S. A. (2009) Balance between synaptic versus extrasynaptic NMDA receptor activity influences inclusions and neurotoxicity of mutant huntingtin. *Nature Medicine*, Vol. 15, No. 12, pp. 1407-1413, ISSN 1078-8956

Olney J. W. & Sharpe L. G. (1969) Brain lesions in an infant rhesus monkey treated with monsodium glutamate. *Science*, Vol. 166, No. 903, pp. 386-388, ISSN 0036-8075

Oyama T., Goto S., Nishi T., Sato K., Yamada K., Yoshikawa M. & Ushio Y. (1995) Immunocytochemical localization of the striatal enriched protein tyrosine phosphatase in the rat striatum: a light and electron microscopic study with a complementary DNA-generated polyclonal antibody. *Neuroscience*, Vol. 69, No. 3, pp. 869-880, ISSN 0306-4522

Ozawa S., Kamiya H. & Tsuzuki K. (1998) Glutamate receptors in the mammalian central nervous system. *Progress in Neurobiology*, Vol. 54, No. 5, pp. 581-618, ISSN 0301-0082

Pardo R., Colin E., Regulier E., Aebischer P., Deglon N., Humbert S. & Saudou F. (2006) Inhibition of calcineurin by FK506 protects against polyglutamine-huntingtin toxicity through an increase of huntingtin phosphorylation at S421. *Journal of Neuroscience*, Vol. 26, No. 5, pp. 1635-1645, ISSN 0270-6474

Paul R., Zhang Z. G., Eliceiri B. P., Jiang Q., Boccia A. D., Zhang R. L., Chopp M. & Cheresh D. A. (2001) Src deficiency or blockade of Src activity in mice provides cerebral protection following stroke. *Nature Medicine*, Vol. 7, No. 2, pp. 222-227, ISSN 1078-8956

Paul S. & Lombroso P. J. (2003) Receptor and nonreceptor protein tyrosine phosphatases in the nervous system. *Cellular and Molecular Life Sciences*, Vol. 60, No. 11, pp. 2465-2482, ISSN 1421-682X

Paul S., Nairn A. C., Wang P. & Lombroso P. J. (2003) NMDA-mediated activation of the tyrosine phosphatase STEP regulates the duration of ERK signaling. *Nature Neuroscience*, Vol. 6, No. 1, pp. 34-42, ISSN 1097-6256

Paul S., Snyder G. L., Yokakura H., Picciotto M. R., Nairn A. C. & Lombroso P. J. (2000) The Dopamine/D1 receptor mediates the phosphorylation and inactivation of the protein tyrosine phosphatase STEP via a PKA-dependent pathway. *Journal of Neuroscience*, Vol. 20, No. 15, pp. 5630-5638, ISSN 0270-6474

Pearce L. R., Komander D. & Alessi D. R. (2010) The nuts and bolts of AGC protein kinases. *Nature Reviews Molecular Cell Biology*, Vol. 11, No. 1, pp. 9-22, ISSN 1471-0080

Pelkey K. A., Askalan R., Paul S., Kalia L. V., Nguyen T. H., Pitcher G. M., Salter M. W. & Lombroso P. J. (2002) Tyrosine phosphatase STEP is a tonic brake on induction of long-term potentiation. *Neuron*, Vol. 34, No. 1, pp. 127-138, ISSN 0896-6273

Perez-Navarro E., Canals J. M., Gines S. & Alberch J. (2006) Cellular and molecular mechanisms involved in the selective vulnerability of striatal projection neurons in Huntington's disease. *Histology and Histopathology*, Vol. 21, No. 11, pp. 1217-1232, ISSN 0213- 3911

Pineda J. R., Pardo R., Zala D., Yu H., Humbert S. & Saudou F. (2009) Genetic and pharmacological inhibition of calcineurin corrects the BDNF transport defect in Huntington's disease. *Molecular Brain*, Vol. 2, pp. 33, ISSN 1756-6606

Poddar R., Deb I., Mukherjee S. & Paul S. (2010) NR2B-NMDA receptor mediated modulation of the tyrosine phosphatase STEP regulates glutamate induced neuronal cell death. *Journal of Neurochemistry*, Vol. 115, No. 6, pp. 1350-1362, ISSN 0022-3042

Pulido R., Zuniga A. & Ullrich A. (1998) PTP-SL and STEP protein tyrosine phosphatases regulate the activation of the extracellular signal-regulated kinases ERK1 and ERK2 by association through a kinase interaction motif. *EMBO Journal*, Vol. 17, No. 24, pp. 7337-7350, ISSN 0261-4189

Rangone H., Poizat G., Troncoso J., Ross C. A., MacDonald M. E., Saudou F. & Humbert S. (2004) The serum- and glucocorticoid-induced kinase SGK inhibits mutant huntingtin-induced toxicity by phosphorylating serine 421 of huntingtin. *European Journal of Neuroscience*, Vol. 19, No. 2, pp. 273-279, ISSN 0953-816X

Ravikumar B., Vacher C., Berger Z., Davies J. E., Luo S., Oroz L. G., Scaravilli F., Easton D. F., Duden R., O'Kane C. J. & Rubinsztein D. C. (2004) Inhibition of mTOR induces autophagy and reduces toxicity of polyglutamine expansions in fly and mouse models of Huntington disease. *Nature Genetics*, Vol. 36, No. 6, pp. 585-595, ISSN 1061-4036

Renna M., Jimenez-Sanchez M., Sarkar S. & Rubinsztein D. C. (2010) Chemical inducers of autophagy that enhance the clearance of mutant proteins in neurodegenerative diseases. *Journal of Biological Chemistry*, Vol. 285, No. 15, pp. 11061-11067, ISSN 0021-9258

Rosenstock T. R., Duarte A. I. & Rego A. C. (2010) Mitochondrial-associated metabolic changes and neurodegeneration in Huntington's disease - from clinical features to the bench. *Current Drug Targets*, Vol. 11, No. 10, pp. 1218-1236, ISSN 1389-4501

Runne H., Regulier E., Kuhn A., Zala D., Gokce O., Perrin V., Sick B., Aebischer P., Deglon N. & Luthi-Carter R. (2008) Dysregulation of gene expression in primary neuron models of Huntington's disease shows that polyglutamine-related effects on the striatal transcriptome may not be dependent on brain circuitry. *Journal of Neuroscience*, Vol. 28, No. 39, pp. 9723-9731, ISSN 0270-6474

Saavedra A., Garcia-Martinez J. M., Xifro X., Giralt A., Torres-Peraza J. F., Canals J. M., Diaz-Hernandez M., Lucas J. J., Alberch J. & Perez-Navarro E. (2010) PH domain leucine-rich repeat protein phosphatase 1 contributes to maintain the activation of the PI3K/Akt pro-survival pathway in Huntington's disease striatum. *Cell Death & Differentiation*, Vol. 17, No. 2, pp. 324-335, ISSN 1350-9047

Saavedra A., Giralt A., Rue L., Xifro X., Xu J., Ortega Z., Lucas J. J., Lombroso P. J., Alberch J. & Perez-Navarro E. (2011) Striatal-enriched protein tyrosine phosphatase expression and activity in Huntington's disease: a STEP in the resistance to excitotoxicity. *Journal of Neuroscience*, Vol. 31, No. 22, pp. 8150-8162, ISSN 0270-6474

Sancak Y., Peterson T. R., Shaul Y. D., Lindquist R. A., Thoreen C. C., Bar-Peled L. & Sabatini D. M. (2008) The Rag GTPases bind raptor and mediate amino acid signaling to mTORC1. *Science*, Vol. 320, No. 5882, pp. 1496-1501, ISSN 0036-8075

Sanna P. P., Berton F., Cammalleri M., Tallent M. K., Siggins G. R., Bloom F. E., Francesconi W. (2000) A role for Src kinase in spontaneous epileptiform activity in the CA3 region of the hippocampus. *Proceedings of the National Academy of Sciences USA*, Vol. 97, No. 15, pp. 8653-8657, ISSN 0027-8424

Sarbassov D. D., Guertin D. A., Ali S. M. & Sabatini D. M. (2005) Phosphorylation and regulation of Akt/PKB by the rictor-mTOR complex. *Science*, Vol. 307, No. 5712, pp. 1098-1101, ISSN 0036-8075

Sarbassov D. D., Ali S. M., Kim D. H., Guertin D. A., Latek R. R., Erdjument-Bromage H., Tempst P. & Sabatini D. M. (2004) Rictor, a novel binding partner of mTOR, defines a rapamycin-insensitive and raptor-independent pathway that regulates the cytoskeleton. *Current Biology*, Vol. 14, No. 14, pp. 1296-1302, ISSN 0960-9822

Schilling B., Gafni J., Torcassi C., Cong X., Row R. H., LaFevre-Bernt M. A., Cusack M. P., Ratovitski T., Hirschhorn R., Ross C. A., Gibson B. W. & Ellerby L. M. (2006) Huntingtin phosphorylation sites mapped by mass spectrometry. Modulation of cleavage and toxicity. *Journal of Biological Chemistry*, Vol. 281, No. 33, pp. 23686-23697, ISSN 0021-9258

Seta K. A., Kim R., Kim H. W., Millhorn D. E. & Beitner-Johnson D. (2001) Hypoxia-induced regulation of MAPK phosphatase-1 as identified by subtractive suppression hybridization and cDNA microarray analysis. *Journal of Biological Chemistry*, Vol. 276, No. 48, pp. 44405-44412, ISSN 0021-9258

Shamloo M., Soriano L., Wieloch T., Nikolich K., Urfer R. & Oksenberg D. (2005) Death-associated protein kinase is activated by dephosphorylation in response to cerebral ischemia. *Journal of Biological Chemistry*, Vol. 280, No. 51, pp. 42290-42299, ISSN 0021-9258

Sharma E., Zhao F., Bult A. & Lombroso P. J. (1995) Identification of two alternatively spliced transcripts of STEP: a subfamily of brain-enriched protein tyrosine phosphatases. *Brain Research Molecular Brain Research*, Vol. 32, No. 1, pp. 87-93, ISSN 0169-328X

Shehadeh J., Fernandes H. B., Zeron Mullins M. M., Graham R. K., Leavitt B. R., Hayden M. R. & Raymond L. A. (2006) Striatal neuronal apoptosis is preferentially enhanced by NMDA receptor activation in YAC transgenic mouse model of Huntington disease. *Neurobiology of Disease*, Vol. 21, No. 2, pp. 392-403, ISSN 0969-9961

Sheppeck J. E., Gauss C. M. & Chamberlin A. R. (1997) Inhibition of the Ser-Thr phosphatases PP1 and PP2A by naturally occurring toxins. *Bioorganic & Medicinal Chemistry*, Vol. 5, No. 9, pp. 1739-1750, ISSN 0968-0896

Shi Y. (2009) Serine/threonine phosphatases: mechanism through structure. *Cell*, Vol. 139, No. 3, pp. 468-484, ISSN 0092-8674

Shibasaki F. & McKeon F. (1995) Calcineurin functions in Ca(2+)-activated cell death in mammalian cells. *Journal of Cell Biology*, Vol. 131, No. 3, pp. 735-743, ISSN 0021-9525

Shibasaki F., Hallin U. & Uchino H. (2002) Calcineurin as a multifunctional regulator. *Journal of Biochemistry*, Vol. 131, No. 1, pp. 1-15, ISSN 0021-924X

Shields S. M., Ingebritsen T. S. & Kelly P. T. (1985) Identification of protein phosphatase 1 in synaptic junctions: dephosphorylation of endogenous calmodulin-dependent kinase II and synapse-enriched phosphoproteins. *Journal of Neuroscience*, Vol. 5, No. 12, pp. 3414-3422, ISSN 0270-6474

Shimizu K., Okada M., Takano A. & Nagai K. (1999) SCOP, a novel gene product expressed in a circadian manner in rat suprachiasmatic nucleus. *FEBS Letters*, Vol. 458, No. 3, pp. 363-369, ISSN 0014-5793

Shimizu K., Okada M., Nagai K. & Fukada Y. (2003) Suprachiasmatic nucleus circadian oscillatory protein, a novel binding partner of K-Ras in the membrane rafts, negatively regulates MAPK pathway. *Journal of Biological Chemistry*, Vol. 278, No. 17, pp. 14920-14925, ISSN 0021-9258

Shimizu K., Phan T., Mansuy I. M. & Storm D. R. (2007) Proteolytic degradation of SCOP in the hippocampus contributes to activation of MAP kinase and memory. *Cell*, Vol. 128, No. 6, pp. 1219-1229, ISSN 0092-8674

Shin D. Y., Ishibashi T., Choi T. S., Chung E., Chung I. Y., Aaronson S. A. & Bottaro D. P. (1997) A novel human ERK phosphatase regulates H-ras and v-raf signal transduction. *Oncogene*, Vol. 14, No. 22, pp. 2633-2639, ISSN 0950-9232

Snyder E. M., Nong Y., Almeida C. G., Paul S., Moran T., Choi E. Y., Nairn A. C., Salter M. W., Lombroso P. J., Gouras G. K. & Greengard P. (2005) Regulation of NMDA receptor trafficking by amyloid-beta. *Nature Neuroscience*, Vol. 8, No. 8, pp. 1051-1058, ISSN 1097-6256

Song C., Zhang Y., Parsons C. G. & Liu Y. F. (2003) Expression of polyglutamine-expanded huntingtin induces tyrosine phosphorylation of N-methyl-D-aspartate receptors. *Journal of Biological Chemistry*, Vol. 278, No. 35, pp. 33364-33369, ISSN 0021-9258

Springer J. E., Azbill R. D., Nottingham S. A. & Kennedy S. E. (2000) Calcineurin-mediated BAD dephosphorylation activates the caspase-3 apoptotic cascade in traumatic spinal cord injury. *Journal of Neuroscience*, Vol. 20, No. 19, pp. 7246-7251, ISSN 0270-6474

Stoof J. C. & Kebabian J. W. (1981) Opposing roles for D-1 and D-2 dopamine receptors in efflux of cyclic AMP from rat neostriatum. *Nature*, Vol. 294, No. 5839, pp. 366-368, ISSN 0028-0836

Strack S., Choi S., Lovinger D. M. & Colbran R. J. (1997) Translocation of autophosphorylated calcium/calmodulin-dependent protein kinase II to the postsynaptic density. *Journal of Biological Chemistry*, Vol. 272, No. 21, pp. 13467-13470, ISSN 0021-9258

Sun Y., Savanenin A., Reddy P. H. & Liu Y. F. (2001) Polyglutamine-expanded huntingtin promotes sensitization of N-methyl-D-aspartate receptors via post-synaptic density 95. *Journal of Biological Chemistry*, Vol. 276, No. 27, pp. 24713-24718, ISSN 0021-9258

Takaki M., Ujike H., Kodama M., Takehisa Y., Nakata K. & Kuroda S. (2001) Two kinds of mitogen-activated protein kinase phosphatases, MKP-1 and MKP-3, are differentially activated by acute and chronic methamphetamine treatment in the rat brain. *Journal of Neurochemistry*, Vol. 79, No. 3, pp. 679-688, ISSN 0022-3042

Tang T. S., Slow E., Lupu V., Stavrovskaya I. G., Sugimori M., Llinas R., Kristal B. S., Hayden M. R. & Bezprozvanny I. (2005) Disturbed Ca2+ signaling and apoptosis of medium spiny neurons in Huntington's disease. *Proceedings of the National Academy of Sciences USA* , Vol. 102, No. 7, pp. 2602-2607, ISSN 0027-8424

Thompson L. M., Aiken C. T., Kaltenbach L. S., Agrawal N., Illes K., Khoshnan A., Martinez-Vincente M., Arrasate M., O'Rourke J. G., Khashwji H., Lukacsovich T., Zhu Y. Z., Lau A. L., Massey A., Hayden M. R., Zeitlin S. O., Finkbeiner S., Green K. N., LaFerla F. M., Bates G., Huang L., Patterson P. H., Lo D. C., Cuervo A. M., Marsh J. L. & Steffan J. S. (2009) IKK phosphorylates Huntingtin and targets it for degradation by the proteasome and lysosome. *Journal of Cell Biology*, Vol. 187, No. 7, pp. 1083-1099, ISSN 0021-9525

Tian Q. & Wang J. (2002) Role of serine/threonine protein phosphatase in Alzheimer's disease. *Neurosignals*, Vol. 11, No. 5, pp. 262-269, ISSN 1424-862X

Torres-Peraza J. F., Giralt A., Garcia-Martinez J. M., Pedrosa E., Canals J. M. & Alberch J. (2008) Disruption of striatal glutamatergic transmission induced by mutant huntingtin involves remodeling of both postsynaptic density and NMDA receptor signaling. *Neurobiology of Disease*, Vol. 29, No. 3, pp. 409-421, ISSN 0969-9961

Valjent E., Pascoli V., Svenningsson P., Paul S., Enslen H., Corvol J. C., Stipanovich A., Caboche J., Lombroso P. J., Nairn A. C., Greengard P., Herve D. & Girault J. A. (2005) Regulation of a protein phosphatase cascade allows convergent dopamine and glutamate signals to activate ERK in the striatum. *Proceedings of the National Academy of Sciences USA* , Vol. 102, No. 2, pp. 491-496, ISSN 0027-8424

Walaas S. I. & Greengard P. (1991) Protein phosphorylation and neuronal function. *Pharmacological Reviews*, Vol. 43, No. 3, pp. 299-349, ISSN: 0031-6997

Wang H. G., Pathan N., Ethell I. M., Krajewski S., Yamaguchi Y., Shibasaki F., McKeon F., Bobo T., Franke T. F. & Reed J. C. (1999) Ca2+-induced apoptosis through calcineurin dephosphorylation of BAD. *Science*, Vol. 284, No. 5412, pp. 339-343, ISSN 0036-8075

Wang L. Y., Orser B. A., Brautigan D. L. & MacDonald J. F. (1994) Regulation of NMDA receptors in cultured hippocampal neurons by protein phosphatases 1 and 2A. *Nature*, Vol. 369, No. 6477, pp. 230-232, ISSN 0028-0836

Wang X., Zhong P. & Yan Z. (2002) Dopamine D4 receptors modulate GABAergic signaling in pyramidal neurons of prefrontal cortex. *Journal of Neuroscience*, Vol. 22, No. 21, pp. 9185-9193, ISSN 0270-6474

Warby S. C., Chan E. Y., Metzler M., Gan L., Singaraja R. R., Crocker S. F., Robertson H. A. & Hayden M. R. (2005) Huntingtin phosphorylation on serine 421 is significantly reduced in the striatum and by polyglutamine expansion in vivo. *Human Molecular Genetics*, Vol. 14, No. 11, pp. 1569-1577, ISSN 0964-6906

Warby S. C., Doty C. N., Graham R. K., Shively J., Singaraja R. R. & Hayden M. R. (2009) Phosphorylation of huntingtin reduces the accumulation of its nuclear fragments. *Molecular and Cellular Neuroscience*. Vol. 40, No. 2, pp. 121-127, ISSN 1044-7431

Weir D. W., Sturrock A. & Leavitt B. R. (2011) Development of biomarkers for Huntington's disease. *Lancet Neurology*, Vol. 10, No. 6, pp. 573-590, ISSN 1474-4422

Wera S. & Neyts J. (1994) Calcineurin as a possible new target for treatment of Parkinson's disease. *Medical Hypotheses*, Vol. 43, No. 3, pp. 132-134, ISSN 0306-9877

Westphal R. S., Tavalin S. J., Lin J. W., Alto N. M., Fraser I. D., Langeberg L. K., Sheng M. & Scott J. D. (1999) Regulation of NMDA receptors by an associated phosphatase-kinase signaling complex. *Science*, Vol. 285, No. 5424, pp. 93-96, ISSN 0036-8075

Wood A. M. & Bristow D. R. (1998) N-methyl-D-aspartate receptor desensitisation is neuroprotective by inhibiting glutamate-induced apoptotic-like death. *Journal of Neurochemistry*, Vol. 70, No. 2, pp. 677-687, ISSN 0022-3042

Wu H. Y., Tomizawa K., Oda Y., Wei F. Y., Lu Y. F., Matsushita M., Li S. T., Moriwaki A. & Matsui H. (2004) Critical role of calpain-mediated cleavage of calcineurin in excitotoxic neurodegeneration. *Journal of Biological Chemistry*, Vol. 279, No. 6, pp. 4929-4940, ISSN 0021-9258

Wu Z. L., O'Kane T. M., Scott R. W., Savage M. J. & Bozyczko-Coyne D. (2002) Protein tyrosine phosphatases are up-regulated and participate in cell death induced by polyglutamine expansion. *Journal of Biological Chemistry*, Vol. 277, No. 46, pp. 44208-44213, ISSN 0021-9258

Xifro X., Garcia-Martinez J. M., Del Toro D., Alberch J. & Perez-Navarro E. (2008) Calcineurin is involved in the early activation of NMDA-mediated cell death in mutant huntingtin knock-in striatal cells. *Journal of Neurochemistry*, Vol. 105, No. 5, pp. 1596-1612, ISSN 0022-3042

Xifro X., Giralt A., Saavedra A., Garcia-Martinez J. M., Diaz-Hernandez M., Lucas J. J., Alberch J. & Perez-Navarro E. (2009) Reduced calcineurin protein levels and activity in exon-1 mouse models of Huntington's disease: role in excitotoxicity. *Neurobiology of Disease*, Vol. 36, No. 3, pp. 461-469, ISSN 0969-9961

Xu J., Kurup P., Zhang Y., Goebel-Goody S. M., Wu P. H., Hawasli A. H., Baum M. L., Bibb J. A. & Lombroso P. J. (2009) Extrasynaptic NMDA receptors couple preferentially to excitotoxicity via calpain-mediated cleavage of STEP. *Journal of Neuroscience*, Vol. 29, No. 29, pp. 9330-9343, ISSN 0270-6474

Yamanaka T., Miyazaki H., Oyama F., Kurosawa M., Washizu C., Doi H., Nukina N. (2008) Mutant Huntingtin reduces HSP70 expression through the sequestration of NF-Y transcription factor. *EMBO Journal*, Vol. 27, No. 6, pp. 827-839., ISSN 0261-4189

Zala D., Colin E., Rangone H., Liot G., Humbert S. & Saudou F. (2008) Phosphorylation of mutant huntingtin at S421 restores anterograde and retrograde transport in neurons. *Human Molecular Genetics*, Vol. 17, No. 24, pp. 3837-3846, ISSN 0964-6906

Zeron M. M., Chen N., Moshaver A., Lee A. T., Wellington C. L., Hayden M. R. & Raymond L. A. (2001) Mutant huntingtin enhances excitotoxic cell death. *Molecular and Cellular Neuroscience*, Vol. 17, No. 1, pp. 41-53, ISSN 1044-7431

Zeron M. M., Hansson O., Chen N., Wellington C. L., Leavitt B. R., Brundin P., Hayden M. R. & Raymond L. A. (2002) Increased sensitivity to N-methyl-D-aspartate receptor-mediated excitotoxicity in a mouse model of Huntington's disease. *Neuron*, Vol. 33, No. 6, pp. 849-860, ISSN 0896-6273

Zhang Y., Venkitaramani D. V., Gladding C. M., Kurup P., Molnar E., Collingridge G. L. & Lombroso P. J. (2008) The tyrosine phosphatase STEP mediates AMPA receptor endocytosis after metabotropic glutamate receptor stimulation. *Journal of Neuroscience*, Vol. 28, No. 42, pp. 10561-10566, ISSN 0270-6474

Zhang Y., Kurup P., Xu J., Carty N., Fernandez S. M., Nygaard H. B., Pittenger C., Greengard P., Strittmatter S. M., Nairn A. C. & Lombroso P. J. (2010) Genetic reduction of striatal-enriched tyrosine phosphatase (STEP) reverses cognitive and cellular deficits in an Alzheimer's disease mouse model. *Proceedings of the National Academy of Sciences USA* , Vol. 107, No. 44, pp. 19014-19019, ISSN 0027-8424

Zhang Z. Y. (2002) Protein tyrosine phosphatases: structure and function, substrate specificity, and inhibitor development. *Annual Review of Pharmacology and Toxicolology*, Vol. 42, No. pp. 209-234, ISSN 0362-1642

Part 3

Learning to Live with Huntington's Disease

9

Risk and Resilience: Living with a Neurological Condition with a Focus on Health Care Communications

Kerstin Roger and Leslie Penner
University of Manitoba
Canada

1. Introduction

There is little research examining the daily lived experiences of families in which one person is living with a neurological condition. Further, there is no research which examines how patients evolve and adapt in ways that allow them to have their needs met within the complex system of health care provision. This paper explores nine factors that emerged in original, empirical qualitative data, and how these factors are perceived by the participants to contribute towards increasing resilience when communicating with the health care system. The data were collected over a three year period, utilizing focus groups and interviews. Our primary focus in this paper will be on the participants living with Huntington's and Parkinson's, although other participants will be referred to as well.

Communication about care can be shaped by many factors such as a concern about being a burden to others, the proximity of family, family dynamics, personalities, stress related to the illness itself, and, socio-cultural belief systems about health and healthcare (in the example of persons with a collectivist versus more individualistic cultural background). It has become clear (Roger et al., 2010; Roger & Medved, 2010; Zloty et al., 2010) that contradictory and often unspoken expectations of care emerge between professionals, family and individuals. Because of this, errors, poor treatment, and misunderstandings can result, in addition to diminished well-being of caregivers and individuals. Further, the ways in which individuals and family members experience and perceive interactions with health care providers have been shown to affect the level of trust that the patients have in their care providers (Tarrant et al., 2003), and have been demonstrated to impact health care outcomes (Moreau et al., 2006; Safran et al., 1998). These outcomes can result in significant costs to individuals and the health care system. This paper will explore how the nine factors that emerged can contribute towards the development of tools that can be used to facilitate improved communication between patients living with neurological conditions and health care providers.

2. Ecological model

Bronfenbrenner's ecological approach (1979) is a suitable framework. His approach identifies how individuals, small groups and larger groups, as well as institutions, interact systemically and bi-directionally to shape relational patterns, norms and values.

Bronfenbrenner (1979) initially described four nested systems: micro-, meso-, exo-, and macrosystems, with family being the primary microsystem within which the individual develops (Bubloz & Sontag, 1993, p. 424). The mesosystem refers to interactions and relationships between the family and other systems where individual learning takes place. This is an important concept in relation to the current study because there is much health care teaching that individuals and their family members are exposed to when interacting with the health care system. Bronfenbrenner suggested that if the connections between families and the environments where learning takes place are healthy and positive, it would affect the individual in a positive way. For example, according to this theory, if individuals and their family members have open and positive connections with their neurologists, the health of these patients will be improved. The exosystem represents environments that adults participate in which, in turn, affect the individual and the family as a whole (e.g. work settings, recreational organizations, volunteer settings). Finally, the macrosystem, which includes cultural beliefs, customs and laws, is the outermost layer of the linked systems – it envelopes and influences the interactions of all system layers. Later in the development of his theory, Bronfenbrenner (1986) added the chronosystem, which refers to the influence of the person's development of changes over time in the context of the environments in which the person interacts. He suggested that life transitions were the simplest form of chronosystem, with the development of an illness being an example. This transition has the potential to affect the development of the individual (and family members) directly, or indirectly by affecting the interactions and functions of the family. The chronosystem includes the cumulative effects of evolving developmental transitions over the life of an individual. This concept is useful when exploring the impact that a chronic, deteriorating neurological illness has on the development of patients and their family members; despite being a difficult transition, it has the potential to instigate developmental change. This systemic approach is particularly useful here since the stories and narratives between couples and care professionals reflect important aspects of Bronfenbrenner's systems approach. The themes that emerged in this study moved from descriptions of very personal responses to situations, to daily communications and interactions among family members, to interactions with the larger network of resources and organizations.

Human beings are inherently social; they do not generally operate independently and in isolation. Therefore, it follows that the behaviour and responses of individuals cannot be fully understood without considering the environment within which they are embedded. Human ecological theory "….is concerned with interaction and interdependence of humans (as individuals, groups, and societies) with the environment" (Bubolz & Sontag, 1993, p. 421). A key concept in this theory is the process of adaptation — the way in which individuals and families attempt to cope with their ever-changing environments. Particular attention is given to communication and the underlying values which guide these decisions (Bubolz & Sontag, 1993). Resilient couples who interact with the health care system on a regular basis can and do find techniques and strategies which ensure effective and creative adaptation to the challenges they face. In this way, Bronfenbrenner's model is a helpful framework for the data to be discussed in this paper.

3. Background

The National Health Charities of Canada (NHCC) is an umbrella organization that works with government, researchers and the community to promote and support services and research to a number of related neurological disease conditions such as neurotrauma (e.g., acquired brain injury and spinal cord injury), neuromuscular disorders (e.g., cerebral palsy, epilepsy and spina bifida), degenerative demyelinating conditions (e.g., multiple sclerosis, Guillian-Barre syndrome), and movement and other neurodegenerative disorders (e.g., Parkinson's Disease, Huntington's Disease, Alzheimer's Disease and Amyotrophic Lateral Sclerosis [ALS]). This study recruited participants from conditions under this umbrella: to be discussed in this paper are participants with Parkinson's Disease (the majority of our sample) and Huntington's.

Huntington's Disease is an inherited neuropsychiatric disorder that causes brain cells to die, resulting in clinical features which present in a triad of movement disorder, cognitive dysfunction and psychiatric or behavioral disturbance (Sturrock & Leavitt, 2010). Because the disease is inherited as an autosomal dominant trait, each child of an affected individual has a 50% chance of inheriting the gene (Aubeeluck & Wilson, 2008). The average age of onset of Huntington's Disease is between 35 and 44 years (Paulsen, Ferneyhough Hoth, Nehl & Stierman, 2005), but it can present anytime between ages 2 to 85 years (Roos, 2010). Huntington's is a rare disease with a prevalence rate that varies between 5-10 per 100,000 in the American population (Nance & Myers, 2001) and 4-8 per 100,000 in the European population (Harper, 1992).There is no cure for Huntington's Disease at this time and patients die, on average, 20 years after onset (Paulsen et al., 2005).

Mild cognitive and personality changes can occur in the early stages of the disease (Sturrock & Leavitt, 2010; Walker, 2007). The early symptoms are often first noticed by family, friends and co-workers and may include disinhibited behavior, fidgetiness, irritability, anhedonia, obsessive behaviors, altered executive function, and slowed processing speed which manifests in decreased productivity (Sturrock & Leavitt, 2010). As the disease progresses, motor disturbances such as chorea, speech and swallowing difficulties, rigidity, bradykinesia and akinesia develop (Roos, 2010). Eventually, mobility is lost (Sturrock & Leavitt, 2010) and oral motor dysfunction leads to incoherence of speech and inability to eat (Sturrock & Leavitt, 2010).

Cognitive deterioration is progressive in Huntington's Disease (Sturrock & Leavitt, 2010). There is a decline in executive functioning that affects judgment, insight, and ability to organize (Roos, 2010; Sturrock & Leavitt, 2010) and there is a progressive deterioration in recall and complex intellectual functioning (Sturrock & Leavitt, 2010). Eventually, cognitive decline becomes global and all aspects of cognition become impaired (Sturrock & Leavitt, 2010). Psychiatric symptoms such as depression and anxiety are often present during the disease trajectory and are relatively independent of the motor and cognitive aspects of the disease (Paulsen, Ready, Hamilton, Mega & Cummings, 2001). As well, although less common, delusions and hallucinations can also as emerge during the course of the illness (Paulsen et al., 2001). There is an increase in suicidal ideation in individuals at risk for, and diagnosed with Huntington's Disease, particularly in the period immediately before receiving a diagnosis ,and in then again in the period where independence begins to diminish (Paulsen et al., 2005).

Parkinson's Disease is the second most common neurodegenerative disorder worldwide, second only to Alzheimer's Disease (de Lau & Breteler, 2006). It is commonly diagnosed in individuals over the age of fifty, with its prevalence affecting approximately three percent of the Canadian population over the age of 65 (Public Health Agency of Canada, 2000). Recent

Canadian research has shown that the prevalence of Parkinson's Disease is increasing, perhaps due to an aging population (Guttman, Slaughter, Theriault, DeBoer, & Naylor, 2003; Lix et al., 2010).

The most common symptoms of Parkinson's Disease are tremor, muscle rigidity and stiffness and psychomotor retardation (bradykinesia) (Clark, 2007; Heisters, 2011). As the disease progresses, postural abnormalities and instability can emerge (Clark, 2007; Nutt, & Wooten, 2005). These symptoms can interfere with ambulation and increase the risk of falls. There is a wide range of non-motor symptoms which pain, dementia, mood disorder, psychosis, apathy, sleep disorder and excessive daytime sleepiness, bowel and bladder dysfunction, excessive sweating, and sexual dysfunction (Clark, 2007; Heisters, 2011). Dementia is common, affecting approximately 30% of patients with Parkinson's Disease (Aarsland & Kurz, 2010). The severity and presentation of Parkinson's related dementia varies between individuals, but common characteristics are impairment in attention, memory, ability to plan, organize and problem solve, and impaired recall, personality changes, behavioral symptoms and hallucinations (Emre, 2003). Because non-motor symptoms affect several domains of functioning, and because they are difficult to treat, the impact on the patient's quality of life can be profound.

Both HD and PD are chronic neurodegenerative and progressive in nature (National Institute of Neurological Disorders and Stroke, 2008; Public Health Agency of Canada, 2000). As well, symptoms can affect all domains of functioning: physical, cognitive and emotional, resulting in complex health care needs.

Although each of these neurological conditions has their own etiology, they share symptoms which can impact everyday activities and the health and well-being of individuals and family members. Shared experiences include disrupted relationships and a reduction in participation in personally meaningful activities (e.g., employment, shared family activities) (Statistics Canada, 2007). While there has been some attention paid to the illness experience (Brody, 1987; Charmaz, 1991), little research was found that examines communication and the daily experiences of persons with neurological conditions in relation to their families and health care providers. The impacts in this context are multi-faceted including multiple changes to couples' roles and responsibilities over years, every day routines, marital relationships and financial status.

4. Methods

This was a qualitative pilot study conducted over three years using interviews and focus groups. Initially, community consultations were held with affiliated staff and organizations (see Table 1) to better understand organizational needs regarding care services to families and couples with long term neurodegenerative conditions (e.g. Huntington's, Alzheimer's, ALS, Multiple Sclerosis, and Parkinson's). This led to a clarification of the need for research on people's daily lived experiences and especially a need to better understand their interactions with the health care system. The research team was then successful in receiving funding to conduct Phase II in 2009. This explored decision-making between couples and care professionals. We received funding for Phase III where we were able to explore in more depth, given the same sample of participants, what had changed for them given their daily lived experiences in the last year. The data to be described in this paper emerged from this last sample in Phase III collected in 2010.

	2007-08	2009	2010
Event	PHASE I: Community-based consultations (3)	PHASE II: Interviews (16)	PHASE III: Follow-up interviews (8) and focus groups (2)

Table 1. Research Phases.

4.1 Ethics approval

The authors prepared an ethics protocol for the most suitable ethics review committee at the local university and this was approved. Components of this protocol included: i. a script for the research assistant to be used when discussing possible recruitment with relevant organizations and a script to be used when discussing the study with potential future participants; ii. a list of the interview questions; iii. a pledge of confidentiality for the research assistant and the transcriber; and, iv. a consent form that described the study, it identified the process that ensured the participant's confidentiality and how this would be maintained over time. The consent form addressed the treatment of the data once the study was to be completed, how the data will be stored, and when and how the data will be discarded.

4.2 Interview and focus group sample

We aimed for equal representation of individuals in the three proposed categories: the individual with a selected neurological condition, a familial support person, as well as a professional care provider (see Table 2). Fifteen people were interviewed in total over three time periods in the three years. Over the three years, some changes did occur to our sample due to divorce, moves out of province, and a willingness to participate in the study. We held two focus groups once the interviews were conducted and themes were analyzed. They were recruited in the same manner as described below for the individual interviews. The focus groups were comprised of six participants each (not the same persons as the interview sample) who were all formal caregivers working in any one of the affiliated organizations. Diversity for the focus group participation was sought in regards to the type of professional (e.g. nurses, social workers, administrators).

Participants with an interest to participate in the study were eligible if they met the following inclusion criteria:

i. They understood the primary goal of the study and were able to articulate their thoughts verbally on the topic;
ii. They fit on of the disease categories;
iii. They were able to provide consent at the beginning of the study by reading the consent form, asking questions about the study, and signing the consent forms;
iv. They were able to hold a full conversation in English;
v. They or a family support was affiliated with one of the selected and recognized institutions. Or, for the focus groups/consultations, they were a staff person in one of the affiliated organizations;
vi. A primary diagnosis of one of the conditions under the NHCC umbrella had occurred as confirmed by a key familial support person, a physician, social worker, nurse or patient care manager familiar with the participant's history;

vii. Participants for the interviews had engaged in communications regarding health care involving a person with a selected condition in the last 6 months; viii. Participants had to be over 18 years of age.

	PSEUDONYM	RELATIONSHIP	AGE	PROFESSIONAL BACKGROUND	PROFESSIONAL/ PATIENT WITH CONDITION
1	Neil	Married to 2			PD
2	Flora	*	65	SW	Support
3	Len	Brother to 4	79	Business	PD
4	Frieda	*	83	Secretary	Support
5	Estrella		2003 began	OT with MS	Prof
6	Sophie		1986 began	SW with HD/PD	Prof
7	Daniel	*	55	Welder	Support
8	Doreen		50	Computer analyst	MS
9	Jane	Married to Ken	59		MS
10	Ivan		1997 began	Warden/vol pall care	Prof
11	Leila		1999 began	nurse	Prof
12	Nettie		2005 began	Health care/MS	prof
13	Janelle	Married to 7	54	Bakery manager	PD
14	Margareta	*	81	banker	PD
15	Friederich	Married to 14	83	Power engineer	support

Table 2. Interview Sample.

Individuals for the interviews were asked whether they would provide one key family support person. A person with one of the selected neurological conditions could take part in this study even if they had no key family support person and wanted to select a second health care provider, or their key family support person declined but someone else was willing to be interviewed. The definition of the family support person was quite broad including family members, common law partners, neighbors who provide significant frequent care, or another relative doing the same. This individual would sign a consent form prior to being interviewed. Both the individual and their family support person received an honorarium for their participation. Confidentiality agreements as documented through the consent form applied to each participant. Professionals working in related areas and with populations who fit the criteria were recruited as well.

Once the consent forms were signed by participants, the interviews were held individually at a site selected by the participant, and lasted approximately two hours. A demographic section began the interview process including basic questions about a person's age, gender, professional affiliation if appropriate and so on. Semi-structured interview questions were then used to investigate the primary objectives of the study. Questions included asking about the wished for and perceived role of health care providers communicating on their behalf, the wished for and perceived impact of family members making decisions on their behalf, and the perceived changes and role of their own independence as their condition was diagnosed and as it progressed. New probes were developed as data was collected based on the findings in the ongoing interviews. All interviews were audio taped and then transcribed verbatim.

Once the consent forms were signed by the participants, two focus groups were held at locations convenient for the participants and lasted approximately two hours. Themes from the individual interviews had been compiled and were presented to the focus group members. Similarities between the themes and the participant's experiences, identified gaps and differences were discussed. Probes had been developed in the ethics protocol for this purpose. Detailed notes were taken in these two focus groups by a research assistant.

4.3 Analytic process

NVIVO8, a qualitative data management program, was used to code all transcribed interviews. Content analysis was used as a framework (Graneheim & Lundman, 2004) where constant comparison is possible between themes and sub-themes as they emerged. Once the researchers coded the transcripts and assessed the main and sub-themes, selected experts were provided with a sample of transcripts in order to code them. By applying the principles of qualitative content analysis, further exploration of the data was performed to encourage trustworthiness and credibility of the research findings. This approach allowed the researcher to "condense" the data into additional and/or comparative codes, followed by "aggregation" or the progressive interpretive process of thematic abstraction. The themes were then compared and similarities noted while differences will be documented in subsequent papers.

Rigor was determined according to principles set out for conducting qualitative research (Morse et al., 2002). For example, *consistency* was ensured by choosing participants who have experiences with the research topic and a genuine interest in taking part in the interviews. *Transferability* will be fulfilled by making certain that detailed information will be provided in future papers so that readers would be able to identify a similar situation in a similar context. *Credibility* was attained through editing of the interview transcripts as well as integration of field notes in line with what does exist in the literature. Inter-rater reliability throughout all phases of analysis solidified credibility. Results and interpretations were checked by members of the research team who then reviewed the analysis, obtaining consensual validation.

5. Findings

Three levels of the Bronfenbrenner ecological model were most apparent in our emerging nine factors: the microsystem, the mesosystem, and the chronosystem. The findings will be presented in two parts – the interview data first and the focus group discussions second.

5.1 Microsystem

Individual and family characteristics were included to represent the microsystem.

1. Manner of Communicating: Ability to Push the System
2. Self-Reflection about Characteristics Prior to Condition
3. Existing Social Supports
4. Education Levels
5. Gender of Primary Caregiver/ Professional

5.2 Mesosystem

The mesosystem includes the connections and interactions between the family and other systems where individual learning takes place. Here, the system where learning takes place is the health care system.

1. Health Care Literacy

5.3 Chronosystem

Bronfenbrenner's chronosystem is useful for examining the impact that the passage of time has on the individual. For example, the passage of time can impact the individual's physical state (eg. children maturing, individual's with chronic illness deteriorating), and this in turn, can affect the way in which they interact with the environment. As well, the passage of time can allow individuals to gain mastery and experience in coping with a difficult situation, for example. The chronosystem encompasses anything that has to do with the passage of time.

1. Length of Relationship to Primary Caregiver
2. Stage of the Illness
3. Age

5.4 Findings from interview data

5.4.1 Microsystem

5.4.1.1 Manner of communicating

Resilience research has often sought to understand specific personality traits or characteristics inherent in an individual - qualities which were described as being protective in nature (Earvolino, 2007; Johnson & Wiechelt, 2004; Richardson, 2002).The participants in this sample demonstrate personality traits that reflect their individual abilities regarding communication. For example, communicating about their care needs in a clear and articulate manner was for some a new skill and for others an existing long standing trait. Not being able to communicate well with care professionals in many cases reduced their ability to interact in effective and beneficial ways with the health care system.

It was evident that the manner in which a patient, family or professional caregiver communicated with others shaped how they perceived their care plans developed. Janelle talks about her ability to communicate to 'push' the system:

Janelle: *And the Pharmacare system out here is a lot stricter as well, and at first they weren't gonna cover me for a couple of my main medications. I had to, this is quite funny. Well it's funny but it wasn't. They made me get a letter from my doctor saying that it was absolutely necessary that I have these medications. And I said, well, of course I do, I have Parkinson's. So they said, well, isn't there something else you could use? And I said no, and I had to get a note from my doctor in order to have those two medications covered.* (Int.: "So you really had to push the system?") *Yes – I really had to work hard to get those medications!*

Janelle described that her ability to be persistent and forthright in her communications with care professionals was a skill she needed to learn, that she had previously been less assertive and unable to express her needs when interacting with professionals in larger institutions or organizations. Her illness 'taught' her this skill. Upon being diagnosed, she learned that her new found ability to 'push' the system by being more assertive was useful when advocating for herself. People are also aware that their ability to communicate on their own behalf will change as their condition progresses. Ironically, participants talked about how important it was to be polite and nice when interacting with health care professionals, to be courteous with care professionals in order to get ones care needs met. However, participants also spoke proudly about their ability to push the system and get what they needed when they were less polite. At times, they enlisted the support of health care professionals to achieve their goals. In cases where a care professional was not able to assist them in successfully 'pushing the system', it was clear that disappointment in the care professional occurred. There was an expectation that when patients had allies in health care, the patients felt better able to communicate within the system. This theme persists throughout the study and becomes important to our broader theme of social support promoting individual resilience. Those who felt supported by a social service professional also expressed higher levels of satisfaction with communications with health care professionals.

Troubling communications with people with neurological conditions are often attributed to the disease itself, while Janelle is articulate in stating that some of her characteristics, which may in another person be seen as a symptom of her condition, are part of her old normal self. Medicalizing personality traits that existed prior to the onset of an illness can lead to mis-understandings and inadequate care plans. In this sense, people's ability to communicate with health care professionals may be interpreted as part of their condition, but in fact, may be describing personal traits and qualities they have always had.

5.4.1.2 Self-reflection about personal characteristics prior to condition

The participants in this study demonstrated resilience in the example of adaptation and coping with extraordinary circumstances. While these may appear as minor or simple reflections of resilience, they must be understood in the context of challenging and usually complex lives. One approach to resilience research has been to seek out adaptive processes or a means of coping with various adversities and defining these as an opportunity to learn or improve upon an individual's protective qualities (Richardson, 2002). Research in this realm has helped to broaden the predominant mindset of problem-oriented approaches, where one would focus on the importance of prevention, encourage strengths and value human fortitude; ultimately, focusing on the basics of a strength-based lens (Krawlik et al., 2006).

For example, Neil says he has always had an optimistic attitude and that this now serves him well as he begins to live with some of his early limitations. He says it could have been anyone who received this diagnosis, so 'why not me?', and he states that he is fine even though he now has this additional condition in his life. His wife Flora also underlines how optimistic he remains after receiving his diagnosis. Janelle describes herself here:

Well, for instance, I'm terribly, terribly disorganized and always have been. Now, I don't write things down and I forget my appointments and like it causes everybody a lot of stress because I'm scrambling at the last minute to make arrangements and what have you, and she'll say to me, get a book. I'll buy you a book and write these things down and I'll help you with your appointments. I'll help you arrange them and I'll help you get there, you know, but you've got to make the effort to write them down and take note of them so, you know, we're not doing things at the last minute. And she said, I'm quite willing to take you and do anything you want, but you've got to at least be a little bit more organized. And it's true, like I need a kick in the butt. Its always been that way.

We know that self-reflection about personal characteristics can fade as disease trajectories of neurological conditions progress. A fading ability to recognize one's own style or interactions with others can lead to challenges for health care professionals with the goal of determining where a person with a neurological condition is at. Certainly, when health care providers have known an individual over years as their condition progresses, they are in a much stronger position to assess how an individual is doing – especially as they become less able to reflect on their own processes.

5.4.1.3 Existing social supports

While this factor (#3) does fit with other levels in the Bronfenbrenner system, it is being placed here as the primary location. Traditional research on resilience was rooted in psychiatric literature and focused primarily on children and adolescents capable of dealing with great difficulty (Garmezy, 1985, 1993; Masten, 1999; Werner, 1990; Werner & Smith, 1977). More current examples reflect essential components of social support when developing qualities associated with that traditional literature on resilience. It appears that social support is highly correlated to resilience and that networks are critical for a positive description of social support. A better understanding of how couples might experience or express resilience can directly and indirectly impact care provision, and a professional's inclination to provide better care for a particular dyad. If social supports result in a more resilient patient, it would be helpful to be able to assess this at intake.

It was clear that participants with strong and reliable family or friendship supports were more able to interact effectively with the health care system. Flora states,

We have a lot of friends who have Parkinson's, by coincidence, not that we've acquired them later on. A lot of people have Parkinson's. And the Parkinson's community now, we've seen it developed. When Nick was first seeing his doctor for Parkinson's, the specialist, there's one neurologist that was looking after it, it was him. Now you've got the Movement Disorders Clinic.....

Flora and Neil were among the most resilient couples, expressing satisfaction with each other and their communications with the health care system, stating in no uncertain terms that they were happy and getting their needs met. Their social network within the PD community contributed in particular to their perception of resilience, and this is mirrored in other research as well (Roger, 2007a,b; 2006a,b; Roger et al., 2010; Roger & Medved, 2010).

Jack lives in an intergenerational home that led to more supports than he would otherwise have: his wife's mother was living with him, and as an older senior who was cognitively well was supporting Jack in the care of her daughter (his wife with early onset dementia). Jack's grown daughter, who is now a mother as well, comes regularly to bathe and care for her own grandmother. This pattern of intergenerational supports clearly reduces the caregiving stress Jack has experienced.

However, alternately, another participant had a very different experience. Margareta, whom her husband described as quite a formidable force, did not find support in her own family. She said:

(Int.: "Do you talk to your kids about it at all?") No...No, they don't want to hear about it...They've got families of their own and they're all busy.

Margareta expressed disappointment that 'one must always do everything for oneself' in regards to her family. She also spoke disparagingly of the health care system as an institution.

Although Len did have a sister who lived near him, he was reluctant to over-rely on her for support. His children did not live in the same province, so when he went for what is typically a day surgery, he demanded extra support from the system to compensate for absent family support:

If I needed it, I'd damn well go after it...I would insist, as I did with the nurses 4 times a day. I told the doctor and his secretary, look, I don't have anybody. If I had somebody, I might not be here. I don't have nobody to do this for me. When I had my surgery, they want someone to stay with you overnight. You shouldn't be alone. I don't have anybody to stay overnight. No family. No relatives. Nobody that can stay the night. I want to stay in the hospital the first night cause I have nobody at home and that's what I want. (Int.:"And what did they do?") They gave it to me...I told them I want it, that's it.

It was apparent that when family supports were not available that participants depended much more strongly on the health care system and in this way also, our data suggests that they did not always feel the health care system was providing for them. Perhaps their expectation of imagined family assistance was superimposed onto the health care system in a way that could only disappoint. Furthermore, the health care system utilizes an individualistic approach which often leaves family support people "out of the loop". Over time, the rigid boundary which exists between the health care system and the family many have reinforced the tendency of individuals to over-rely on health care professionals, with expectations that the system should provide supports which are not possible in all circumstances.

5.4.1.4 Education levels

A study by Berkman and Syme (1979) identified that a greater social network and frequency of contact lead to decreased mortality of men and women across all ages, even when controlling for socioeconomic status, health status and health practices. However, interestingly, we found participants stated a perception that education and financial resources in fact would significantly improve their interactions with health care professionals. Neil suggests:

Yeah, probably. Cause I know how to write a letter. You know, that's the thing, when you're submitting your resume, you put a covering letter. The first 5 sentences determine where you're gonna go. I got good writing letters when I was a department head of science. There are ways of writing a letter of recommendation which are positive, and there are negative ways.

Later, he describes:

Well you know when you start speaking with an educated person or an uneducated person, you'll notice things in their conversation, grammatical structures and the like, that are more middle class or upper middle class, if you listen carefully, the subjunctive case if you were. If I were instead of if I was. That's what makes a more educated or less educated conversationalist. Now I don't want to be pedantic, but one, so I do make some really simple conversions, but there's different classes of language in English. If you listen carefully, you can tell a person's grade level.

Janelle's partner (who became her ex in the course of the study), was a skilled labourer and was intimidated not only of the health care system (as he said) but also by engaging with us as researchers in this study. He initially felt he had nothing important to say, which changed as he began to engage with us in the interviews.

It was apparent that other participants who felt confident about their ability to articulate their needs clearly and those with higher levels of education felt more confident in getting their needs met from the health care system.

5.4.1.5 Gender of primary caregiver/ professional

Upon examining ageing women with MS, Harrison and colleagues (2008) identified that women with higher levels of social support experienced higher levels of positive attitude towards their condition even when measured over a period of seven years. Janelle reflects here on her very close care relationships with her daughter:

My daughter and I...As close as you can get to a caregiver. (Int. "Okay. So I'm gonna just sort of, like the boys, are they more sort of a peripheral role?") *Yes.* (Int. "Okay. Okay. But your daughter is the one who is more primary?") *Yes, absolutely.* (Int. "Okay. Alright. So I'm just curious. Do you think that's a function of her being a woman or a nurse?") *Actually I think, it's hard to say, but I'd say as a daughter. More as a daughter.*

Another participant, Margareta, exclaimed in no uncertain terms that her girlfriends were her best supports, and regrettably she added, that may include ruling out her husband. Even Jack reflects on gender when he describes that he did not feel comfortable with the quick advice he received from his younger and male doctors:

Oh, the males were stereotypic doctors. They knew, they had all the answers and attitude and whatever. And the women were there to find out what was wrong with you.

Later, Jack says that his son was much less involved and even interested in the kinds of care needs he has with his wife and mother-in-law. Evidently, he thought gender played a role in how caregiving occurred and who was hands on in his household. It appears that the gender of the primary caregiver or the care professional shaped how communication occurred, in the minds of our participants.

5.4.2 Mesosystem

5.4.2.1 Health care literacy

Couples who had good 'health care literacy' were most able to effectively get their needs met. The relationship between health care provision and the couples we interviewed was described in particular in relation to the participant's ability to confidently interact with the system. Couples who were the most familiar with the health care system also appeared to have the most effective tools of communication.

For example, Flora and Neil had several experiences with illnesses (each) before Neil was diagnosed with Parkinson's Disease. This meant that they had had a previous entry into the health care system and how it worked and they were more able to translate this into assistance. In Flora's case, her ability to maneuver within the health care system was compounded by the fact that she had been a Social Worker and had firsthand knowledge of how 'care systems' and institutions operate. She speaks proudly of her high level of health care literacy, acknowledging that this has supported Neil's care plan over the years.

On the other hand, Janelle had not had previous health care concerns or interactions with health care, and so when she was diagnosed, she states in no uncertain terms that she found it very difficult to begin to understand the health care system in a way that provided her with the resources. She stressed that she had been a very independent person prior to being diagnosed, and that this new condition left her feeling more vulnerable and needy than previously. Her husband at the time similarly felt overwhelmed by potential interactions with health care professionals. It appears that being new to 'illness' and 'health care' was an additional challenge (and form of literacy) that some participants were less able to deal with.

In another example, Friedrich had been deaf for years, and that now that his elderly wife Margareta had Parkinson's, he said they just 'carried on as usual'. He said they were already familiar with health concerns and the health care system, they were older and had been married over 50 years, and he felt that they were simply able to step into the system and communicate their needs well within it.

In another similar example, Jack described that one of his parents had had a declining neurological condition and that he had grown up with awareness of this condition and the kinds of care and interactions with care professionals that it required. Now, he was caring for his wife and his mother-in-law. He stated that this gave him some insight and even potentially positive perspectives on how now to deal with his wife's young diagnosis in the context of the health care system.

A study by Wallace and colleagues (2001) suggested that resilience improved among individuals who had a sense of purpose and opportunities for communication particularly during times of personal duress. It was found that providing opportunities for communication could impact a person's compliance to medication, reduce errors in communication, and generally improve the experience of the disease trajectory. Further, those who had previous experience of stressful situations and had a sense of purpose might be better able to maximize previous successful social supports as new situations arose. It was evident that those participants in our study who had experienced previous health crises in their lives, and had already become familiar with the health care system, were much better equipped to handle changes now related to the new diagnosis. Clearly, health care literacy improved participant's interactions with health care providers.

5.4.3 Chronosystem

5.4.3.1 Length of relationship to primary caregiver

Weak social ties have been shown to be correlated with poor health and premature death (Berkman et al., 2000).This may be due to the fact that healthy support systems encourage good self-care. For example, men in happy marriages are less likely to have health problems, and both men and women in happy marriages are more likely to access health care services when required (Sandburg et al., 2009). Kiecolt-Glaser and Newton (2001) reviewed evidence from 64 articles published from 1991 to 2001, and concluded that poor marital quality negatively impacts health of individuals both directly and indirectly, through poor health habits and depression.

Papadatou (2009) states that social support shapes well-being between people over time, especially when they are dealing with exceptionally difficult life processes, and these may include: a long time committed and shared trajectory; shared responsibility; reinforcement of communication and involvement between committed partners; continuity in times of uncertainty and distress; and allowing for shared learning throughout the defining life process. Certainly, those participants who could be described as strong in their committed relationships appeared to be more resilient and excelled at interacting with the health care system. Thus, evidence suggests that the bond that couples have with each other can contribute to health-related benefits and improve upon an individual's capacity for resilience.

An important factor was how long couples had been together and whether they were married and had raised children together. It was clear that couples who had raised children together and/or had been married for a longer time, were more resilient in handling the issues that now arose. In fact, one of the younger (in age) couples who had only been together a few years and that we interviewed in the first Phase of the study, were no longer together in the second Phase of the study. It became clear in the second interview in Phase II, when we only interviewed one person in the couple, that the progression of the condition had contributed towards the ending of their relationship. In another case, however, a long time marriage led to a deepened sense of commitment to the husband who had one of the selected conditions.

I don't have trouble with that really. Well if anything's bothering me, I tell her right out. I don't care how they feel about it. In my mind, my concern is my husband. I don't care what you're doing with anybody else, but my husband, I want him looked after too. And they've been very, very good. (Marlene)

Marlene stresses that she knows her husband well and what his needs are and that this aids her in communicating more effectively with the health care professionals. She acknowledges that the long term care unit her husband is on is chronically lacking enough staff to adequately meet the residents' needs. However, her loyalty and commitment to her husband ensure she advocates for him so that he gets his needs met, despite a lack of resources:

I don't have trouble with that really. Well if anything's bothering me, I tell her right out. I don't care how they feel about it. In my mind, my concern is my husband. I don't care what you're doing with anybody else, but my husband, I want him looked after too. And they've been very, very good. (Marlene)

Length of time together is an indicator of relationship commitment and loyalty, and even when the patients cannot advocate for themselves, a committed and assertive partner can ensure they have their needs met, even in an overburdened healthcare system.

Margareta and Friedrich also stressed that their 50 + years of marriage had allowed them to grow more resilient as a couple over time in a way that was demonstrated by their ability to now cope. This length of time together, according to Friedrich, has positively impacted their ability to communicate with health care professionals.

5.4.3.2 Stage of the illness

It became evident over the three years of collecting data that the patient's stage of illness in tandem with existing social supports largely contributed to their sense of resilience (or lack thereof) and (in)ability to communicate well with health care professionals. Research has shown a consistent positive relationship between social connectedness, integration and stages of physical health (Cohen, 2004). Janelle became much less able to engage with the health care system after her relationship ended and her condition deteriorated. However, she then made the decision to move to another province where her children were living and this dramatically improved her health – as evidenced in her second interview with us. She felt more able to communicate about her needs, and she certainly had social supports around her.

Flora on the other hand, suggested that you need to prepare for times ahead when you know a condition will be deteriorating:

I think it's partly communication. Sometimes people just don't know what to ask for even in the beginning. Like you haven't been trained to know what to ask for. You know, people vary. Sometimes they just think, oh I'll just keep managing, or I'll just keep going. They wait until there's a crisis instead of saying, okay, we're on this path anyways now. But this is a chronic illness. What is it's path? What do we expect? You can't predict. You know, you could have Parkinson's and die of a heart attack. You have to start early and prepare for things down the road.

Other participants reflected on a 'future' when they may not be able to communicate as well as they do now. They were developing an awareness of the kinds of supports they might need to put into place for that point in time. When people are living with a neurological condition, a fact which clearly demarcates them from examples such as cancer, they know that their condition may progress over sixteen or more years. Their ability to consider a distant future means that they have a lot of time to consider changes that might occur to them. This makes their situation unique from other conditions. Their engagement with health care professionals will also remain in a more 'chronic' phase for many years, with room for many discussions about possible later stages. This can both be a strength and a vulnerability where people can prepare and plan, but also may become overwhelmed with realities. Health care professionals must have a clear understanding of this trajectory which includes emotional, cognitive and physical realms.

5.4.3.3 Age

While there were few quotes that specifically explored participant's reflections on age, it was apparent that 'age' was a constant presence in the discussions regarding health care communications. Jack stated how much he did not appreciate 'the younger physicians', who he felt had less experience and fewer insights into situations he might have questions about. Age shone through in another way as well - it was clear that the older couples in our sample were more resilient than the younger couples and that they were more prepared for eventualities related to neurological decline. They appeared to have more capacity when interacting with and communicating with the health care system as well. It was apparent that younger folk had a much harder time with their diagnosis, such as Janelle. She would not have anticipated this diagnosis at such a young age, and her stories indicate that she was having a harder time in general. Age also intersected with the long term couples to create a bond that promoted not just their social supports developed over time, but also their sense of resilience as individuals and a couple.

5.5 Findings from focus group data

The focus group data consolidated the importance of the nine factors found in the interviews that have been discussed above – bringing together key elements to this study and the emerging data. The above nine factors were presented in summary form to the focus groups to ascertain the extent to which these findings reflected the participant professional's experiences. Each of our focus group participants confirmed that these factors were highly relevant in their experience of intake with new individuals in order to determine how couples were handling difficult situations related to their diagnosis. They stated that the nine factors were central to how well the couples (and families) were doing and thus also how they would benefit from health care communications.

However, focus group participants also expressed concern that there was not a standard form or approach to this kind of intake assessment. Few tools if any existed to refine or better understand these nine factors. They underlined how relevant this information would be if it were being collected and analyzed more effectively by individual organizations / researchers.

One of the key discussions in the focus groups thus revolved around the preparation, implementation and compilation of their organization's intake forms. The participants in our focus groups stated that while intake forms were used to collect information related to the nine factors, the process of collecting information and the forms themselves were limited. For example, there were several different forms to be used at intake. Little training existed in how best to fill out the intake forms and what to do with the information professionals had collected. Further, our focus group participants described that any number of forms developed by their organizations might be used at intake and then filed away without being compiled or analyzed. Therefore, the information being collected was fragmented and lacked a cohesive structure or purpose after collection.

The focus group participants stressed that developing a unified form, and a comprehensive analysis of the data on these forms, could result in an important source of information for developing not only better assessment tools for intake, but also towards improved services for patients. Professionals stated they could better assess couples at risk and also provide more catered and effective care services if this information was made analyzed and compiled and then available to them. However, care professionals in our focus groups stated they had neither the time nor the skills to compile and analyze the data available to them through their own organizational intake forms.

6. Discussion

Since we know so little about interactions between family care providers and their loved ones in terms of health communications, and we know equally little about their interactions with health care professionals, it is even more significant that we also know so little about a large group of persons living with neurological decline. Living with a neurological condition is a reality which can affect individuals and their caregivers for well over fifteen years. The unique medical realities associated with the etiology of the neurological conditions encompassed within the mandate of the NHCC must be better understood.

Firstly, the value of social support has emerged in this data as central to the couples interactions with health care professionals, and this in turn, matches what the literature suggests about resilience. Assessing for social support and resilience early on in the intake procedure will benefit a well implemented care plan and improved well-being for all concerned. Social support has been shown to emerge not only through personal family and friendship relationships but also through professionals who have had a continuous relationship with the patient over time. When there is a high turnover and professionals have little education and training in dealing with neurological conditions, patients are impacted with less than optimal care conditions. Compliance to treatment plans and general well-being are affected.

In the context of Bronfenbrenner's ecological model, we can presume that a care professional's ability to communicate clearly with couples in a health care context depends on an understanding of factors that go beyond the medical condition itself. A couple's level of social support appears to be important to building their perception of their own resilience. Likely, social support is critical when we consider communication issues with health care providers as well - potential errors in developing care plans, misjudgment of what is required, and the patient's ability to successfully carry out what has been suggested. If professionals have a good understanding of social factors that surround a patient's daily life, these could be articulated and understood in order to benefit the medical aspects of the treatment. To separate out medical aspects of a condition from daily lived experiences (e.g. social support) may be setting the stage for poor care plans that may not be implemented properly – leading to potential for further crisis and poor health down the road.

The participant narratives demonstrate that the couples' perception of resilience was intertwined with factors associated with social support. Participants who were less able to 'push the system' also appeared to have fewer social supports in their life, they had less familiarity with the health care system, they appeared to have lower levels of education, or, they were simply farther along on the disease trajectory and depended on others to advocate on their behalf. A better understanding of the intersection of these nine factors is imperative.

The goal of this study has been to better understand how couples living with a neurological condition communicate and how they do so in the context of health care communications. In particular, the data discussed in this paper are intended to assist the development of tools that can also assist professionals in improving their understanding of individuals (e.g. couples and families who provide care) living with neurological conditions. Recommendations towards this goal follow.

7. Recommendations

Several recommendations are highlighted as a result of this study (see Table 3). It was evident that social support can be seen to improve the participant's sense of their own resilience when communicating about health and with the health care system. Intake could also be improved to assess for levels of social support and resilience in couples. The nine factors found in our sample reflect important aspects of social support and resilience. This information can lead the way to the development of a new tool that would provide more insight into how couples experience resilience and how this can benefit their communication with health care professionals and the health care system. This data leads to the recommendation that the nine factors be used to develop a new form which could be piloted in a selected set of organizations. These organizations could then participate in a second phase where the data collected over a specified period of time be compiled and analyzed with 'social supports as promoting resilience' in mind. This would have in mind a third phase with the purpose of establishing improved communication training (e.g. developing new training and education) between professionals and clients.

PILOT NEW FORM	NEW DATA COLLECTION UPON INTAKE	NEW TRAINING FOR PROFESSIONALS AND FAMILY
1. To develop a pilot of a new form that encompasses the nine factors identified here.	2. To collect data on each of the nine factors as these relate to patient intake. To support inhouse compilation and analysis of these data.	3a. This would include training for professionals in order to identify levels of risk and resilience.
		3b. Selected mentors, advocates, andor a buddy system within health care could be created to train family members upon intake.

Table 3. Recommendations for New Research and Organizational Interventions.

8. Conclusion

This paper has discussed original, empirical data highly critical for health service provision given the anticipated increased diagnoses of persons with neurological conditions. Since we know that little research has been found examining the daily lived experience of families, where one person is living with a neurological condition, this study contributes to knowledge in this area. The paper has explored nine factors that emerged from the data. The authors suggest that communication about care, and the many factors that shape it, must be better integrated into our daily health care provision – expanding on what we know about medical aspects of conditions such as Huntington's and Parkinson's. Since contradictory and often unspoken expectations of care emerge between professionals, family and individuals, a better understanding of social factors that influence communication might reduce errors in care, poor treatment, and misunderstandings. These outcomes can result in significant cost savings for the health care system but also improved well-being of families and those affected by neurological conditions.

9. Acknowledgements

The authors would like to acknowledge the University Start-up Grant (University of Manitoba) and the University Research Grants Program each for funding this study over the three years.

10. References

Aarsland, D. & Kurz, M. (2010). The epidemiology of dementia associated with Parkinson disease. *Journal of the Neurological Sciences,* 289, pp. 18-22

Aubeeluck, A. & Wilson, E. (2008). Huntington's disease. Part 1: Essential background and management. *British Journal of Nursing,* 17, pp. 146-151

Berkman L. & Syme L. (1979). Social networks, host resistance, and mortality: A nine-year follow up study of Alameda County residents. *American Journal of Epidemiology,* 109, 2, pp. 186-204

Berkman, L., Glass, T., Brissette, I., & Seeman, T. (2000). From social integration to health: Durkheim in the new millennium. *Social Science & Medicine,* 51, pp. 843- 857

Brody, H. (1987). *Stories of Sickness,* Yale University Press, New York, USA

Bronfenbrenner, U. (1979). *The Ecology of Human Development: Experiments by Nature and Design,* Harvard University Press, ISBN 978-067-4224-57-5, Cambridge, Massachusetts, USA

Bronfenbrenner U. (1986). Ecology of the family as a context for human development research perspectives. *Developmental Psychology,* 22, pp. 723–742.

Bubolz, M. & Sontag, M. (1993). Human ecology theory, In: *Sourcebook of family theories and methods: A contextual approach,* P. G. Boss, W. J. Doherty, R. LaRossa, W. R. Schumm, & S. K. Steinmetz (Eds.), pp. 419-450, Plenum Press, New York

Charmaz, K. (1991). *Good Days, Bad Days: The Self in Chronic Illness and Time,* Rutgers University Press, ISBN 978-081-3519-67-8, New Jersey, USA

Clark, C. (2007). Parkinson's disease. *British Medical Journal,* 335, pp. 441-445

Cohen, S. (2004). Social relationships and health. *American Psychologist,* 59, pp. 676-684

Earvolino-Ramirez, M. (2007). Resilience: A concept analysis. *Nurse Forum,* 42, 2, pp. 73-82

Garmezy, N. (1985). Stress-resistant children: The search for protective factors, In: *Recent Research in Developmental Psychopathology,* J. Stevenson (Ed.), pp. Pergamon Press, ISBN 978-008-0308-28-9, Oxford, UK

Garmezy, N. (1993). Children in poverty: Resilience despite risk. *Psychiatry,* 56, 1, pp. 127-136

Graneheim U. & Lundman B. (2004). Qualitative content analysis in nursing research: Concepts, procedures and measures to achieve trustworthiness. *Nurse Educ Today,* 24, pp. 105-112

Guttman, M. Slaughter, P., Theriault, M., DeBoer, D., & Naylor, C. (2003). Burden of Parkinsonism: A population-based study. *Movement Disorders*, 18, pp. 313-336

Harper, P. (1992). The epidemiology of Huntington's disease. *Human Genetics*, 89, pp. 365-376

Harrison, T., Blozis, S., & Stuifbergen, A. (2008). Longitudinal predictors of attitude towards aging among women with multiple sclerosis. *Psychology of Aging*, 23, 4, pp. 823-832

Heisters, D. (2011). Parkinson's: Symptoms, treatments and research. *British Journal of Nursing*, 20, pp. 548-554

Johnson, J. & Wiechelt, S. (2004). Introduction to the special issue on resilience. *Substance Use and Misuse*, 39, 5, pp. 657-670

Kiecolt-Glaser, J. & Newton, T. (2001). Marriage and health: His and hers. *Psychological Bulletin*, 127, pp. 472-503

Krawlik, D., van Loon, A., & Visentin, K. (2006). Resilience in the chronic illness experience. *Educational Action Research*, 14, 2, pp. 187-201

Lix, L., Hobson, D., Azimaee, M., Leslie, W., Burchill, C., & Hobson, S. (2010). Socioeconomic variations in the prevalence and incidence of Parkinson's disease: A population-based analysis. *Journal of Epidemiology and Community Health*, 64, pp. 335-340

Masten, A. (1999). Resilience comes of age: Reflections on the past and outlook for the next generation of research, In: *Resilience and Development: Positive Life Adaptations*, M. Glantz & J. Johnson (Eds.), pp. 281-296, Kluwer Academic/Plenum Publishers, ISBN 978-030-6461-23-1, New York, USA

Moreau, A., Boussageon, R., Girier, P., & Figon, S. (2006). The "doctor" effect in primary care. *La Presse Medicale*, 35, pp. 967-973

Morse, J., Barrett, M., Mayan, M., Olson, K., & Spiers J. (2002). Verification strategies for establishing reliability and validity in qualitative research. *International Journal of Qualitative Methods*, 1, pp. 1-19

Nance, M. & Myers, R. (2001). Juvenile onset Huntington's disease—Clinical and research perspectives. *Mental Retardation and Developmental Disabilities Research Reviews*, 7, pp. 153-157

National Institute of Neurological Disorders and Stroke. (2008). NINDS Huntington's disease information page, 19.07.2008, Available from: http://www.ninds.nih.gov/disorders/huntington/huntington.htm

Nutt, J. & Wooten, F. (2005). Diagnosis and initial management of Parkinson's disease. *The New England Journal of Medicine*, 353, pp. 1021-1213

Papadatou, D. (2009). *In the face of death: Professionals who care for the dying and the bereaved*, Springer Publishing Company, ISBN *978-082-6102-56-0*, New York, USA

Paulsen, J., Ready, R., Hamilton, J., Mega, M., & Cummins, J. (2001). Neuropsychiatric aspects of Huntington's disease. *Journal of Neurology, Neurosurgery and Psychiatry*, 71, pp. 310-314.

Public Health Agency of Canada. (2000). Research on Alzheimer's care giving in Canada: Current status and future directions, *Chronic Diseases in Canada (CDIC)*, 25, 3/4,, Available from:
www.phac-aspc.gc.ca/publicat/cdic-mcc/25-3/c_e.html

Richardson, G. (2002). The metatheory of resilience and resiliency. *Journal of Clinical Psychology*, 58, 3, pp. 307-321

Roger, K., Mary-Quigley, L., & Medved, M. (2010). Perceptions of Health Care and Familial in the Context of Parkinson's Disease and Multiple Sclerosis. *Journal of Communication in Healthcare*, 3, 2, pp. 124-137

Roger, K. & Medved, M. (2010). Couples manage change in the case of terminal medical conditions including neurological decline. *International Journal of Qualitative Studies on Health and Well-being*, 5, 2, pp. 5129

Roger, K. (2007a). It's a problem for other people, because I am seen as a Nuisance: Hearing the voices of people with dementia. *Alzheimer Care Quarterly*, 8, 1, pp. 17-25

Roger, K. (2007b). End-of-life care and dementia. *Geriatrics and Aging*, 10, 6, pp. 380-384

Roger, K. (2006a). Understanding social changes and the experience of dementia. *Alzheimer Care Quarterly*, 7, pp. 185-193

Roger, K. (2006b). Literature review on palliative care, end of life, and dementia. *Palliative and Supportive Care*, 4, pp. 1-10

Roos, R. (2010). Huntington's disease: A clinical review. *Orphanet Journal of Rare Diseases*, 5, 40

Safran, D., Taira, D., Rogers, W., Kosinski, M., Ware, L., & Tarlov, A. (1998). Linking primary care performance to outcomes of care. *The Journal of family practice*, 47, 3, pp. 213-220

Sandburg, G., Miller, R., Harper, J., Robila, M., & Davey, A. (2009). The impact of marital conflict on health and health care utilization in older couples. *Journal of Health Psychology*, 14, pp. 9-17

Statistics Canada. (2007). *Participation and Activity Limitation Survey 2006: Analytical Report*. Ministry of Industry, Catalogue no. 89-628-XIE, Ottawa, Ontario, Canada

Sturrock, A., & Leavitt, B. (2010). The clinical and genetic features of Huntington disease. *Journal of Geriatric Psychiatry and Neurology*, 23, pp. 243-259

Tarrant, C., Stokes, T., & Baker, R. (2003). Factors associated with patients' trust in their General practitioner: A cross-sectional survey. *British Journal of General Practice*, 53, pp. 798-800

Walker, F. (2007). Huntington's Disease. *The Lancet*, 369, 9557, pp. 218–228

Wallace K., Bisconti T., & Bergman C. (2001). The mediational effect of hardiness on social support and optimal outcomes in later life. *Basic Applied Social Psychology*, 23, 4, pp. 269- 279

Werner, E., & Smith, R. (1977). *Kauai's children come of age*, University of Hawaii Press, ISBN 978-0824804756, Honolulu, Hawaii, USA

Werner, E. (1990). Protective factors and individual resilience, In: *Handbook of Early Intervention*, S. Meisels & J. Shonkoff (Eds.), pp. 97-116, Cambridge University Press, 978-052-1387-77-4, Cambridge, UK

Zloty, A., Lobchuk, M., & Roger, K. (2010). A model for the development of caregiver networks. *WORK: A Journal of Prevention, Assessment & Rehabilitation,* in press.

10

Communication Between Huntington's Disease Patients, Their Support Persons and the Dental Hygienist Using Talking Mats

Ulrika Ferm[1], Pernilla Eckerholm Wallfur[2],
Elina Gelfgren[2] and Lena Hartelius[2]
*[1]DART Centre for Augmentative and Alternative
Communication and Assistive Technology, Regional Rehabilitation Centre,
Queen Silvia Children's Hospital, Sahlgrenska University Hospital,
[2]Institute of Neuroscience and Physiology,
Division of Speech and Language Pathology, University of Gothenburg,
Sweden*

1. Introduction

Communication is at the heart of any health care situation and individuals, who have difficulties describing their problems and expressing their needs, are in danger of being misunderstood or mistreated (Bartlett et al., 2008). Persons with Huntington's Disease (HD) have cognitive, emotional and motor problems which affect their communication and they frequently need support to be able to communicate in their daily life in general and in health care situations in particular. This chapter describes an effort to enhance communicative effectiveness in a dental and oral health care situation using Talking Mats. Eleven individuals, their support persons and a dental hygienist volunteered to help in exploring the use of this method in a clinical situation.

2. Background

Several of the changes associated with the progression of HD affect communication. Cognitive and emotional changes lead to fewer communicative initiatives, word finding difficulties, grammatical errors and difficulties in keeping track of what is being said in a conversation (Jensen et al., 2006; Yorkston et al., 2004). Furthermore, difficulties in managing complex discourse, tasks that involve interpretation of ambiguous, figurative and inferential meaning, are common and can appear early in disease progression (Chenery et al., 2002; Saldert et al., 2010; Saldert & Hartelius, 2011). Changes in motor function affect speech and articulation and symptoms of dysarthria are common (Hartelius et al., 2003; Yorkston, et al., 2004). The most frequently occurring perceptual deviations found in continuous speech in the study by Hartelius, et al., were mainly related to speech timing and phonation and reflected the underlying excessive and involuntary movement pattern. Deviation related to speech timing were variations in speech rate, shortened phrase length, and prolongation of interword and intersyllable intervals. Phonation-related aspects included increased pitch, harsh and strained-strangled phonation, and decreased pitch variation. Imprecise consonant articulation was also prominent, but to a less severe degree (Hartelius et al., 2003).

Individuals with HD report that communication demands more concentration and is more tiring than before they had the disease (Hartelius et al., 2010). In the same interview study, family members and carers reported that the persons with HD had increased difficulties understanding complex information and that their personality changes also had led to decreased quality of communication with lack of in-depth talk, difficulties shifting focus in conversation, etc. One action to take to meet the communicative difficulties is to introduce different kinds of augmentative and alternative communication (AAC) strategies and tools. It is important that AAC, and communication aids in particular, are introduced early in the disease process, that they are simple to use and that a conversation partner is actively present to create structure and support in the use of the aid in real-life communication (Yorkston et al., 2004). Attitudes, skills and knowledge in conversation partners influence communication (Allwood, 2000; Kagan et al., 2004) and AAC-interventions relating to persons with HD should take the experiences of conversation partners into consideration (cf. Saldert et al., 2010).

Huntington's Disease is, in every sense of the word, a family disease, and significant others are often closely involved in care and communication surrounding the afflicted family member. The disease eventually leads to increasing need of health care and a multitude of health care contacts (McGarva, 2001; Roos, 2010). One of the health care professionals frequently in contact with persons with HD is the dental hygienist. Dental and oral health is of vital importance because of its effects on chewing, swallowing and speech and essential to avoid the increased risk of caries, gingivitis and periodontitis that comes with dental and oral care neglect (Kidd, 2005; Klinge & Gustavsson, 2011). Individuals with HD often need to increase the number of daily meals and the energy content in their food, they have decreased flow of saliva and frequently also anti depressant medication which create dry mouth. These factors all contribute to a danger of oral and dental health problems.

In dealing with dental and oral health care, significant others play an important role. Problems with fine motor control makes it more difficult for the person with HD to manage toothbrush, dental floss, fluoride tablets etc. and the cognitive problems are challenging when trying to follow instructions and remembering the appropriate use of different items (Gabre, 2009). The visit to the dental hygienist is not unique in this sense. Murphy (2006) investigated communication between health care personnel and persons with aphasia or cognitive disabilities. Both patients and personnel experienced misunderstandings because of communication difficulties. The patients had problems remembering what they wanted to say and following instructions from the doctor. Doctors also used words that the patients didn't understand. The patients expressed the need to have information given in writing and with supporting pictures. All social activities are related to certain procedures, goals and roles that influence communication in different ways. As far as the support of persons with cognitive and communicative disabilities is concerned, it is important to take these activity factors into consideration (cf. Ahlsén, 1995; Allwood, 2000).

Talking Mats™, TM (Murphy & Cameron, 2006) is a method used to enable persons with cognitive and communicative difficulties to express their opinions (see Figure 1). Talking Mats does not replace a person's communication aid but can be used without or together with a communication aid. The method consists of a textured mat on which relevant pictures are stuck in a structured way. There are three sets of pictures: a visual evaluation scale, a picture describing a topic and pictures associated with the different questions relating to the topic. The conversation partner (the person responsible for the TM conversation, e.g. a nurse, a speech-language pathologist, or as in this case, a dental hygienist) formulates open questions such as: "How does it work to use…?", "What to you think of…?" etc. In addition to the prepared picture-based questions, new issues written down on pieces of note paper or empty cards can also be added. The person answering the questions (the person with difficulties expressing themselves, in this case individuals with HD) places the picture representing a specific question below the picture in the visual evaluation scale that best matches his or her opinion, but can also point to the part of the evaluation scale where the picture should be put. At the end of the conversation, the conversation partner recapitulates the discussion and seeks confirmation regarding the opinions expressed by the person being interviewed (Murphy & Cameron, 2006).

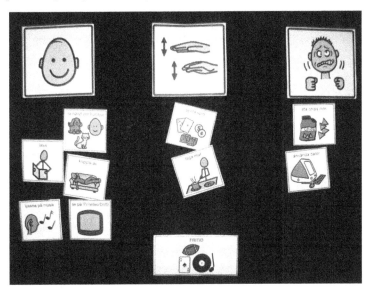

Fig. 1. A mat (Talking Mats) including a visual evaluation scale at the top, a picture for the conversational topic at the bottom, and pictures for different questions relating to the topic in the middle. The figure includes Picture Communication Symbols © 1981-2011 by Mayer-Johnson LLC.

One aim of conversations using TM is increased communicative involvement. Murphy et al. (2010b) conducted a study where individuals with dementia and their significant partners were engaged in two types of conversation, with and without TM. The conversations were on everyday topics such as personal care and household work. Results showed that persons with dementia as well as their partners felt significantly more involved in the conversations using TM and the increase was significantly higher for the partners compared to the participants with dementia. Communication effectiveness was assessed to be significantly higher in the conversation using TM compared to without TM.

Ferm et al. (2010) compared unstructured and structured conversations with conversations using TM with five individuals in different stages of HD. Conversations were compared with respect to communication effectiveness as measured by EFFC (Effectiveness Framework for Functional Communication, Murphy & Cameron, 2008). Communication effectiveness was significantly higher in the structured conversation as compared to the unstructured and highest in the conversation using TM. The conversation partner expressed the view that the persons with HD showed a greater involvement in the conversation and also that it felt more natural to wait quietly for the participant's answer when using TM. Talking Mats as a communication support has also been tried successfully in group discussions for persons with HD (Hallberg et al., 2011) but not yet in real health care situations. The participants in the discussion group studied by Hallberg et al. were more effective communicating about diet and health when TM was used than when the questions around these topics were discussed without TM. The difference in communicative effectiveness between the conditions was significant on both individual and group levels. Another interesting finding of this study was that the group leader and some of the individuals with HD asked significantly more follow-up questions when using TM than when the group discussion was unaided. Over all the group members with HD were positive about using TM.

As mentioned earlier, one of the health care situations that persons with HD encounter is dental and oral care. In Gothenburg, Sweden, most individuals with HD visit the dental hygienist between once a month and once every third month, to create or to keep a good dental and oral health. During a typical visit, a good part of the communication is done when the patient receives his or her treatment, lying down in the dental chair. The dental hygienist starts by talking about general things to make the patient feel at ease and continues on to give instructions, frequently with the support of pictures. When the ability to care for their own dental and oral hygiene is decreased, the instructions are given to the person supporting the patient during the visit (e.g. family member, assistant or carer). Communicative support in the dental and oral health care situation is of great value (Lewis et al., 2008) and the development and evaluation of appropriate support methods is important.

The aim of the present study was to explore the use of Talking Mats in conversations with individuals with HD in the dental and oral health care situation. The specific research questions asked were: 1) is there a significant difference in communicative effectiveness between conversations where Talking Mats is used compared to conversations where TM is not used?, 2) Is there a significant difference in perceived communicative involvement between the two types of conversation on the part of the individuals with HD?, 3) Is there a difference in perceived communicative involvement between the two types of conversation on the part of the support persons? And 4) Does the dental hygienist perceive the use of TM as a beneficial support in the dental and oral health care consultation?

3. Method

The study was designed to compare two different types of conversations between persons with HD, their support persons and a dental hygienist using both quantitative and qualitative methodology. Data was collected during naturally occurring dental and oral health care consultations.

3.1 Participants

Twenty four persons participated in the study; eleven individuals with HD (seven men and
four women, mean age = 52 years, range 24 – 75 years), twelve support persons and a dental
hygienist. The same dental hygienist carried out all conversations. The individuals with HD
and their partners formed eleven dyads. As can be seen in Table 1, dyad 1 included two
assistants which meant it really was a triad (i.e., included three individuals). For the sake of
simplicity, we will call it a dyad. The support persons were relatives and professionals that
accompanied the person with HD to the dental hygienist. Ten of the participants with HD
had continuous contact with the dental hygienist; one participant had met the dental
hygienist a couple of times. The dental hygienist was trained in TM but had limited
experience in its use.

Dyad	Participants	Age	Onset HD	Phase	Education	Used TM before	Length of relationship (years)
F1	F1	53	40	4	compulsory school	yes	
	F1(A)ass	55			high school	no	10 months
	F1(B)ass	28			high school	no	1 year
F2	F2	75	57	5	university	yes	>50 yrs
	F2husband	77			university	no	
F3	F3	64	58	3-4	university	yes	3.5 yrs
	F3ass	59			university	no	
F4	F4	58	50	4-5	university	no	5 months
	F4ass	19			high school	no	
M1	M1	24	20	4	high school	yes	6 months
	M1ass	45			high school	no	
M2	M2	28	22	3	high school	yes	3.5 years
	M2ass	57			compulsory school	no	
M3	M3	57	47	4	university	no	3 years
	M3ass	22			high school	no	
M4	M4	46	30	3	university	yes	2.5 years
	M4ass	50			high school	no	
M5	M5	52	50	3	compulsory school	no	1.5 years
	M5support person	46			university	no	
M6	M6	57	52	no info	compulsory school	no	a couple of years
	M6counselor	43			university	no	
M7	M7	57	54-55	2	compulsory school	no	29 years
	M7daughter	29			high school	no	

Table 1. Participant characteristics. F = female; M = male; Onset HD = Age of first symptoms
of HD, Phase = TFC-phase (Shoulson et al., 1989) for the participant with HD according to
the dental hygienist, Education = highest completed education, ass = personal assistant;
Length of relationship = number of months or years the participants had known each other.

Invitation of participants was done by the dental hygienist. All participants were registered as clients at Mun-H-Center[1]. Inclusion criteria were HD, contact with the dental hygienist and interest and willingness to participate in a study about communication support. No formal cognitive or linguistic assessments were made. However, persons in the late stage of the disease were not invited to participate. All participants communicated through speech and no one used personal communication aids during the visit at the dental hygienist's. The participants' speech varied in intelligibility.

3.2 Ethical considerations

The study built on relevant research and was led by professionals with expert knowledge within the fields of HD and augmentative and alternative communication. Participation was voluntary and built on informed consent. The individuals with HD and their support persons all signed consent forms. Due to the cognitive and linguistic difficulties accompanying HD particular attention was given to the process of informing the participants with HD. The study was described in detail by the dental hygienist and the researchers on three different occasions. Simplified written information with pictures was also supplied. The participants were informed that they could withdraw from the study at any time without specific reasons and without personal consequences. They were also informed that their data would be treated with integrity and that no names would be used in the dissemination of the results. All participants were informed about the results of the study and participants with HD received photographs of their mats.

3.3 Material

Black textured mats (37 x 58 cm), five pictures (6 x 6 cm) representing a visual evaluation scale, a picture (5 x 5 cm) for the conversational topic oral hygiene and prophylaxis, and pictures (5 x 5 cm) of the questions relating to the topic were used. Velcro on the back of the pictures allowed these to be placed and moved around on the mat. Digital photographs and Picture Communication Symbols PCS (Mayer-Johnson™, 1981-2011) were used.

Fig. 2. The visual evaluation scale used with Talking Mats. The figure includes Picture Communication Symbols © 1981-2011 by Mayer Johnson LLC.

Twenty questions about oral hygiene and prophylaxis were developed by the dental hygienist and the researchers (Table 2). The questions formed two sets which included ten questions each. The questions were designed to be equivalent with regard to content and level of difficulty. Each dyad received both sets of questions; one set in the condition where TM was used and the other set in the condition where TM was not used. The order of the

[1]Swedish national oro-facial centre of expertise for rare disorders and national resource centre for oro-facial assistive devices, Gothenburg, Sweden.

question sets and conditions (TM and nonTM) were counter balanced (Table 3). The purpose of using two different but equal sets of questions in the two conditions was to create different but yet content wise similar conversations. In this way, the effects of TM, rather than of different questions, could be evaluated.

Question	Set 1	Set 2
1	How does teeth brushing work?	What would you say about getting help with teeth brushing?
2	How does it work brushing the inside of your teeth?	How does it work brushing exactly where you intend to?
3	How does it work using a regular toothbrush?	How does it work using a double toothbrush?
4	What would you say about getting help cleaning between your teeth?	How does it work cleaning in between your teeth?
5	How does it work using an interspace toothbrush?	How does it work using dental floss?
6	How does self cleaning work?	How does it work rinsing the mouth after the meal?
7	How does it work using toothpaste with extra fluoride?	How does it work rinsing the mouth with fluoride?
8	How does it work using fluoride chewing gum?	How does it work using fluoride tablets?
9	How does it work using gel against mouth dryness?	How does it work using spray against mouth dryness?
10	How does it work sitting in the chair?	How does it work lying in the chair?

Table 2. The two sets of questions used in the two conditions, TM and nonTM.

The participant with HD and the support person each filled out two questionnaires about the two different conditions. The questionnaire regarding the nonTM condition included seven questions (1 to 7 below). The questionnaire regarding the TM condition included the same seven questions (1 to 7 below) and one additional question (8). Questions 1 to 5 and 7 were similar to the questions used by Murphy et al. (2010b). Questions 6 and 8 were constructed for this study. The questions were: (1) Do you think that the questions asked were relevant for you? (2) Did the others listen to you in the conversation? (3) Were you able to express your opinions? (4) Did you have enough time to express your opinions? (5) Did you feel involved in the conversation? (6) Did it work well doing this together with NN? (7) How well do you think the conversation went? Circle the picture that best suits your opinion! (8) What do you think about using Talking Mats? Describe with your own words! A visual scale including four pictures of the concepts all/always, most/usually, a few/occasionally and none/never was used for questions 1 to 6. A seven point scale representing the continuum bad to excellent was used for question 7. The scales included pictures (Mayer-Johnsson™, 1981-2011) and were similar to the ones used by Murphy et al. (2010b).

The dental hygienist filled out two questionnaires for each dyad; one for the nonTM condition and one for the TM condition. The questionnaires included seven identical questions: (1) To what degree did the person with HD understand the questions? (2) To what degree did you get carefully considered answers to the questions? (3) To what degree did you feel listened to in the conversation? (4) How natural was the conversation? (5) How easy was it to stay on topic in this conversation? (6) How involved did you feel in the conversation? (7) How well do you think the conversation went? Circle the picture that best suits your opinion! Questions 1 to 6 and 7 were answered according to the same four and seven point scales that were used by the participants with HD and by the support persons.

After each consultation, a semi-structured interview was carried out with the dental hygienist. The interview included six open questions about the two conditions and about TM.

The consultations, with and without TM, were recorded using a Canon HD Legria HF S11 camera and the mats were photographed using a Panasonic Lumix DMC-TZ8.

The Effectiveness Framework of Functional Communication EFFC (Murphy & Cameron, 2008) was used to measure communicative effectiveness in the two conditions.

3.4 Procedure

Data collection was done during regular consultations with the dental hygienist at Mun-H-Center (9 dyads), at one participant's home (1 dyad), and at an activity centre (1 dyad) from November 2010 to February 2011. There were totally eleven consultations, one for each dyad. During each consultation two different conversations were carried out; one with Talking Mats (TM) and one without Talking Mats (nonTM). Consequently, there were 22 conversations in total. Each consultation started with repeated information about the study by the researchers and the signing of consent forms. A short conversation with TM was demonstrated. Thereafter the main researchers (second and third authors) left the room and the dental hygienist carried out the TM and nonTM conditions with the dyad. The dental hygienist was informed about the order of conditions and question sets for each dyad (Table 3) and about the fact that additional questions were allowed. The ten questions within each set were asked in the same order. Both conversations were recorded with a digital video camera. Towards the end of each session, some of the participants received dental treatment by the hygienist.

Dyad	Condition	Question set
M1, F2, M6	TM	1
	nonTM	2
M2, M4, M7	nonTM	2
	TM	1
M3, F3, F4	TM	2
	nonTM	1
F1, M5	nonTM	1
	TM	2

Table 3. Order of conditions and question sets for the eleven dyads.

After the completion of the two conversations the participants filled out the questionnaires. One researcher assisted the persons with HD who needed it by reading the questions aloud and by noting which picture in the visual scale the person pointed to. For question 8, the persons with HD were encouraged to describe their opinions about TM. These were written down by the researcher. The support persons filled out the questionnaires independently but a researcher was close by in case any of them had questions. The two questionnaires were answered in the same order as the two conditions had been carried out. The dental hygienist filled out the questionnaire on her own after the completion of the two conversations. The interview was carried out at the end of the consultation, that is, after the dental treatment. One researcher asked the questions and the other researcher took notes.

Data was compiled and communicative effectiveness as well as the participants' feelings of communicative involvement and satisfaction in the two conditions were examined and compared on group and individual levels.

3.5 Analysis

The communicative effectiveness of the persons with HD in the two conditions was evaluated by the two researchers who also assisted with data collection during the consultations. The evaluation was done using EFFC (Murphy & Cameron, 2008). Each conversation was evaluated according to four factors namely (a) the participant's understanding of the questions, (b) the participant's engagement in the conversation, (c) the participant's ability to keep to the questions discussed, and (d) the interviewer's (dental hygienist) understanding of the participant's views. The evaluations were based on the criteria set out by Murphy et al. (2010b), Murphy et al. (2010a) and Ferm et al. (2010) but also depended on thorough discussions taking place between all the researchers in this particular study. Each conversation was evaluated according to the four factors and using a 5-point scale representing low (0) to high (4) effectiveness. The evaluation of the *participant's understanding of the questions* was based on both verbal answers and body communication. To get a high score it should be obvious that the person with HD understood the questions. Lack of answers, irrelevant or inadequate answers resulted in low scores as did misunderstandings. A lower score was also given if it was difficult to understand the person's answers and hence to make the evaluation. The *participant's engagement in the conversation* concerned the social closeness that is a result of social interaction and which is maintained through different kinds of feedback and shared attention. Facial gestures and other body communication as well as verbal feedback were observed. High scores depended on active engagement and interest shown through eye contact, explicit feedback, and humour or by the participant's development of a topic. It was decided that to get one or more points, more than a short answer was needed. The *participant's ability to keep to the questions discussed* was based on the relevance of the participant's answers and on his or her ability to stay on track when answering and discussing the questions. A lower score was given if the participant changed or drifted away from the topic and if it, considering the person's communicative contributions, was difficult to make an evaluation of the factor. The *interviewer's understanding of the participant's views* was evaluated on the basis of the dental hygienist's reactions, verbal and through body communication, to the participant's answers.

The two researchers were trained in EFFC by evaluating video-recordings of conversations involving persons with HD that were not used in the study. Thereafter, the films of the 22 conversations were evaluated in a randomized order. First, the two researchers rated each recording independently. This meant that they looked at the recording together but did their own rating. Subsequently, the researchers discussed their ratings and reached a consensus score for each factor in each recording. The maximum score for each conversation was 16. Twelve points is the cut-off for an acceptable level of effectiveness (Murphy et al., 2010a). To check for interrater reliability, two independent external raters evaluated 30 % of the data using the same procedure. To check for intra-rater reliability, the two main researchers did a second evaluation of 30 % of the data a week after the first evaluation. The two conditions were also compared with respect to time and with respect to number of questions and follow-up questions that were asked.

The answers to the questionnaire items were transferred to a descriptive scale as follows: all/always (4), most/usually (3), a few/occasionally (2), and none/never (1). The individual scores for the six questions were added to form a total involvement score for each condition and participant. Means were calculated as well. Written comments in questionnaires were analysed and categorised with regard to content.

Statistical calculations were done using SPSS (version 19). Internal interrater reliability, measured using intra-class correlation (ICC) was 0.85. External interrater reliability, between the main two researchers and the external raters, was 0.64. The reliability between the researchers was higher (0.91) for the nonTM condition than for the TM condition (0.78). Intrarater reliability calculated on the basis of the researchers' consensus scores was 0.96. Differences in scores of communicative effectiveness and involvement as well as differences in the duration of the two conditions were analysed using Wilcoxon Signed Ranks Test (p<0.05).

4. Results

The inherent differences between the two types of conversations, with and without TM, had a few consequences that need to be kept in mind when interpreting the results. In the conversations using TM, the questions were introduced visibly using pictures presented to the participant. Also, in these conversations the participants had an opportunity to delete or add questions, while this was not an option in the conversation without TM. Several of the participants, particularly support persons, deleted as well as added questions both before the conversation started and during the conversations. Support persons were also more active in giving support during conversations using TM. After the TM conversations, the dental hygienist went through the answers together with the participants, who had an opportunity to change the answers. Some of the participants with HD chose to do so. In the conversations without TM, the questions were put to the participants with HD in the predetermined order, and the answers were not documented/written down, albeit recorded.

In the following, results will be presented according to the research questions being asked.

4.1 Is there a significant difference in communicative effectiveness between conversations where Talking Mats is used compared to conversations where TM is not used?

No statistically significant difference between the two types of conversation was found in this group (see Figure 3). Mean effectiveness score without TM (nonTM) was 12.27 (SD 3,26) and mean effectiveness score with TM was 11.45 (SD 2.98).

Individual ratings on the four different parameters of EFFC, together with the total score, are shown in Table 4. Six of the 11 participants with HD, were rated as more effective in their communication in conversations without TM and 3 were rated as equally effective in both conditions. Two individuals communicated more effectively using TM.

Additional qualitatively important aspects of communicative effectiveness are time (duration of the conversations) and number of questions and follow-up questions being asked. Table 5 shows that conversations where TM were used were significantly longer than conversations without TM. This is in part due to the fact that the TM conversations included significantly more follow-up questions, see Table 6.

Research questions number 2 and 3 concerned the perceived communicative involvement on the part of the individuals with HD and the support persons. These questions were answered using the previously described questionnaires.

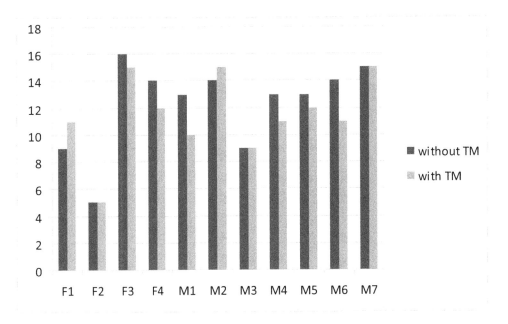

Fig. 3. Communicative effectiveness, as measured by EFFC, in conversations with (grey bars) and without Talking Mats (black bars). Acceptable communicative effectiveness cut-off value is 12 points.

Participant	Condition	Understanding	Engagement	Stick to the topic/questions	Interviewer's understanding	Effectiveness score
F1	nonTM	2	2	2	3	9
	TM	3	2	2	4	11
F2	TM	1	1	1	2	5
	nonTM	1	1	1	2	5
F3	TM	4	3	4	4	15
	nonTM	4	4	4	4	16
F4	TM	3	2	3	4	12
	nonTM	4	2	4	4	14
M1	TM	3	1	3	3	10
	nonTM	3	2	4	4	13
M2	nonTM	4	2	4	4	14
	TM	4	3	4	4	15
M3	TM	2	2	2	3	9
	nonTM	2	2	2	3	9
M4	nonTM	3	3	3	4	13
	TM	2	3	3	3	11
M5	nonTM	3	2	4	4	13
	TM	3	2	3	4	12
M6	TM	2	2	3	4	11
	nonTM	3	3	4	4	14
M7	nonTM	4	3	4	4	15
	TM	4	3	4	4	15

Table 4. Individual ratings and effectiveness scores of the eleven participants with HD. N.B.: nonTM = without Talking Mats, TM = with Talking Mats.

	nonTM	TM
Mean (SD)	3.7 (0.89)	12.8 (4.01)
Max	5.78	19.38
Min	2.47	7.68

Table 5. Duration of conversations in minutes, without (nonTM) and with (TM) Talking Mats. The difference is statistically significant (Wilcoxon Signed Rank test, p= .003).

	nonTM		TM	
	Questions	Follow-up questions	Questions	Follow-up questions
Mean (SD)	9.82 (0.41)	3.55 (2.12)	10.09 (0.83)	9.64 (4.23)
Max	10	7	11	15
Min	9	1	9	3

Table 6. Number of questions and follow-up questions being asked by the dental hygienist during the two different types of conversations, without (nonTM) and with (TM) Talking Mats. The difference is statistically significant (Wilcoxon Signed Rank test, p= .005).

4.2 Is there a significant difference in perceived communicative involvement between the two types of conversation on the part of the individuals with HD? And is there a difference in perceived communicative involvement between the two types of conversation on the part of the support persons?

The participants with HD rated their communicative involvement significantly higher in conversations using TM compared to conversations without TM (nonTM). Differences between the two conditions were not statistically significant for the support persons or the dental hygienist, see Table 7.

	Participants with HD		Support persons		Dental hygienist	
Conversation type	nonTM	TM	nonTM	TM	nonTM	TM
Mean(SD)	21 (2.37)	22.45 (1.51)	21.25 (3.05)	21.50 (2.58)	20.27 (2.61)	20.82 (2.14)
Max	24	24	24	24	23	24
Min	18	20	15	15	16	16

Table 7. Ratings of perceived communicative involvement during the two different types of conversations, without (nonTM) and with (TM) Talking Mats. The difference is statistically significant for the participants with HD (Wilcoxon Signed Rank test, p= .048) but not for the support persons or the dental hygienist.

The participants' reactions to the use of TM were also collected and a general finding was that participants with HD as well as support persons were positive. A qualitative analysis of the notes generated four themes: *Understanding, Thinking and memory, Expressive function* and *The use of Talking Mats*. Themes and associated quotes are included in Table 8.

Theme	Illustrative quotes from participants with HD	Illustrative quotes from support persons
Understanding	*"people who do not understand sometimes people do not understand, then it would be good"* (M3) *"easier if you find yourself in a conflict situation, which I avoid, then it would be good"* (M3)	*"you don't always understand what he says, in that case he can show and point out"* (assistant to M4) *"I think the pictures are good, they help with understanding and being able to express oneself"* (assistant to F1) *"She understood more with the pictures"* (assistant to F1)
Thinking and memory	*"it's easier to think and understand when there are pictures"* (M7) *"made me think some more about the different stuff with oral care, that can be good"* (M5)	*"he has a fairly poor memory, and then you can take out the mat and show what we agreed on"* (assistant to M4) *"it can be useful to remember what you talked about even if the verbal communication does work"* (assistant to F3) *"she has difficulties making decisions and form opinions"* (husband to F2)

Expressive function	"you can express feelings just by pointing to a face" (M4) "it is a bit easier to find the words with the mat" (M2) "it is a bit easier to talk about it with the mat" (M2)	"it clarifies when the words get muddy" (assistant to M1) "he talked more with the help from the Talking Mats" (counselor M6)
The use of Talking Mats	"damn good with pictures" (M3) "I didn't think it was going to be so easy" (M3) "it became a bit slow with the mat and better flow in the conversation without the mat" (F4)	"it was easier than I thought, and I don't think she had any difficulties with it either" (assistant to F4) "to think about using it during the right phase of the illness. To not be offended" (support person to M5) "a good "tool" to use in the future should it be necessary" (daughter of M7) "the mat was very good used like that regularly it will be great" (assistant to M3) "maybe clearer instruction before the interview about the use of Talking Mats about the pictures that was graded and the questions/conversation topic words" (counselor to M6) "felt a bit conflicting at times – several things in one picture that were opposites" (assistant to F3) "it is a bit difficult to say, I didn't know if I could expand, I was afraid to take over too much, I wanted to add more questions but didn't really know how much I was allowed to ask" (assistant to M2) "I didn't really know how much I was supposed to interfere in the conversation" (assistant to K3)

Table 8. Themes and quotes from the interviews with participants with HD and support persons, concerning the use of Talking Mats.

The last research question concerned the perceived benefit of the use of TM as reported by the dental hygienist in the interview conducted after the consultation had been completed and both types of conversations implemented.

4.3 Does the dental hygienist perceive the use of TM as a beneficial support in the dental and oral health care consultation?

In the interview, the dental hygienist expressed the general view that the use of TM supported the counseling and treatment of persons with HD. Her opinion was, that all conversations using TM were superior to the conversations without TM. The qualitative analysis of her answers to the interview questions yielded six different themes: *Talking Mats as a method, Information and intervention, Individual adjustments, Memory, Understanding,* and *Naturalness.*

Talking Mats as a method. TM made the conversation obvious, transparent and concrete. One particular advantage of the method was that you were able to review the answers afterwards: *"the possibility to go back, add and comment on things in the conversation"*. The use of TM also gave a visible overview of the conversation. The pictures served as support for the memory both for the dental hygienist and the patient and they made the conversation concrete: *"easier to talk and discuss with the pictures as a support"*. The method Talking Mats and the mat in itself created a joint focus for the participants *"you have the whole conversation in front of you, it's there on the table"*. At times, the dental hygienist found it difficult to stick to the preset wordings of the questions: *"the questions are a bit tricky sometimes"*. It was evident from her answers to the questionnaire, that she found it difficult to engage in the conversations without TM – *"it feels as though you only want to get it over with"*, particularly if it was the second conversation: *"I don't feel as engaged when I'm going to ask almost the same questions again"*.

Information and intervention. One other positive aspect of the use of TM in conversation was that new and more in-depth information about several of the participants' oral and dental care appeared: *"I found out that she has difficulties remembering to brush her teeth but that she wants to be reminded"*, *"you can go deeper into the questions"*. Three participants with HD wanted to try new products or methods when they communicated using TM: *"it became apparent that the patient was interested in cleaning between his teeth, I thought this was impossible before, he has a strong sense of integrity"*. The dental hygienist experienced that two support persons contributed with new thoughts in the TM conversation: *"new thoughts appeared from the assistants"*.

Individual adjustments. The dental hygienist described that she would have wanted the opportunity to adjust the questions to particular individuals. In the present study, for the sake of consistency, she had to ask questions that were not relevant to all participants with HD: *"you have to individualize the picture material so that you can adjust the questions/pictures to the patients"*, *"I know that patient so it feels a bit silly to ask about things that are not relevant for that person"*.

Memory, Understanding and *Naturalness.* The dental hygienist saw TM as a support for her own memory: *"it supports the memory, you remember what the conversation has been about, what you have talked about"*, *"good when you go through the answers afterwards you remember what you talked about"*. Talking Mats seemed to make things more visible and clear both for her and for the participant with HD: *"easier for me to understand and probably also for the patient"*, *"it's good because it's difficult to understand what he says, you have to ask again, and in that case the mat helps"*. In two conversations using TM, with F4 and M7, the dental hygienist experienced that TM affected naturalness: *"it felt a bit repetitive, it did not have the same flow as earlier conversations using TM"*, *"it (the TM conversation) is not an ordinary conversation"*.

5. Discussion

We examined communicative effectiveness in conversations between persons with HD, their support persons and a dental hygienist, with and without Talking Mats. We also examined the participants' experiences from the two conditions as well as the dental hygienist's experiences from using TM in dental and oral health care consultations. To summarise, there was no increase in communicative effectiveness for the group when TM was used. Two individuals communicated more effectively with TM but more than half of the participants were evaluated as more effective when TM was not used. Three individuals were evaluated as equally effective in the two conditions. Importantly, the participants with HD experienced a significantly higher degree of communicative involvement when TM was used than when conversation was unaided. The support persons also experienced a higher degree of communicative involvement with TM than without TM but this difference between conditions was not significant. The dental hygienist was very positive about TM. In her view, conversations with TM worked better than those without TM. She received new and more comprehensive information when TM was used.

Previous studies have shown that TM leads to more effective communication for persons with dementia and for persons with HD in dyadic as well as group conversations (Ferm et al., 2010; Hallberg et al., 2011; Murphy et al., 2010a, 2010b). A number of differences between this and previous studies regarding the way data was collected, goals, roles and procedures of activities may have contributed to the different results obtained.

Individuals with HD have many medical and health related contacts in which communication is of central importance. A purpose of the present study was to examine if TM could be helpful in such consultations. Thus, it was important to collect data in situations that were as natural as possible. It was believed that it was more natural if all data from each participant was collected during one and the same consultation than if the participant had to come back to the dental hygienist a second time, just to finish data collection. Hence, all data from each participant was collected on one occasion. This procedure is different from that of previous TM studies of effectiveness and could have influenced the participants' behaviours and the rating of effectiveness. For example, it may have been unnatural as well as tiring for the participants to answer similar questions twice during one and the same visit. However, four of the six participants that were scored as more effective without the mat carried out this condition after they had used the mat. Perhaps it was even positive for these individuals, with varying levels of cognitive functioning, to hear the questions twice. The fact that the participants had answered questions before may have contributed to less hesitation and more concise answers. It is possible that these answers were seen as efficient and informative and thus rated as more effective by the outside observers.

Another important difference between this and previous studies is that previous studies examined activities where communication was a main goal. It has also been the case in previous studies, at least in the study by Ferm et al. (2010), that the activity was constructed for the study. Although communication is important in dental and oral health care consultations it typically is not the main goal of the activity and although the present activity was natural for the participants and not constructed, it was slightly changed as far as procedure and goals are concerned. Communication usually takes place when the patient lies in the treatment chair and the goal is to promote good oral health; the patient gives information about his or her dental and oral status upon questions and requests from the dental hygienist who, based on the information given by the patient, gives advice about care routines, aids and products. In this study, the consultation started by the table. Communication about dental and oral health was "lifted out" from the more "practical" dental treatment and in this sense got a different and somewhat more prominent function than the participants were used to. The change of the activity, and the fact that communication was more in focus than is often the case at the dental hygienist's, may have led to increased demands on the person with HD to, for example, give more nuanced answers than yes and no when TM was not used. Such changes in communication may have influenced the observers' ratings.

Dental hygienist consultations are typically associated with different roles which were slightly changed in this study. These changes, pertaining to the rights and obligations of support persons in particular (cf. Allwood, 2000), may have influenced the participants' communicative behaviours in ways that had effects on the ratings. The dental hygienist usually leads the activity and the patient, in this case the participant with HD, is supposed to do what the dental hygienist suggests. The support person usually does not accompany the person with HD into the treatment room but a prerequisite for participation in this study was that both the person with HD and a partner participated in the consultation. It is possible that the role of the partner was unclear. It was an unfamiliar situation for the partner both to discuss dental and oral health care and to participate actively in the conversation. Eight of the support persons were personal assistants whose role, apart from assisting the person they work for in relation to practical issues, involves promoting independence in that person. To argue against and even question the opinions of the person with HD during his or her "private" consultation was perhaps difficult. The analysis showed that overall, the support persons participated little in the conversations but the personal assistants interfered more often than others. The support person was supposed to have knowledge about the dental and oral health of the person with HD. This was not the case in all dyads. Some of the support persons managed everything that had to do with oral care in the person with HD; others didn't know anything about this daily issue. Not having the knowledge needed for participation in the study probably affected the support persons' behaviour and communication negatively. The dental hygienist's role was also changed. She would usually ask questions as she performed the actual treatment. In this study she talked with the patient before the treatment. She also used a communication method that was new to her.

All of the above mentioned factors could have influenced the participants' behaviours and, hence, the outside observers' rating of communicative effectiveness in the persons with HD. In future analyses, we will look more closely into these factors.

For two participants, F1 and M2, communicative effectiveness increased when TM was used. It is important to note that both of them had used TM before. For some people at least, communicative effectiveness with TM may be related to amount of experience as well. Both F1's own and the dental hygienist's understanding was higher in the TM condition. The TM conversation took a longer time which meant that F1's conversational space increased and, as a result, her and the dental hygienist's understanding. The dental hygienist asked F1 fewer clarifying questions (e.g., *And that works well?*) when TM was used which was interpreted as a sign for her better understanding. The situation was similar for M2. The TM conversation took a longer time and M2 had more room for developing his answers and showing humour, factors which, according to the criteria used, can have been a reason for why M2 was assessed as engaged in the TM conversation.

TM was assessed in three different ways; through outside observers' rating of communicative effectiveness, through the participants' responses to questionnaires about communicative involvement in the two conditions and through interviews with the dental hygienist. A most significant finding of the study is that the majority of the participants with HD and their support persons appreciated TM. Even if only two participants were more effective in conversations with TM, many participants appreciated the mat and thought it supported memory and word finding. Talking Mats also supported understanding in interaction. It was easier for the participants to make themselves understood and to understand others when TM was used. Interaction with other people is problematic for persons with HD who become less talkative and more isolated with the progression of the disease (Hartelius et al., 2010; Power et al., 2011). Finding ways to support participation in different social activities is important and the individual's ability to communicate in activities relating to own health should be prioritized. This study indicates that TM is one possible way of supporting communication between persons with HD and their conversational partners. The participants with HD felt significantly more involved, that is, experienced greater communicative involvement, when TM was used than when conversation was unaided. The support persons also experienced increased communicative involvement with TM but for them the difference between the two conditions was not significant. The support persons interfered more in the mat conversations. Some of them even assisted the person with HD, physically and psychologically, placing the pictures on the mat. Again, unclear instructions from the researchers and contradictions between the typical rights and obligations of assistants to promote independence in the person they work for and the expectations on assistants in this study, to converse with the person with HD on equal terms, may have contributed to the lack of significance between conditions as far as the support persons' feelings of communicative involvement is concerned. Still, the present findings are similar to those of Murphy et al. (2010b) where individuals with dementia and in particular their partners felt more involved in conversation when TM was used.

An all-embracing purpose of the study was to explore the use and function of TM for individuals with HD at the dental hygienist's and perhaps the most interesting finding is the fact that the dental hygienist experienced that TM conversations were better than conversations in which TM was not used. The dental hygienist also asked more follow-up questions when TM was used, indicating that TM stimulated conversation. A similar pattern was found in the study by Hallberg et al. (2011): In this study both the leader of the group discussions and the participants with HD asked more follow-up questions when they used TM than when they didn't have this support. By asking follow-up questions the dental hygienist could get more information about the dental and oral care situation of the person who has HD and as a result, she appreciated the situation. In her view, she got new and more comprehensive information from the dyads when TM was used, information that could lead to improved counselling and individual treatments of individuals who have HD. The dental hygienist's comment about individualizing questions and pictures is in line with the methodology of TM and would not be a problem in her future clinical work. For more comprehensive discussions in relation to follow-up questions and other queries that arise during conversations, she could use sub-mats (Murphy & Cameron, 2006).

Measuring communicative effectiveness is not easy and as has been shown in this study, ratings by outside observers must be complemented with measurements of the interlocutors own experiences. What then, is the difference between communicative involvement and communicative effectiveness? The questions about involvement used in this study were developed from Murphy et al. (2010b). It is possible that they reflect not only involvement but also effectiveness. Questions number 2, 3 and 4 in the questionnaire used in this study relate to communicative effectiveness; to be able to convey a message in an effective way and to be able to influence other people (Hustad, 1999). Question 4 focuses on time for expression of opinions. Perhaps the participants, in answering this question, considered both how much time they got from others and to what degree they were able to take their time in the conversations. In fact, it is reasonable to believe that the participants' rating of communicative involvement mirrored their perceptions of how effective they had been in the conversations.

5.1 Using the EFFC

Despite lots of training and discussion of criteria the researchers experienced difficulties using the EFFC in relation to these data. A re-analysis of consensus discussions, recordings and final scores shows that there were more disagreement between the raters in relation to the TM conversations than in relation to the unaided conversations, suggesting the former were more difficult to rate. Lack of experience in TM and EFFC as well as too vague criteria were obvious threats to agreement. The researchers' experiences and ideas about an ideal "effective" dental hygienist consultation also may have influenced their rating of the participants' communicative effectiveness. It also may have been the case, that the raters favoured oral expressions and treated these differently from body communication in their ratings. For example, the criteria used for rating of the participant's *understanding of the questions* and ability to *keep to the questions discussed* meant that higher points were given if the person was very explicit in her or his oral expression. It is possible that, unconsciously of course, a very short, adequate and concise utterance by a participant was valued higher and accordingly rated higher than a quiet placement of a picture on the mat. Some individuals with HD had less eye contact with their support persons and the dental hygienist when using TM. This seems to have influenced the observers rating of the participants' *engagement*.

5.2 Limitations

The conversations examined in this study were conducted by a dental hygienist who had limited experience in using TM. She was instructed about the order of question sets, conditions and individual questions but was free to formulate follow-up questions. Treatment integrity (Schlosser, 2003), that is, the degree to which the dental hygienist followed the procedure as planned, was considerable. Each participant received most of the questions and she was consequent in using the open question format. It is important to remember that this study was carried out in an authentic clinical situation and that time pressure and the dental hygienist's previous knowledge about the participants' dental and oral health may have influenced the conversations. Several of the participants had to catch transportation service at scheduled times which may have been stressful for both them and the dental hygienist. The dental hygienist's enthusiasm over TM and participation in the study certainly constituted threats to validity but were difficult to control and did not lead to higher ratings of TM conversations. Rather, it is possible that her enthusiasm affected her communicative behaviours in ways which had negative effects on the rating of effectiveness in participants with HD. Her satisfaction and hope in TM as a resource in her future clinical work may have influenced her ability to behave equally in the two conditions and to overestimate the benefits of TM in the interview.

A limitation of the study which, considering the purpose of exploring communication support in real life also is its strength, relates to the fact that each participant's data was collected on one occasion.

5.3 Strengths and clinical implications

The strengths of the study outweigh its limitations by far. A considerable set of interaction data involving as many as eleven individuals in different phases of HD and their support persons has been examined. The investigation of interaction in a natural health care situation is in itself unique. The fact that the intervention focused on the situation of individuals with HD, for whom communication is often complicated and related to the many other difficulties that come with the disease, makes the study even more interesting.

Both quantitative and qualitative methods were used and the fact the participants' own experiences were taken into consideration strengthens the ecological validity of the study.

Talking Mats is used by speech language pathologists (SLP), teachers and others who know of its benefits. The present findings suggest that TM could function as a communication support not only in dental and oral health care but also in other clinical care situations that are important for individuals with HD and those who care for them, for example in conversations with the physician, the dietician, the physiotherapist, the occupational therapist and the psychologist. With training and careful instruction to all people involved, TM could lead to increased communicative effectiveness and a feeling of communicative involvement for the person with disability as well as for conversation partners. Considering the strategies and experiences of conversation partners to individuals with communication difficulties is important (cf. Saldert et al., 2010).

More studies focusing the communication of individuals with cognitive and communicative disability in naturally occurring activities are needed. The present researchers' future contributions to the field include more comprehensive interaction analyses of the present data (Ferm & Saldert, 2011) as well as evaluations of TM in interactions between persons that have Parkinson's Disease and their partners at home.

6. Conclusion

Interactions between individuals with HD, their support persons and a dental hygienist have been examined regarding communicative effectiveness and perceived communicative involvement with and without Talking Mats (Murphy & Cameron, 2006). According to outside observers, TM may not lead to more effective communication for persons with HD during dental and oral health care consultations. However, a most significant finding is that the participants found it valuable using the mat. Both the participants with HD and their partners felt more involved in the TM condition than when conversation was unaided. For example, the participants commented that it was easier expressing feelings with the mat, that it was a good method for reflecting on oral health and that it was easier thinking and understanding with the mat than without it. Participants also reported that the pictures supported memory. The dental hygienist was positive as well. It was easier for her to understand the views of some of the participants when she used TM. For example, patients, who typically were inflexible as far as oral hygiene and prophylaxis is concerned, were more open minded and positive towards trying new methods and aids when discussing these issues with TM. According to the dental hygienist, TM has the potential to support communication in consultations involving persons with HD and their partners. Clinical activities in which TM could be useful include instruction and treatment planning, individual goal setting and follow up.

To date, few studies have investigated the use and value of augmentative and alternative communication for persons with HD and their partners in different activities. Research focusing communication support in care situations hardly exists. In this sense, and because it was conducted within an ordinary clinical practice, the findings of this study are important for the rehabilitation and treatment of individuals with HD and those who care for them.

7. Acknowledgment

Our greatest appreciation is to the individuals with HD and their support persons who accepted to participate in this research during one of many health consultations. Furthermore, the research had not been possible without the full participation by the dental hygienist. Her support was invaluable for the carrying out of the study. Her enthusiasm as far as communication support is concerned, and Talking Mats in particular, certainly will continue to be very important for families who are affected by HD. The writing of this chapter was partly funded by the Promobilia Foundation.

8. References

Ahlsén, E. (1995). Activity demands and communication ability in aphasia: A protocol and a case study. In: *Papers from the XVth Scandinavian Conference of Linguistics*, I. Moen, H. Gram Simonsen, & H. Lødrup, (Eds.), 1-12, ISBN 8291298025 9788291298023, Oslo: Oslo University, Department of Linguistics

Allwood, J. (2000). An activity based approach to pragmatics. In: *Abduction, Belief and Context in Dialogue: Studies in Computational Pragmatics*, H. Bunt & B. Black (Eds.), 47-80, ISBN 9027249830, Amsterdam: John Benjamins

Bartlett, G.; Blais, R.; Tamblyn, R.; Clermont, R.J. & MacGibbon, B. (2008). Impact of patient communication problems on the risk of preventable adverse events in acute care settings. *Canadian Medical Association Journal CMAJ*, 178(12), pp. 1555-1562, ISSN 0820-3946

Chenery, H. J.; Copland, D. A. & Murdoch B. E. (2002). Complex language functions and subcortical mechanisms: evidence from Huntington's disease and patients with non-thalamic subcortical lesions. *International Journal of Language and Communication Disorders*, 37(4), pp. 459-474, ISSN 1460-6984

Ferm, U.; Sahlin, A.; Sundin, L. & Hartelius, L. (2010). Using Talking Mats to support communication in persons with Huntington's disease. *International Journal of Language & Communication Disorders*, 205, pp. 523-536, ISSN 1460-6984

Ferm, U. & Saldert, C. (2011). Evaluation and revision in interactions with Talking Mats: Conversations between persons with Huntington's disease, their close others and a dental hygienist. *Manuscript in preparation*

Gabre, P. (2009). Strategies for the prevention of dental caries in people with disabilities: a review of risk factors, adapted preventive measures and cognitive support. *Journal of Disability and Oral Health*, 10, pp. 184-192, ISSN 1754-2758

Hallberg, L.; Mellgren, E.; Hartelius, L. & Ferm, U. (in press). Talking Mats in a discussion group for people with Huntington's disease. *Disability and Rehabilitation: Assistive Technology*, ISSN

Hartelius, L.; Carlstedt, A.; Ytterberg, M.; Lillvik, M. & Laakso, K. (2003). Speech disorders in mild and moderate Huntington disease: results of dysarthria assessments of 19 individuals. *Journal of Medical Speech-Language Pathology*, 11, pp. 1-14, ISSN 1065-1438

Hartelius, L.; Jonsson, M.; Rickeberg, A. & Laakso, K. (2010). Communication and Huntington's disease: quality interviews and focus groups with persons with Huntington's disease, family members, and carers. *International Journal of Language & Communication Disorders*, 45, pp. 381-393, ISSN 1460-6984

Hustad, K. C. (1999). Optimizing Communicative Effectiveness: Bringing it together. In: *Management of motor speech disorders in children and adults*, K. M. Yorkston, D. R. Beukelman, E. A. Strand, & K. R. Bell, (Eds.), 483-541, ISSN 0-89079-784-6, Austin, Texas: Proedition

Jensen, A. M.; Chenery, H. J. & Copland, D.A. (2006). A comparison of picture description abilities in individuals with vascular subcortical lesions and Huntington's disease. *Journal of Communication Disorders*, 9(1), pp. 62-77, ISSN 1873-7994

Kagan, A.; Winckel, J.; Black, S.; Felson Duchan, J.; Simmons-Mackie, N. & Square, P. (2004). A set of observational measures for rating support and participation in conversation between adults with aphasia and their conversation partners. *Topics in Stroke Rehabilitation*, 11(1), pp. 67-83, ISSN 1074-9357

Kidd, E. A. M. (2005). *Essentials of Dental Caries* (3d edition) ISBN 978-0198529781, Oxford: Oxford University Press

Klinge, B. & Gustafsson, A. (2011). *Parodontit: en introduktion* (4th edition), ISBN 9789172057609, Stockholm: Gothia Förlag AB

Lewis, D.; Fiske, J. & Dougall, A. (2008). Access to special care dentistry, part 7. special care dentistry services: seamless care for people in their middle years – part 1. *British Dental Journal*, 205, pp. 305-317, ISSN 1476-5373

Mayer-Johnson, 1981–2011, *The Picture Communication Symbols©*, Solana Beach, CA: Mayer-Johnson LLC,
http://www.mayer-johnson.com/

McGarva, K. (2001). Huntington's disease: seldom seen – seldom heard? *Health Bulletin, 59*, pp. 306-308, ISSN 0374-8014

Murphy, J. (2006). Perceptions of communication between people with communication disability and general practice staff. *Health Expectations, 9*, pp. 49–59, ISSN 1369-7625

Murphy, J. & Cameron, L. (2006). *Talking Mats a Resource to Enhance Communication*. Stirling: University of Stirling, Available from info@talkingmats.com

Murhpy, J.; Gray, C.M.; Cox, S.; Van Achterberg, T. & Wyke, S. (2010a). The effectiveness of the Talking Mats framework with people with dementia. *Dementia; International Journal of Social research and Practice* 9(4), pp. 454-472, ISSN 1741-2684

Murphy, J.; Oliver, T. M. & Cox, S. (2010b). *Talking Mats® and involvement in decision making for people with dementia and family carers*. Stirling: University of Stirling, Joseph Rowntree Foundation, Available from
http://www.jrf.org.uk/publications/talking-mats-decision-making

Murphy, J. & Cameron, L. (2008). The effectiveness of Talking Mats with people with intellectual disability. *British Journal of Learning Disabilities, 36*, pp. 232-241, ISSN 1468-3156

Power, E.; Anderson, A. & Togher, L. (2011). Applying the WHO ICF framework to communication assessment and goal setting in Huntington's Disease: A case discussion. *Journal of Communication Disorders*, 44(3), pp. 261-275, ISSN 1873-7994

Roos, R. A. C. (2010). Huntington's disease: a clinical review. *Orphanet Journal of Rare Diseases, 5*, pp. 1-8, ISSN 1750-1172

Saldert, C. & Hartelius, L. (2011). Echolalia or functional repetition in conversation – a case study of an individual with Huntington's disease. *Disability and Rehabilitation, 33* (3), pp. 253-260, ISSN 1464-5165

Saldert, C.; Eriksson, E.; Petersson, K. & Hartelius L. (2010). Interaction in conversation in Huntington´s disease: An activity-based analysis and the conversation partner's view of change. *Journal of Interactional Research in Communication Disorders* 1(2), pp. 169-197, ISSN 2040-512X

Saldert, C.; Fors, A.; Ströberg S. & Hartelius, L. (2010). Comprehension of complex discourse in different stages of Huntington's disease. *International Journal of Language & Communication Disorders, 45*, 656-669, ISSN 1460-6984

Schlosser, R. W. (2003). *The Efficacy of Augmentative and Alternative Communication*, ISBN 978-0126256673, San Diego, CA: Academic Press

Shoulson, I.; Kurlan, R. A.; Rubin, A. J.; Goldblatt, D.; Behr, J.; Miller, C.; Kennedy, J.; Bamford, K. A.; Caine, E. D.; Kido, D. K.; Plumb, S.; Odoroff, C. (1989). Assessment of functional capacity in neurodegenerative movement disorders: Huntington's disease as a prototype. In: *Quantification of Neurologic Deficit*, T. L. Munsat, (Ed.), 271–283, ISBN 9780409901528, Boston: Butterworth

Yorkston, K. M.; Miller, R. M. & Strand, E. A. (2004). *Management of speech and swallowing disorders in degenerative diseases* (2nd edition), ISBN 0-89079-966-0, Austin, Texas: Proed

Permissions

The contributors of this book come from diverse backgrounds, making this book a truly international effort. This book will bring forth new frontiers with its revolutionizing research information and detailed analysis of the nascent developments around the world.

We would like to thank Nagehan Ersoy Tunalı, PhD, for lending her expertise to make the book truly unique. She has played a crucial role in the development of this book. Without her invaluable contribution this book wouldn't have been possible. She has made vital efforts to compile up to date information on the varied aspects of this subject to make this book a valuable addition to the collection of many professionals and students.

This book was conceptualized with the vision of imparting up-to-date information and advanced data in this field. To ensure the same, a matchless editorial board was set up. Every individual on the board went through rigorous rounds of assessment to prove their worth. After which they invested a large part of their time researching and compiling the most relevant data for our readers. Conferences and sessions were held from time to time between the editorial board and the contributing authors to present the data in the most comprehensible form. The editorial team has worked tirelessly to provide valuable and valid information to help people across the globe.

Every chapter published in this book has been scrutinized by our experts. Their significance has been extensively debated. The topics covered herein carry significant findings which will fuel the growth of the discipline. They may even be implemented as practical applications or may be referred to as a beginning point for another development. Chapters in this book were first published by InTech; hereby published with permission under the Creative Commons Attribution License or equivalent.

The editorial board has been involved in producing this book since its inception. They have spent rigorous hours researching and exploring the diverse topics which have resulted in the successful publishing of this book. They have passed on their knowledge of decades through this book. To expedite this challenging task, the publisher supported the team at every step. A small team of assistant editors was also appointed to further simplify the editing procedure and attain best results for the readers.

Our editorial team has been hand-picked from every corner of the world. Their multi-ethnicity adds dynamic inputs to the discussions which result in innovative outcomes. These outcomes are then further discussed with the researchers and contributors who give their valuable feedback and opinion regarding the same. The feedback is then collaborated with the researches and they are edited in a comprehensive manner to aid the understanding of the subject.

Apart from the editorial board, the designing team has also invested a significant amount of their time in understanding the subject and creating the most relevant covers. They scrutinized every image to scout for the most suitable representation of the subject and create an appropriate cover for the book.

The publishing team has been involved in this book since its early stages. They were actively engaged in every process, be it collecting the data, connecting with the contributors or procuring relevant information. The team has been an ardent support to the editorial, designing and production team. Their endless efforts to recruit the best for this project, has resulted in the accomplishment of this book. They are a veteran in the field of academics and their pool of knowledge is as vast as their experience in printing. Their expertise and guidance has proved useful at every step. Their uncompromising quality standards have made this book an exceptional effort. Their encouragement from time to time has been an inspiration for everyone.

The publisher and the editorial board hope that this book will prove to be a valuable piece of knowledge for researchers, students, practitioners and scholars across the globe.

List of Contributors

Fabíola M. Ribeiro, Eduardo A. D. Gervásio-Carvalho and Jader S. Cruz
Department of Biochemistry and Immunology, Universidad Federal de Minas Gerais (UFMG), Brazil

Fernando A. Oliveira
Department of Biological Sciences, Universidad Federal de São Paulo (UNIFESP), Brazil

Tomas Dobransky
DB Biotech, Kosice, Slovakia

Elizabeth Hernández-Echeagaray, Gabriela De la Rosa-López and Ernesto Mendoza-Duarte
Laboratorio de Neurofisiología Del Desarrollo y la Neurodegeneración, Unidad de Biomedicina, FES-Iztacala, Universidad Nacional Autónoma de México, México

Valerio Leoni and Claudio Caccia
IRCCS National Institute of Neurology "C. Besta", Milano, Italy

Ingemar Björkhem
Karolinska Institute, Stockholm, Sweden

Teresa Cunha-Oliveira and Ildete Luísa Ferreira
CNC-Center for Neuroscience and Cell Biology, University of Coimbra, Portugal

A. Cristina Rego
CNC-Center for Neuroscience and Cell Biology, University of Coimbra, Portugal
Faculty of Medicine, University of Coimbra, Portugal

C. M. Kelly and A. E. Rosser
Brain Repair Group, School of Biosciences, Cardiff, UK

Melvin M. Evers and Willeke M. C. van Roon-Mom
Center for Human and Clinical Genetics, Leiden University Medical Center, Leiden, the Netherlands

Rinske Vlamings and Yasin Temel
Departments of Neuroscience and Neurosurgery, Maastricht University Medical Center, Maastricht, the Netherlands
European Graduate School of Neuroscience (EURON), the Netherlands

Maryna Baydyuk and Baoji Xu
Georgetown University, USA

Ana Saavedra, Jordi Alberch and Esther Pérez-Navarro
Departament de Biologia Cellular, Immunologia i Neurociències, Facultat de Medicina, Universitat de Barcelona, Barcelona, Spain
Institut d'Investigacions Biomèdiques August Pi i Sunyer (IDIBAPS), Barcelona, Spain
Centro de Investigación Biomédica en Red sobre, Enfermedades Neurodegenerativas (CIBERNED), Spain

Kerstin Roger and Leslie Penner
University of Manitoba, Canada

Ulrika Ferm
DART Centre for Augmentative and Alternative Communication and Assistive Technology, Regional Rehabilitation Centre, Queen Silvia Children's Hospital, Sahlgrenska University Hospital, Sweden

Pernilla Eckerholm Wallfur, Elina Gelfgren and Lena Hartelius
Institute of Neuroscience and Physiology, Division of Speech and Language Pathology, University of Gothenburg, Sweden

Printed in the USA
CPSIA information can be obtained
at www.ICGtesting.com
JSHW011428221024
72173JS00004B/719